Hanns Hippius

Hans-Jürgen Möller

Norbert Müller

Gabriele Neundörfer-Kohl

The University Department of Psychiatry in Munich

From Kraepelin and his predecessors to molecular psychiatry

Hanns Hippius

Hans-Jürgen Möller

Norbert Müller

Gabriele Neundörfer-Kohl

The University Department of Psychiatry in Munich

From Kraepelin and his predecessors to molecular psychiatry

With 219 figures

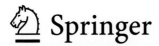 Springer

Prof. Dr. Hanns Hippius

Prof. Dr. Hans-Jürgen Möller

Prof. Dr. Dipl.-Psych. Norbert Müller

Dr. Gabriele Neundörfer-Kohl

Klinik für Psychiatrie und Psychotherapie
Klinikum der Universität München – Innenstadt
Nußbaumstraße 7
D-80336 München

ISBN 978-3-540-74016-2 Springer Medizin Verlag Heidelberg

Bibliografische Information der Deutschen Bibliothek
The Deutsche Bibliothek lists this publication in Deutsche Nationalbibliographie;
detailed bibliographic data is available in the internet at http://dnb.ddb.de.

Springer Medizin Verlag
springer.com
© Springer Medizin Verlag Heidelberg 2008

Planning: Hanna Hensler-Fritton, Heidelberg
Project management: Barbara Knüchel, Heidelberg
Typesetting: TypoStudio Tobias Schaedla, Heidelberg
Printing: Stürtz GmbH, Würzburg

SPIN 12067718

18/5135/BK – 5 4 3 2 1 0

Preface

This book first appeared in Germany in 2004. In response to the great amount of interest in the book expressed by colleagues from all over the world, we subsequently decided to produce this English version. We have also taken this opportunity to update the information on the Department of Psychiatry since 1994 to include further developments up to the present day (see Chapter 15). One can look at a hospital from all kinds of different perspectives. For psychiatrists with the daily medical task of dealing with the life histories of their patients, it is understandable that they are interested in the development of their hospital from a historical perspective.

To do this for the University Department of Psychiatry of Munich an introduction can be made by reminding the reader of a date: just over 100 years ago, on November 7, 1904, the newly constructed »Royal Psychiatric Hospital of the University of Munich« was inaugurated with a ceremonial act and handed over to the public. Emil Kraepelin gave a ceremonial speech on the occasion.

Our book was first published for the 100-year celebration of the hospital. To begin with it was intended to give the history with emphasis on the building history of the hospital (most people from Munich and abroad refer to the hospital as the »Nervenklinik« (»hospital for nervous disorders«)). This would have been justified, since every hospital exists first as a building followed by the history; and the building history of the Munich hospital reflects the changes and metamorphoses in the concept of clinical psychiatry.

The hospital building was planned at the beginning of the 20th century by Kraepelin's predecessor, Anton Bumm, together with the architect, Max Littmann. The building was erected right next to the old hospital »Links der Isar« (on the left bank of the river Isar) and was designed as a psychiatric hospital, which should not only offer patient care and student training, but also put an emphasis on scientific research. In the 1920s Oswald Bumke changed the hospital into a hospital for nervous disorders (psychiatric and neurological hospital); after the 2nd World War Georg Stertz and then Kurt Kolle managed it again as a hospital for nervous disorders.

In 1971 the hospital was subdivided into a psychiatric and a neurological department. Instead of the previous chair for »psychiatry and neurology« two separate chairs for »psychiatry« and »neurology« each were established.

The neurological department was opened at the Hospital Grosshadern. The hospital for nervous disorders became once again a psychiatric department.

From 1969 onwards plans were developed for considerable rebuilding and extension, which were slowly carried out, once the neurological department had moved out. On completion of all construction work in 1998 the new hospital kept its historical core, but had all the equipment for modern, psychiatric in- and out-patient care, rooms for student training and other training activities and considerable research facilities.

The hospital was built as a university hospital, the professorship of the university department and the directorship of the hospital both were and still are today owned by the same person. Therefore the terms ,department of psychiatry', ,psychiatric hospital', and ,psychiatric clinic' (according to the German tradition) are more or less used identically. The term ,hospital' is more related tot he building, ,department' to the academic, and ,clinic' to the medical aspects.

Due to their merits in the field of psychiatry, two heads of the department, August Solbrig and Bernhard Gudden were ennobled by the Bavarian King. After the ennoblement, in the respective chapters Solbrig and Gudden are named von Solbrig and von Gudden.

The **building history** of the Munich hospital substantiates the developments in psychiatry during the past 100 years, but an illustration of the constructional aspects alone would be dull and impersonal. The development of a hospital should be understood as a **life story**, in which not only the building and organisation structure itself, but also the patients treated in the hospital and the people working there should be taken into consideration: Doctors from the Munich hospital have always enhanced the development of clinical psychiatry and psychiatric science decisively. As such, the names of Emil Kraepelin and Alois Alzheimer are known to all psychiatrists all over the world nowadays – even to those who do not realize that the scientific work of these names is closely linked to the Munich hospital. Many of the names of doctors from the Munich hospital have been long forgotten and a book about the hospital will remind us of some of them. This was our aim, but we realize that we have not achieved this entirely and it is even less possible to mention all the names and give credit to the many staff, who have supported the doctors right from the beginning and who as such have contributed considerably to the reputation of the hospital; in particular to be mentioned here are the nursing staff. Of course, not only does the workforce belong to a hospital, but most importantly the patients! The work and atmosphere of a hospital is reflected in the patients' lives and their opinion of the hospital. Obviously it is not possible to give details on patients' lives, but we have tried to show this side of hospital life with a few examples.

In our portrayal of the many facetted developments of the Munich hospital we have not only covered the period as of 1904. The **hospital's roots** stem from the beginning of the 19th century, when the first in-patient facilities for psychiatric patients were created. In the middle of the 19th century efforts were made to turn psychiatry – within the medical faculty – into a clinical subject with equal rights like the other clinical disciplines. These developments also belong to the history of the hospital.

When taking a look at the early history of the hospital, it is necessary to also illuminate the role and the importance of the hospital for the psychiatric **care** of the citizens of Munich and its surroundings.

Of course the **research activities** of the hospital need to be shown in detail and given proper appreciation. However, in most of the chapters these are only referred to in a more general sense.

In order to give a completely satisfactory and detailed account of the above points, it would have been necessary to write a real opus on the history of psychiatry, which was not possible.

All the same we hope that the book will find interested and appreciative readers in present and past hospital staff, colleagues and doctors, the historically interested and also the one or other patient who has been treated at the hospital.

Kurt Kolle, one of the previous directors of the Munich hospital, once complained that historical interest and historical conscience has disappeared nowadays, but this seems to have changed during the past decades. We therefore hope that our cursory account of the history of the »University Department of Psychiatry in Munich« may animate others to follow up on life or work histories of past researchers at the hospital and to systematically study the effect they may have had on the hospital.

But before thinking of a future with potentially rich contributions to psychiatric-historical research, we would like to thank all those, who contributed to the compilation and publishing of this book!

With Professor Dr. Norbert Müller and Dr. Gabriele Neundörfer-Kohl we wrote the text for chapters 1 to 14 of the book and compiled the illustrations. The manuscripts (and the corrections) were taken care of by Mrs Karin Koelbert in an immaculate fashion.

Furthermore, we owe special thanks to certain persons:

Mrs Alma Kreuter, who worked as secretary from 1924–1970, the librarians, Mrs E. Wolf and Mrs E. Sund, as well as Mrs F. Hostalka, who compiled the various illustrative material. There were also many former staff of the hospital as well as relations and friends of former staff, who let us have their documents and photos.

We are greatly indebted to Ms Cheryl Wooding-Deane, who took on the enormous task of translating the whole book. Without her professional and highly motivated work, this book would never have been realised. Our thanks also go to Ms Mije Hartmann, Ms Jacqueline Klesing and Ms Sindy Lehwald for their assistance with various preparatory, administrative and editorial tasks.

Last but not least we would like to mention the publisher »Springer« in Heidelberg (Mrs. H. Hensler-Fritton), who proved to be most competent and reliable partner.

Munich, September 2007
H. Hippius
H.-J. Möller

Materials – Sources – Literature

The book follows the brochure by H. Hippius and P. Hoff on the »Psychiatric Hospital of the Ludwig-Maximilians University of Munich – Documents of a Building History«, which was published on the occasion of the celebration of the first section of the rebuilding and extension of the hospital.

For the hospital's »Psychiatry-History Workgroup« Dr. Gabriele Neundörfer-Kohl, as of 1997, supported by Mrs E. Sund, compiled and filed all documents and material. This »Psychiatry-Historical Collection of the Psychiatric Hospital of the Ludwig-Maximilians University of Munich« is not yet published, but is available as a collection in the Psychiatry-Historical Museum in the Alzheimer hall.

On various occasions since 1976, psychiatry-historical exhibitions have taken place (1976: 50th anniversary of the day of death of E. Kraepelin; 1986: 100th anniversary of the day of death of B. von Gudden; 1988: International Congress for Neuropsychopharmacology (CINP); 1989: celebration of the first section of the rebuilding and extension of the hospital.

The opening (1998) of the restored, historical Emil Kraepelin-building was celebrated by a first exhibition in the Alois Alzheimer hall, in which particularly interesting parts of the psychiatry-historical collection can be seen in 11 display cabinets. Dr. Gabriele Neundörfer-Kohl prepared a catalogue for this exhibition, which is now available in a re-worked and graphically newly designed edition prepared by Mr Josef Christan and Mrs Karin Koelbert.

Mrs Alma Kreuter (born 1906) is to be given special thanks for the existence of the psychiatry-historical collection; she started work as a secretary at the hospital during Kraepelin's lifetime and later became executive secretary to O. Bumke, G. Stertz and K. Kolle. Mrs Kreuter edited the manuscripts of the three volumes published by K. Kolle on »Famous Psychiatrists«. In connection with this work she systematically collected biographies and bibliographies of German-speaking psychiatrists and neurologists. She used this material as a basis for a 3-volume lexicon she published in 1996 on »German-Speaking Neurologists and Psychiatrists – from the Forerunners to the Middle of the 20th Century« (Saur, Munich, 1996).

Mrs Kreuter's lexicon assisted us when we wrote this book and proved to be an exceptionally informative and important source of information. Furthermore, Mrs Kreuter brought us into contact with numerous, previous staff of the hospital and other persons, who gave us further information.

Many documents were put at our disposal by the Bavarian State Archive, the City of Munich Archive and the Archive of the Ludwig-Maximilians University, the Archive of the Max-Planck Institute and the Historical Krupp Archive (Alfried Krupp von Bohlen and Halbach Foundation). We thank the very helpful staff of these archives and everyone else, who gave us details on former times.

However, most of the documents and photos published in this book stem from the psychiatry-historical inventory of the hospital; for this material we did not mention the origin in the texts and legends.

When looking through the material in the hospital, we located originals and copies of letters, manuscripts, draft lectures and newspaper articles, as well as a lot of photos. These include the entire estate of M. Mikorey. In particular to be mentioned amongst the correspondence are the letters from E. Kraepelin to his brother Karl, to Gustav Krupp von Bohlen and Halbach, to Wilhelm Wundt, as well as correspondence between Oswald Bumke and Alfred Hoche, and between Georg Stertz and Alfred Hoche, between Heinrich Laehr and Fritz Siemens. In the collection we located many handwritten documents, which reflect E. Kraepelin's methods (including detailed, handwritten records on James Loeb's illness).

Some of the sources are mentioned at the end of each chapter but detailed literature references have not been included.

Contents

Early Psychiatric Institutions in Munich

Psychiatry did not become a medical discipline until the end of the 18th century and before this time the mentally ill, if at all, were isolated as »mentally disturbed« in prison-like asylums and mad houses. They were even kept in penitentiaries and mad houses together with common criminals where no medical attention was available. There were, however, a few exceptions to the usual practise of isolation and discrimination of the »mentally disturbed« in Germany, such as at the Julius Hospital in Wurzburg and, understandably, the Julius Hospital was considered one of the first medical institutions in the Free State of Bavaria, where the mentally ill were given medical care. The Julius Hospital was built in 1576 during the reign of the prince bishop Julius Echter von Mespelbrunn. Right from the beginning of its existence, 30 to 40 psychiatric patients were admitted for care.

Nothing similar existed in Munich until the beginning of the 19th century, although with respect to medical institutions there had been some attempts to set up something prior to the opening of the first independent psychiatric hospital in 1803. Some psychiatric patients were admitted for care to the existing hospitals for internal medicine and infectious diseases. At the city gates (near the fruit and vegetable market) the Hospital of the Holy Ghost (□ Fig. 1.1–1.3) had already been founded in the 13th century with a couple of separate cells for the mentally disturbed (so-called »pits for fools

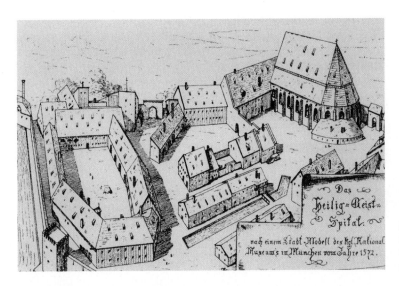

□ **Fig. 1.1.**
Hospital of the Holy Ghost in Munich, 1572 (from H. Kerschensteiner, 1913)

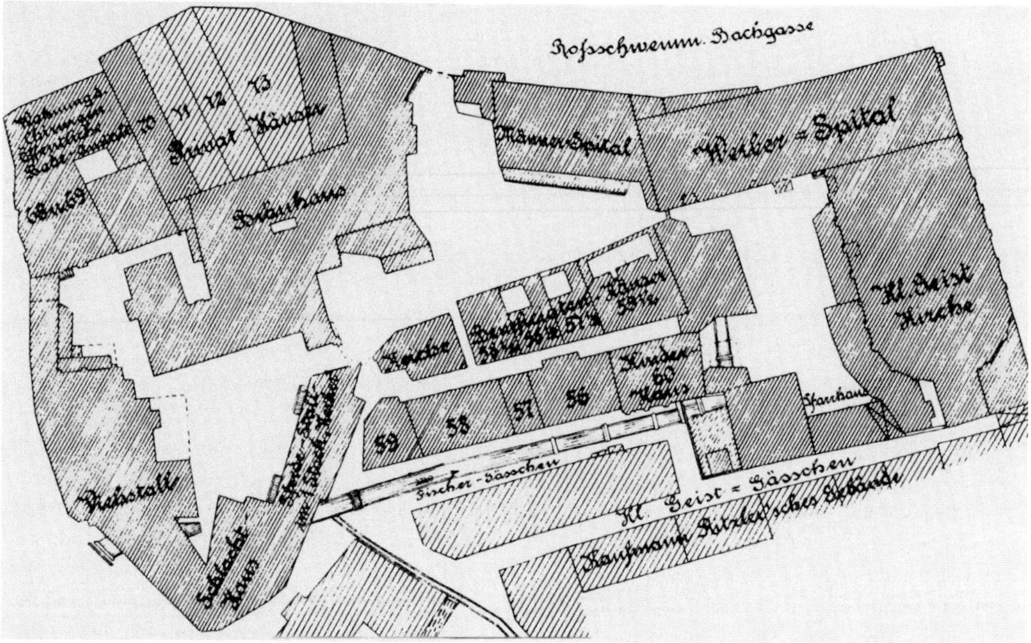

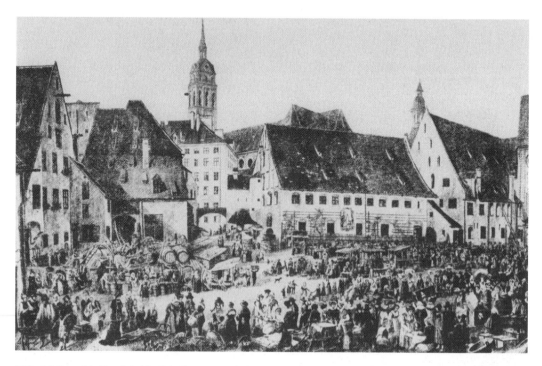

Fig. 1.2. Overview plan of the Hospital of the Holy Ghost (re-sketched and amended according to the plan of Huhn) from H. Kerschensteiner (1913)

Fig. 1.3. View of the Hospital of the Holy Ghost in Munich (from H. Kerschensteiner, 1913). On the right-hand side of the picture: end of the nave of the Holy Ghost Church; the view over today's fruit and vegetable market shows the tower of the old town hall and the old St. Peter's church. In front were the units for men and for women. Approx. at the position of the observer were the »idiot pits«.

and idiots«). For a long time (until 1822) the Hospital of the Holy Ghost was a care establishment for the poor and aged as well as an institute for parturition; between 1498 and 1783 it also functioned as a foundling house and from 1664 as »fumigation chamber« for contagious diseases. Single cells for psychiatric patients and later even a special »house for madmen« made up the fifth part of the Hospital of the Holy Ghost. Rooms for 30 »madmen« were available. In 1803, the »house for madmen« actually had 64 in-patients.

Apart from the Hospital of the Holy Ghost, the mentally ill were also admitted to the Herzogsspital, which opened in 1601, and the St. Josephs-Spital (◘ Fig. 1.4).

However, the conditions for the mentally ill in the Hospital of the Holy Ghost were inhumane. One visitor in 1786 even mentioned the »awful accommodation for madmen«. Around 1800, chains were to be seen on the walls of the so-called pits for fools. On June 9, 1802 a report was made in a Munich newspaper, the Tageblatt, about a visit to the Hospital of the Holy Ghost. With the title »Something about the public institution for the mentally ill« it describes his impressions: »….. in the hope of seeing wide, light rooms, I entered the cellar; instead of fresh, healthy air a repugnant vapour hit me and instead of dry cleanliness I met damp dirtiness. No separate and freestanding beds, but human stalls made of wooden slats were to be seen. These areas were the pits.« The overseers of the fools' pits were called the »strikers«.

In his famous book, written in 1917 »A Hundred Years of Psychiatry«, Kraepelin included a picture originating from Kaulbach (◘ Fig. 1.5) at the beginning of the 19th century, which showed why he found »the situation of the mentally ill« at this time to be »appalling«. In this picture, standing behind the patients is a guard who rightfully

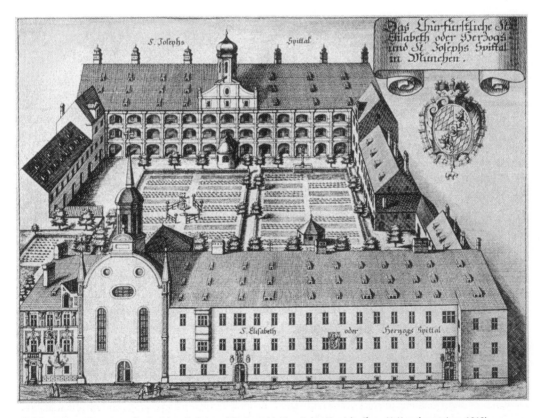

◘ **Fig. 1.4.** The »Elector's St. Elisabeth's or Duke's and St. Joseph's Hospital in Munich« (from H. Kerschensteiner, 1913)

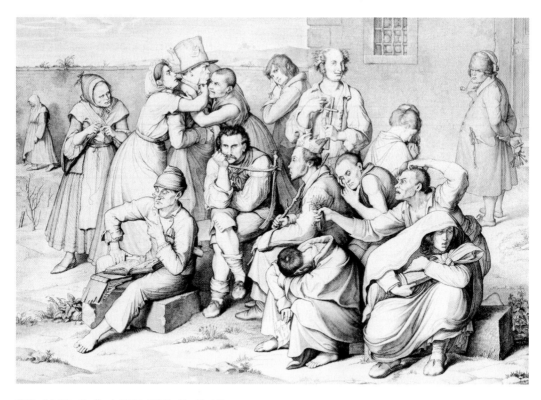

▣ Fig. 1.5. W. v. Kaulbach (1805 –1874): »The Mad House«

looks exactly like what at that time was considered a »striker«.

All together in Munich – as in the rest of Bavaria – the care facilities for the mentally ill, annexed to hospitals, were completely insufficient. As described in the report to the Munich newspaper, »Tageblatt«, in 1802 about a visit to the Hospital of the Holy Ghost, the public conscience was gradually becoming aware of the situation.

Furthermore, not only was a critical report on the conditions in the hospital printed in the Munich »Tageblatt«, but it was clearly and distinctly – although, with care and diplomatic skill – printed that improvements must be made: »….. Bavaria can be proud to have made good progress with all kinds of public institutions and although they are not all together perfect, they cover the most important needs. The present government, which is so aware of the public well-being, tries every now and then to introduce improvements in spite of the costs and to complete its institutions to perfection. All kinds

of unlucky souls find help and support in Bavaria. Only the most unfortunate class of humans, the mentally ill, has been comparatively neglected until now……. After being given an anonymous draft, for which he is grateful, His Electoral Highness has given the general government orders to check the proposal and to ensure the building of a good mental institution as soon as possible.«

This public demand was fulfilled in 1803: The Giesing »Madhouse« (also known as the »Mental Ayslum of Giesing«, ▣ Fig. 1.6) was opened as the Royal Hospital in 1901 »half an hour away from Munich«. The Royal Hospital had been opened in 1746 in Giesing on the Auermühlbach (Auermühl stream), which is today known as Kolombus Square (Kolumbusplatz) for the treatment of »high fevers«, originally intended for ill officials, servants and pages from the electoral court. After the opening of the two-storied building the windows on the ground floor were walled up and on the first floor they were barred. On the ground floor there were

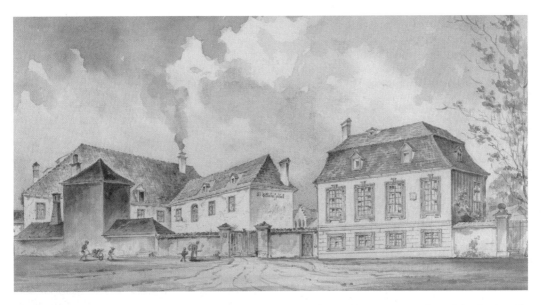

◻ Fig. 1.6. Munich-Giesing, »Mad House«; opened 1803 in the former Royal Hospital; water-colour and pencil drawing from Ch. Steinicken 1880 (owned by the Munich Municipal Museum)

13 cells for the »really mad« and a room for a guard; on the upper floor there were 9 further cells for the calmer »madmen« who were also monitored by a guard. »….. The duties of the guards were not only surveillance and cleanliness of the madmen, since the humane treatment of the institution meant that the inhabitants were not treated with means of coercion, except perhaps with a strait jacket …… each room had a toilet, which could be emptied from the corridor. The heating and lighting were indirect from the central corridor. The ventilation system (although useless) developed by Franz Xaver von Häberl at the General Hospital in Munich was installed. In the bathroom two wooden tubs were ready for use, although the patients were washed in the courtyard in the summer.«

The »Giesing Mental Asylum« had room for 25 patients, but often there were more than 50 patients, since all patients, who would have been admitted previously to the Hospital of the Holy Ghost, were now admitted here. Since the »Giesing Mental Asylum« also had to serve right from the start as a care institution for the »incurable«, its over-occupancy grew from year to year. Furthermore, the rapid increase in Munich's population during the first decade of the 19th century contrib-

uted to the continuous lack of space, which also meant that female and male patients could not be given separate accommodation.

At the »Giesing Mental Asylum« only one doctor was responsible for all patients; and this doctor had other jobs apart from his work at the hospital. For example Dr. Christlmüller, who worked at the »Asylum« from 1837 to 1859, also had his own practice in Giesing. Soon after starting to work there, Dr. Christlmüller considered the conditions at the »Giesing Mental Asylum« to be unbearable for the patients and therefore suggested in 1839 that Munich urgently needed a »larger mental asylum«. And, although means of coercion had been applied less at the »Giesing Mental Asylum« than in the past, the overcrowding was »dreadful« and led to such means of coercion being used more often.

Christlmüller made his demands public and a law laid down during the reign of King Ludwig the First (on initiative of Johann Nepomuk Ringseis) (see Chaper 2) became the basis of a development, which first led to the building of an »Upper Bavarian District Mental Asylum« in the middle of the century and then the building of the Royal Psychiatric Clinic in Munich on the Nussbaumstrasse at the beginning of the 20th century.

Literature

Jetter, D. (1966): Geschichte des Hospitals. Vol. 1, Franz-Steiner-Verlage: Wiesbaden

Kerschensteiner, H. (1913): Geschichte der Münchener Krankenanstalten insbesondere des Krankenhauses Links der Isar. Lehmanns-Verlag: Munich-Berlin

Kraepelin, E. (1917): 100 Jahre Psychiatrie. Z.f.d.ges. Neur. & Psych. 38, p. 161-275

Martin, A. (1934): Geschichtliche Darstellung der Kranken- und Versorgungsanstalten zu München mit medizinisch-administrativen Bemerkungen aus dem Gebiet der Nosokomialpflege. Georg-Franz-Verlag: Munich

Psychiatric Care in Bavaria in the 19th Century

In 1837, a law was made in Bavaria with a title difficult to understand nowadays: »The elimination of district encumbrances from the state encumbrances and formation of district funds« (November 17, 1837; revised May 23, 1846) (☐ Fig. 2.1a,b). From the title of the law it is not possible to realise what an important role it would play in psychiatric care.

Based on this law the »districts« (nowadays known under a different term in German) of the kingdom of Bavaria formed »district funds«; and one of the tasks to be financed by the district fund was the duty to build »mental asylums«. At the time the law was very progressive, compared to the situation in other German states. In German-speaking territories in Austria and later on Prussia there were similar processes, which could be considered key.

When the law was made in 1837, there were only few independent institutions where the mentally ill could be admitted and which could be considered a real, or at least conceptual basis for the building of a »district mental asylum«. In the district of Upper Bavaria the »Giesing Mental Asylum«, opened in 1803, was one of them (▶ Chapter 1).

Once the law had been made, developments in Bavaria, however, were very slow and it was for this reason that Heinrich Damerow (1798–1866) declared in 1844 that »the public handling of the mentally ill in Bavaria is still notoriously backwards«. At that time, Damerow's opinion was quite important because, as together with Chr. F. W. Roller (1802–1878), they were the most prominent and influential psychiatrists of their time the idea

☐ Fig. 2.1a,b. Title page and paragraph K of the law from 1837

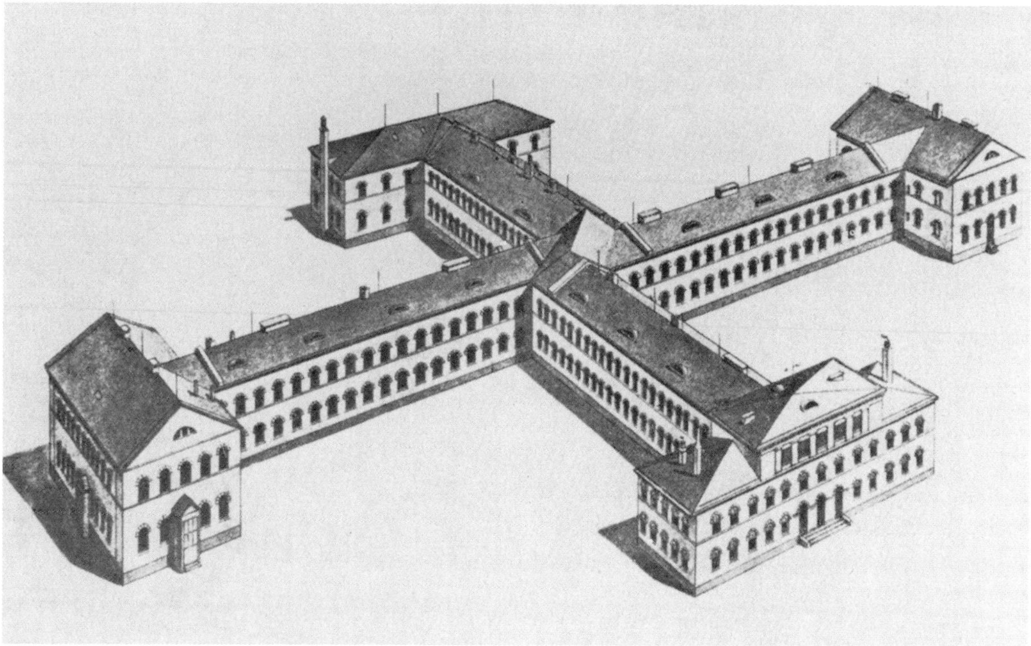

Fig. 2.2. Panoptical building style of the Middle Franconian District Mental Hospital in Erlangen, 1846

of combined cure and care institutions for the mentally ill.

With this form of organisation it was intended to avoid the stark separation of the so-called »cure institutions« (for the mentally ill with potential for recovery) and »care institutions« (for the incurably ill).

In Bavaria it took a further 9 years after the law had been made in 1837 before finally in Erlangen the first Bavarian district mental asylum could be opened in 1846 (Fig. 2.2) (for the district of Middle Franconia). Nothing was built in any of the other districts, although already existing buildings (e.g. monasteries during the secularization) were adapted as district mental asylums. In this manner the previous monastery, Irsee, was opened in Swabia as a district mental asylum in 1849. In 1852 it was followed by Karthaus/Prull, near Regensburg, for the district of Upper Palatinate; Upper Franconia had its district mental asylum in 1855 at Werneck Castle (Fig. 2.3). Following the opening in Erlangen, the next new building to be constructed was that in Klingenmuenster in 1857; at that time the Palatinate belonged to Bavaria. In

Munich it took longer, in spite of public demand during the first decades of the century, following the law of 1837 and Christlmüller's urgent requests from his daily experience at the Giesing Mental Asylum. Finally in 1859, the new building of the District Mental Asylum for Upper Bavaria took shape, whilst the district mental asylum for Upper Franconia was built in Bayreuth in 1870 and for Lower Bavaria in Deggendorf in 1869.

The plans for the first, new institution building in Bavaria (Erlangen) came from Johann Michael Leupoldt (1794–1874), who had studied medicine, graduated and qualified as a university lecturer in 1818 in Erlangen. He gave lectures on anatomy and physiology and, as one of the first German universities to do so, also lectured on mental diseases. In 1820 the Bavarian government gave him a grant to travel, which he used to visit Berlin and see the department for the mentally ill at the Charité. On his return to Erlangen and his promotion to extraordinary professor (1821), he presented then (and again in 1825) his initiatives to the Bavarian provincial diet to reform the treatment of the mentally ill. In 1825 he proposed an autonomous institution, cut off

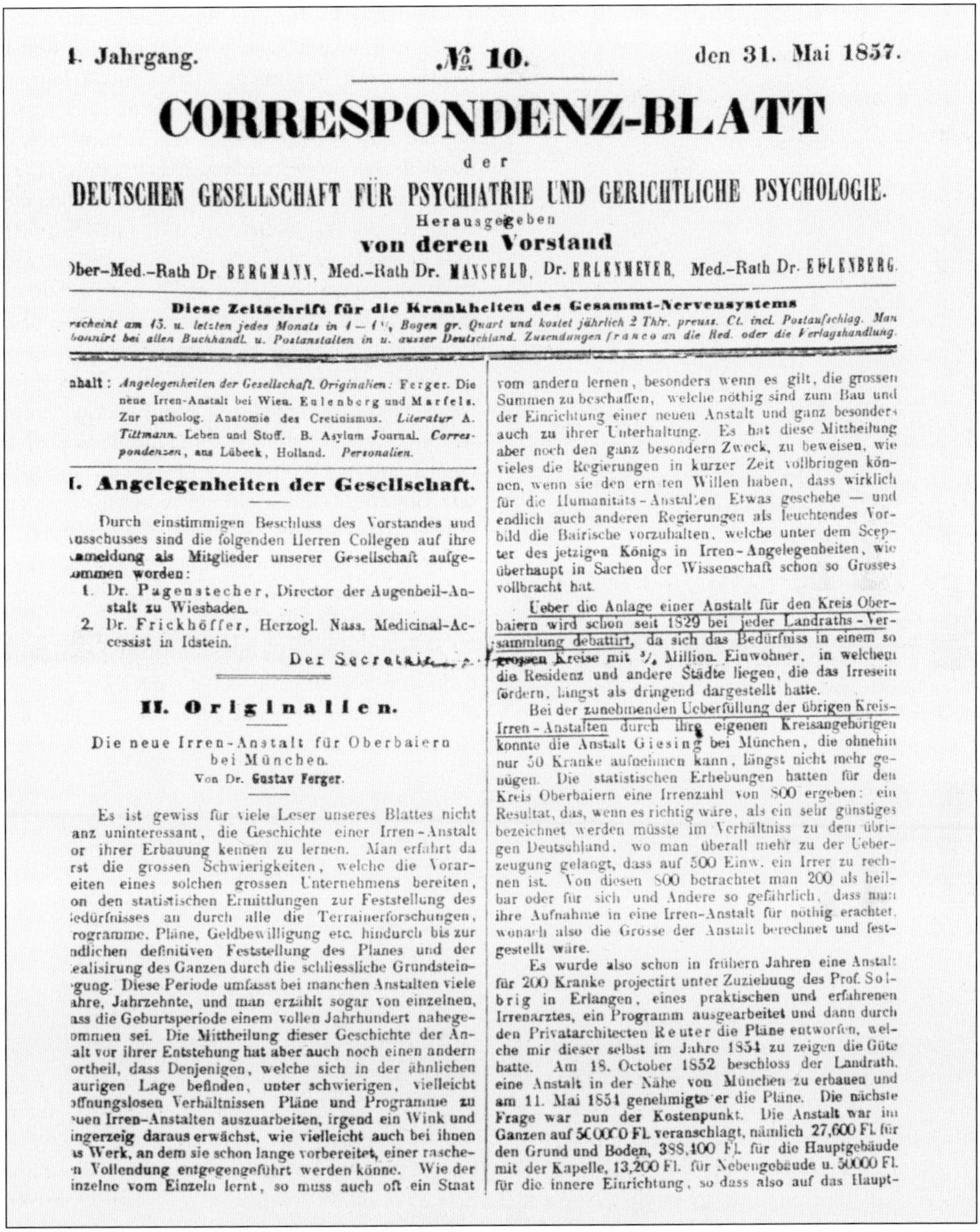

1. Jahrgang.   № 10.   den 31. Mai 1857.

CORRESPONDENZ-BLATT

der

DEUTSCHEN GESELLSCHAFT FÜR PSYCHIATRIE UND GERICHTLICHE PSYCHOLOGIE.

Herausgegeben

von deren Vorstand

Ober-Med.-Rath Dr BERGMANN, Med.-Rath Dr. MANSFELD, Dr. ERLENMEYER, Med.-Rath Dr. EULENBERG.

Diese Zeitschrift für die Krankheiten des Gesammt-Nervensystems

erscheint am 15. u. letzten jedes Monats in 1—1½ Bogen gr. Quart und kostet jährlich 2 Thlr. preuss. Ct. incl. Postaufschlag. Man bonnirt bei allen Buchhandl. u. Postanstalten in u. ausser Deutschland. Zusendungen franco an die Red. oder die Verlagshandlung.

Inhalt: *Angelegenheiten der Gesellschaft. Originalien:* Ferger. Die neue Irren-Anstalt bei Wien. Eulenberg und Marfels. Zur patholog. Anatomie des Cretinismus. *Literatur* A. Tittmann. Leben und Stoff. B. Asylum Journal. *Correspondenzen,* aus Lübeck, Holland. *Personalien.*

I. Angelegenheiten der Gesellschaft.

Durch einstimmigen Beschluss des Vorstandes und Ausschusses sind die folgenden Herren Collegen auf ihre Anmeldung als Mitglieder unserer Gesellschaft aufgenommen worden:

1. Dr. Pagenstecher, Director der Augenheil-Anstalt zu Wiesbaden.
2. Dr. Frickhöffer, Herzogl. Nass. Medicinal-Accessist in Idstein.

Der Secretair.

II. Originalien.

Die neue Irren-Anstalt für Oberbaiern bei München.

Von Dr. Gustav Ferger.

Es ist gewiss für viele Leser unseres Blattes nicht ganz uninteressant, die Geschichte einer Irren-Anstalt vor ihrer Erbauung kennen zu lernen. Man erfährt da erst die grossen Schwierigkeiten, welche die Vorarbeiten eines solchen grossen Unternehmens bereiten, von den statistischen Ermittelungen zur Feststellung des Bedürfnisses an durch alle der Terrainerforschungen, Programme, Pläne, Geldbewilligung etc. hindurch bis zur endlichen definitiven Feststellung des Planes und der Realisirung des Ganzen durch die schliessliche Grundsteinlegung. Diese Periode umfasst bei manchen Anstalten viele Jahre, Jahrzehnte, und man erzählt sogar von einzelnen, dass die Geburtsperiode einem vollen Jahrhundert nahegekommen sei. Die Mittheilung dieser Geschichte der Anstalt vor ihrer Entstehung hat aber auch noch einen andern Vortheil, dass Denjenigen, welche sich in der ähnlichen traurigen Lage befinden, unter schwierigen, vielleicht öffnungslosen Verhältnissen Pläne und Programme zu neuen Irren-Anstalten auszuarbeiten, irgend ein Wink und Fingerzeig daraus erwächst, wie vielleicht auch bei ihnen das Werk, an dem sie schon lange vorbereitet, einer raschen Vollendung entgegengeführt werden könne. Wie der einzelne vom Einzeln lernt, so muss auch oft ein Staat vom andern lernen, besonders wenn es gilt, die grossen Summen zu beschaffen, welche nöthig sind zum Bau und der Einrichtung einer neuen Anstalt und ganz besonders auch zu ihrer Unterhaltung. Es hat diese Mittheilung aber noch den ganz besonderen Zweck, zu beweisen, wie vieles die Regierungen in kurzer Zeit vollbringen können, wenn sie den ernsten Willen haben, dass wirklich für die Humanitäts-Anstalten Etwas geschehe — und endlich auch anderen Regierungen als leuchtendes Vorbild die Bairische vorzuhalten, welche unter dem Scepter des jetzigen Königs in Irren-Angelegenheiten, wie überhaupt in Sachen der Wissenschaft schon so Grosses vollbracht hat.

Ueber die Anlage einer Anstalt für den Kreis Oberbaiern wird schon seit 1829 bei jeder Landraths-Versammlung debattirt, da sich das Bedürfniss in einem so grossen Kreise mit ¾ Million Einwohner, in welchem die Residenz und andere Städte liegen, die das Irresein fördern, längst als dringend dargestellt hatte. Bei der zunehmenden Ueberfüllung der übrigen Kreis-Irren-Anstalten durch ihre eigenen Kreisangehörigen konnte die Anstalt Giesing bei München, die ohnehin nur 50 Kranke aufnehmen kann, längst nicht mehr genügen. Die statistischen Erhebungen hatten für den Kreis Oberbaiern eine Irrenzahl von 800 ergeben: ein Resultat, das, wenn es richtig wäre, als ein sehr günstiges bezeichnet werden müsste im Verhältniss zu dem übrigen Deutschland, wo man überall mehr zu der Ueberzeugung gelangt, dass auf 500 Einw. ein Irrer zu rechnen ist. Von diesen 800 betrachtet man 200 als heilbar oder für sich und Andere so gefährlich, dass man ihre Aufnahme in eine Irren-Anstalt für nöthig erachtet, wonach also die Grösse der Anstalt berechnet und festgestellt wäre.

Es wurde also schon in frühern Jahren eine Anstalt für 200 Kranke projectirt unter Zuziehung des Prof. Solbrig in Erlangen, eines praktischen und erfahrenen Irrenarztes, ein Programm ausgearbeitet und dann durch den Privatarchitecten Reuter die Pläne entworfen, welche mir dieser selbst im Jahre 1854 zu zeigen die Güte hatte. Am 18. October 1852 beschloss der Landrath, eine Anstalt in der Nähe von München zu erbauen und am 11. Mai 1854 genehmigte er die Pläne. Die nächste Frage war nun der Kostenpunkt. Die Anstalt war im Ganzen auf 500000 Fl. veranschlagt, nämlich 27,600 Fl. für den Grund und Boden, 388,400 Fl. für die Hauptgebäude mit der Kapelle, 13,200 Fl. für Nebengebäude u. 50000 Fl. für die innere Einrichtung, so dass also auf das Haupt-

Fig. 2.5. Excerpt from the journal »Correspondenzblatt« of the German Association for Psychiatry and Forensic Psychology, May 31, 1857

»II. News

The new mental hospital for Upper Bavaria in Munich. By Dr. Gustav Ferger

Ever since 1829 there have been debates at the district administrator assemblies about the site for an asylum, as the need in such a large district with ¾ million inhabitants, which promotes mental diseases, has long become an urgent matter. With the *increasing over-crowding in existing district mental asylums*, filled with local inhabitants, the asylum in Giesing, which only caters for 50 patients, has not been able to keep up with demand for a long time now..«

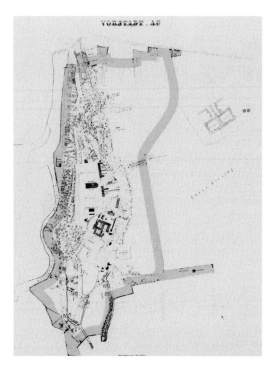

Fig. 2.6. Site plan of the Upper Bavarian District Mental Hospital, ca. 1860

At that time, the most important German scientific journal, published by Damerow and Roller together with Flemming, »The General Journal for Psychiatry« printed an article in 1958 praising the »fast construction of the Munich mental hospital. Half of the building already stands. Three quarters of the walls surrounding the building are complete. All this is the work of the past year. As long as money is available, the entire project will be finished in autumn 1959 and Bavaria will be an institute richer. Bavaria is the most innovative state for mental hospitals in Germany«.

Solbrig did not become director of the new Munich institute immediately. Bernhard Gudden, at that time director of the Lower Franconcian district mental hospital, Werneck, (▶ Chapter 4), was chosen. However, Gudden did not accept the position offered to him and the job was offered to Solbrig.

Solbrig accepted the offer and on November 1, 1859, the institute was opened with great celebrations and with Solbrig as its director.

When it opened its doors in 1859, the institute had room for 280 patients (»curable« and »incurable«) and soon it became necessary to extend the

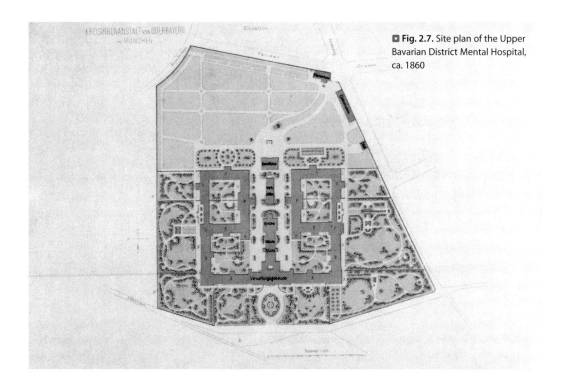

Fig. 2.7. Site plan of the Upper Bavarian District Mental Hospital, ca. 1860

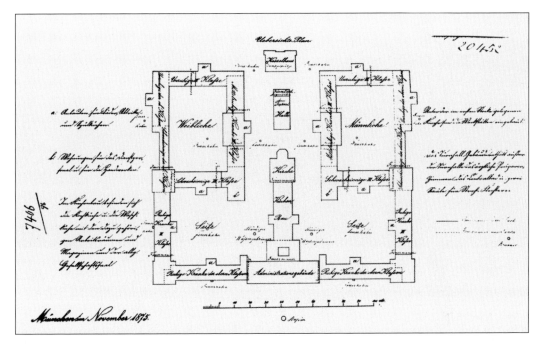

Fig. 2.8. Floor plan of the Upper Bavarian District Mental Hospital from 1875

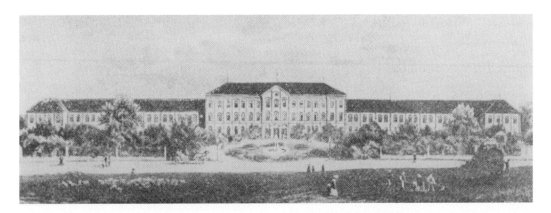

Fig. 2.9. Exterior view of the Upper Bavarian District Mental Hospital »Auf der Auer Lüften«

existing building to accommodate 400 patients. The demand continued and at the beginning of the 1870's the hospital was caring for 500 patients. As it did not seem to be a good idea to make further extensions, in 1873 a further hospital was built in Attel, which did not adhere to the principle of a »relatively combined cure and care institution« and which was purely for men. Yet another district

mental hospital for Upper Bavaria was built in Gabersee, near to Wasserburg, in 1883. Gabersee was constructed in an entirely different manner to the clinics built according to the »Illenau« model; the principle of the »relatively combined cure and care institution« was used, unlike in Attel.

In 1898, the Upper Bavaria provincial diet resolved to close the Munich district mental hos-

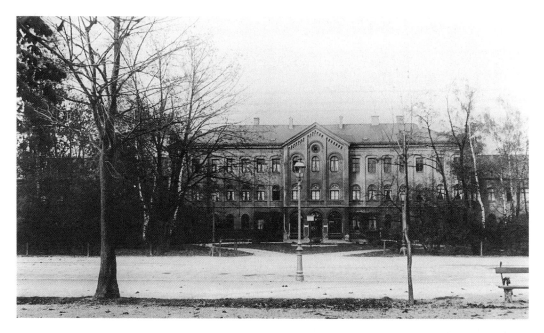

◘ Fig. 2.10. View of the façade of the Upper Bavarian District Mental Hospital, Aufeldstrasse, from 1907 (from the municipal archives in Munich)

pital »In der Au«, which, in spite of extensions and reconstruction, was over-flowing, and to build a new district mental hospital outside Munich in Eglfing. The building was opened in 1905 and soon was over-flowing, too; as a result the next step was planned and directly next to Eglfing the asylum Haar was opened in 1912.

Solbrig did not live to experience these developments, he died in 1872.

However, he had started the proceedings leading to a totally new goal 30 years after his death: During his time in Munich he had not remained a staunch supporter of Roller's concept of the »partly combined cure and care institution«: Roller vehemently maintained this from his position in Illenau. He saw it as an affront to the medical faculty and with it to the psychiatry taught at the university.

Solbrig's importance for psychiatry in Munich was that – compared to many of the other directors – he sought contact to the medical faculty. Solbrig made a considerable contribution to turning psychiatry into a clinical discipline at the Munich medical faculty. His personal engagement in set-

ting up the chair for psychiatry at the medical faculty and in having it included as a subject in clinical tuition was enterprising and exemplary. In the Munich district mental hospital, planned and managed by him from 1859 to 1872, Solbrig started the developments, which finally led to the building of an independent, psychiatric clinic of the university in Munich.

Literature

Ferger, G. (1857): Die neue Irren-Anstalt für Oberbaiern bei München. Corresp. Blatt 4, Nr. 10, p. 73-74

Haisch, E. O. (1975): Historisches zur Entwicklung der Anstalts- und Universitätspsychiatrie. Oeff. Gesundh.-Wesen 37, p. 70-76

The Chair for Psychiatry at the Medical Faculty of the University of Munich

Karl August Solbrig is not only to be merited for developing psychiatry in Munich as well as planning, building and finally managing the Upper Bavarian district mental hospital; Solbrig also achieved the inclusion of psychiatry as a medical discipline at the Munich medical faculty.

Karl August Solbrig (◘ Fig. 3.1) was born in Furth on September 17, 1809, as the son of a »royal forensic doctor« and later »city doctor to Nuremberg«. On leaving school at Ansbach, he studied medicine in Munich and Erlangen and visited the lectures of J.M. Leupoldt (► Chapter 2) on »mental diseases«. In 1831 Solbrig received his doctor title in Erlangen and worked for A.Chr. H. Henke (1775–1843), the full professor in Erlangen for »physiology, pathology and state pharmacy«. From Henke's title doesn't make clear that his position meant that he was primarily occupied with the »forensic judgement of mental disorders for legal reasons«. Under Leupoldt and Henke's influence Solbrig used a travel grant to make a journey in 1834 to psychiatric institutions in Germany, France and Belgium.

> At that time many young scientists were given grants to travel with the intention that on their travels they would have personal contact with well-known researchers and clinicians and would learn from them and be encouraged by them. On return from their journeys the gathered information often prompted them to decide on their future career direction.

Solbrig wrote a report on his »study travel«, which contained proposals on »public mental care« in

Bavaria and the inclusion of psychiatry in the medical curriculum.

Further following his apparently ever increasing interest in psychiatry and after completing his studies in Erlangen (1836), Solbrig spent several months with C.W. Ideler (1795–1860) at the mental health department of the Charité in Berlin. He did not remain in psychiatry, but became a general

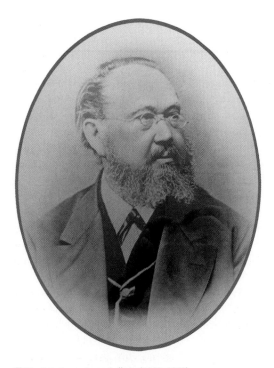

◘ **Fig. 3.1.** August von Solbrig (1809–1872)

practitioner at his home town of Furth and stayed there for 10 years. In 1845 he applied for the position of director of the district mental hospital in Erlangen. He was accepted and became the first director at Erlangen in August 1846. As well as managing the district mental hospital, he also planned to become professor at the medical faculty of Erlangen.

> At this time only few German universities had members of the medical faculty who worked as clinical psychiatrists. Should a university at that time even have a chair for what one would call »psychiatry« nowadays, then the position was usually held by academics trained in philosophy rather than medicine and with almost no understanding of the practice as seen in the cure and care psychiatric institutions.

After complicated negotiations with the medical faculty, Solbrig became »honorary professor« in Erlangen in 1849. He had actually wanted a professorship of psychiatry and was therefore not satisfied with the title »honorary professor«. In his opinion the honorary professorship was attached to him as a person and as such did not do justice to the importance of psychiatry within the medical faculty.

Unlike Solbrig, most of the mental hospital directors at that time were of the opinion that the inclusion of the »mental asylums« into the medical faculty would be detrimental for the further development of psychiatry. In particular, the promoter of the »relatively combined cure and care institutions«, Chr. F. W. Roller strongly defended (until his death in 1878) the opinion that psychiatric clinics should not be connected to universities.

On the other hand, voices demanding chairs for psychiatry and psychiatric training at universities were becoming louder and Solbrig did not let himself be distracted from his goal to establish psychiatry decisively as a discipline at the medical faculty. Because he did not succeed with his intentions in Erlangen, he left and was offered (following the refusal by B. Gudden) the option of taking over the district mental hospital in Munich in 1859, as its first director. However, shortly after taking up office in Munich he was only given an »honorary professor« title and it was not until he turned down

the offer to go to Berlin in 1864 that his demand was fulfilled and he was given the title of »professor of psychiatry« (◻ Fig. 3.2)! He was also given the title of »Privy Councillor« and was raised to the peerage (◻ Fig. 3.3). Solbrig had finally achieved in Munich what had been impossible in Erlangen: With the formation of a full chair for psychiatry it had been put on the same footing as the other clinical disciplines.

As well as being director of the clinic, Solbrig also had extensive responsibilities as forensic doctor and consultant at many of the Munich clinics. Whenever new psychiatric institutions were in planning, he was asked to give his expert advice.

In particular with public lectures, Solbrig tried to give the general public an understanding of the mentally ill and the problems of psychiatry. In 1861, on behalf of the »Association of German Psychiatrists«, Solbrig gave a lecture at the »Assembly of German Scientists« in Speyer on the subject of »psychiatric clinics«. The lecture was one of the main contributing factors why shortly afterwards – based on developments in Bavaria – some other German countries established psychiatry as an academic discipline at the medical faculty.

Shortly before Solbrig took over the district mental hospital in Munich, the academic Senate of the University of Munich had received orders from the Bavarian Ministry of the Interior that psychiatry was to become a subject to be taught. As Solbrig was *only* an honorary professor of the medical faculty at this time, an assistant of the Munich polyclinic, A. von Franque, was given the job to give lectures on psychiatry. A. von Franque had qualified as professor with a thesis on delirium tremens and received the »venia legendi« for psychiatry. At that time von Franque gave lectures to the public on »Disorders of Mental Activity« and to medical students on »Special Pathology and Therapy of Mental Illnesses«. When psychiatry became recognized as an academic subject, Solbrig also began to lecture. From the summer term 1861 onwards, he lectured on the »Psychiatric Clinic«; and only a year later (as of 1862) this student training was also given at the District Hospital for Mental Diseases.

Due to the tradition, initiated by von Solbrig, of giving lectures with the presentation of patients

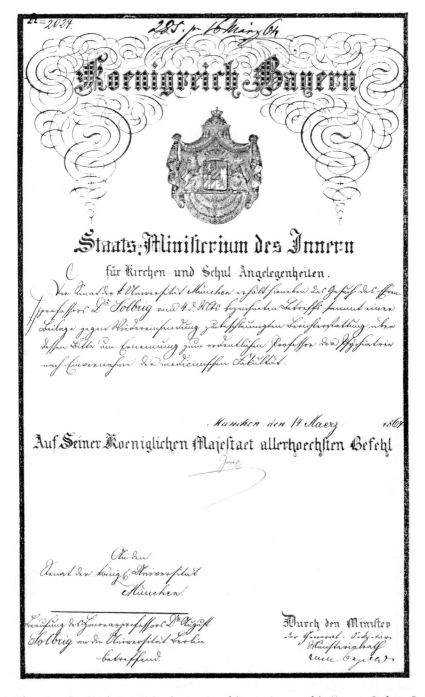

Fig. 3.2. Certificate issued on March 14, 1864 (on the occasion of the appointment of the Honorary Professor Dr. August Solbrig to the University of Berlin): **Kingdom of Bavaria. State Ministry for Church and School Matters. The senate of the Royal University receives hereby the request of the Honorary Professor Dr. Solbrig on the 4th of the month (together with an enclosure) to accelerate the handling of his request on the appointment as ordinary professor of psychiatry on the examination by the medical faculty. Munich, March 14, 1864, by the order of His Royal Majesty.** (from the university archives Munich, signed E-II-526)

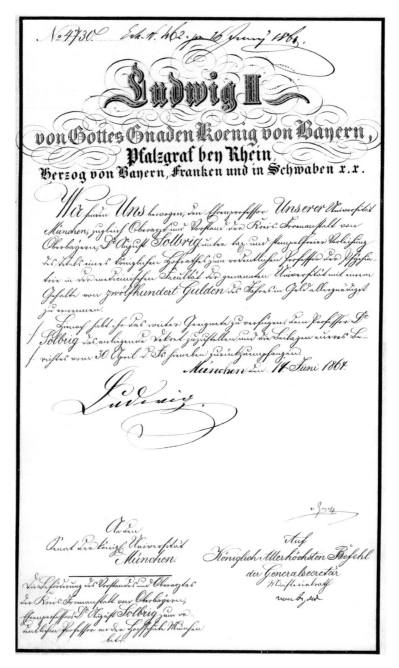

◘ Fig. 3.3. Certificate of June 14, 1864, from King Ludwig the Second (to the Senate of the University): **Ludwig, the Second by God's grace King of Bavaria, Palatinate Count of Rhine, Duke of Bavaria, Franconia and Schwabia. xx We find ourselves disposed to graciously appoint the Honorary Professor of our University in Munich, at the same time Senior Consultant and Head of the District Mental Asylum of Upper Bavaria, Dr. August Solbrig, free from tax and stamp duty the award of the title of Royal Court Councillor to Ordinary Professor of Psychiatry in the medical faculty of the same university with a salary of twelve hundred guilders p.a. in gold. Accordingly, all necessary should be done that the decree is delivered to Professor Dr. Solbrig and that we receive the enclosures to our report of April 30 of the year.** (from the university archives Munich, signed E-II-526)

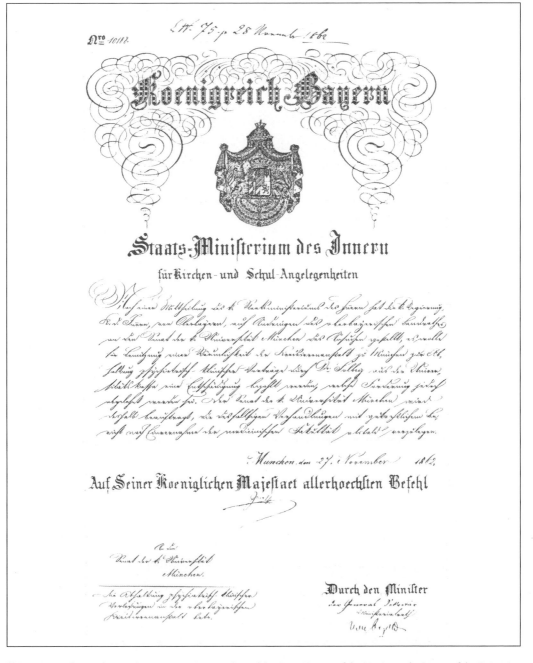

◨ **Fig. 3.4.** Certificate of November 27, 1862. Memorandum of the State Ministry of the Interior to the Senate of the University: **Kingdom of Bavaria, State Ministry of the Interior for Church and School Matters. According to a memorandum from the Royal State Ministry of the Interior, the Royal Government of Upper Bavaria, at the insistence of the Upper Bavarian District Administrator to the Senate of the Royal University Munich, places a plea for the use of rooms at the District Mental Asylum in Munich for psychiatric-clinical lectures by Prof. Solbrig to be paid from the university exchequer, which request, however, has been turned down. The Senate of the Royal University has therefore been commissioned to carry out pragmatic negotiations with expertise reports by the university as soon as possible. Munich, November 27, 1862. By order of His Royal Majesty.** (from the university archives Munich, signed: Sen 308)

themselves (although occasionally administrative difficulties occurred regarding the financing of the tuition (☐ Fig. 3.4)) a lecture theatre was made available in the newly built clinic as of 1904.

Apart from his own specialist subjects von Solbrig was also scientifically interested in »public diseases« and questions of hygiene. In a publication on »Contradictions in Medicine« von Solbrig pointed out the role of mental influences on the development of public diseases and the psychological side of hygiene in the treatment and prophylaxis of these diseases. Under von Solbrig's influence the frequently used »blood-letting« was restricted at the Munich district mental hospital, as he was of the opinion that blood and sufficient circulation of blood was very important for brain function. For von Solbrig good and sufficient food was more important than diets and fasting. In the asylum long, luke-warm, but also cold head baths were performed; for younger, agitated patients cold hip baths were prescribed. Von Solbrig only referred to the effects of medication in very cautious terms; he had not achieved any remarkable results with either opium or ether. In cases of »periodical raving madness« cannabis extracts were administered; chloroform was considered to be effective for »fits of rage«. Straits jackets and fixtures to the beds were seldom used at the Munich district mental hospital. Von Solbrig considered the »caring, always giving and always devotional love« to be the most important basis for dealing with psychiatric patients.

Contemporaries and staff both praised von Solbrig's organizational talent and diplomatic skills. In all matters he gave his opinion with self-confidence, convincingly and kindly, and in this manner achieved a lot for the reputation and position of psychiatry.

Von Solbrig was also a convivial person, who appreciated art and music. He was father of two sons and three daughters.

In the spring of 1872 a typhus epidemic hit Munich; von Solbrig became infected. On May 31, 1872 he died of a typhus pneumonia.

August von Solbrig was responsible for the development of psychiatry in Munich in many ways:
- He planned, built and finally managed the District Mental Hospital for Upper Bavaria in Munich for 13 years (1859–1872).
- As reported by his contemporaries, he was an enthusiastic teacher, who made a considerable contribution by ensuring that as of 1862 the psychiatric training for medical students no longer took place far away from the psychiatric patients themselves, but that it was given in a psychiatric clinic.
- It is the greatest achievement of K. a. von Solbrig that a chair for psychiatry was founded in Munich in 1864, thus giving it equal footing with the other clinical subjects.

Literature

Eberstadt-Kreichgauer, E. (1947): Karl August von Solbrig. Dissertation, Erlangen

Solbrig, A. (1869): Statische Mitteilungen aus der Oberbayerischen Kreisirrenanstalt. Intelligenzblatt 34, p. 369-370

Solbrig, A. (1871): Aus dem Rechnungsbericht 1870 der Oberbayerischen Kreisirrenanstalt. Intelligenzblatt 46, p. 566-568

Bernhard von Gudden, Doctor and Founder of Modern Neuromorphology

Following August von Solbrig's death in May 1872, Bernhard von Gudden took over the chair for psychiatry in Munich. This time, he accepted the position offered (▶ Chapter 2, page 13) and became the second director of the Upper Bavarian District Mental Hospital.

Bernhard von Gudden, Professor of Psychiatry at the University of Munich (1872–1886)

Bernhard von Gudden (◘ Fig. 4.1) was born on June 7, 1824, in Cleves, in what was then a Prussian Rhineland province. He was the third of seven sons of an estate owner from a middle-class family (Gudden used the name Bernhard Gudden until 1874 when he was gentrified in Bavaria and was known in psychiatric history as Bernhard von Gudden).

After attending school in Cleves and at the age of 18, he went to the university of Bonn which had been founded in 1818 in the Rhineland province, and began to study philosophy. After one term, he changed to medicine in 1844 and continued in Halle and Berlin, finally completing his studies with state exams and graduation. Following a year at the army, he returned home and became »assistant doctor« to Karl Wigand Maximilian Jacobi (1775–1858) at the Rhineland mental asylum »Siegburg«. It was here that he met Jacobi's granddaughter, Clarissa, to whom he became engaged in 1851. Once he had left the hospital at Siegburg, Gudden and Clarissa married in 1855 when he become director of the District Mental Hospital Werneck in Lower Franconia, and it was here that their nine children were born.

Before taking over Werneck in 1855, Gudden worked from 1851 to 1855 – after a short period as general practitioner in Cleves – as assistant to Chr. F. W. Roller at the mental asylum Illenau. Then he was director at Werneck for 14 years (1855–1869)

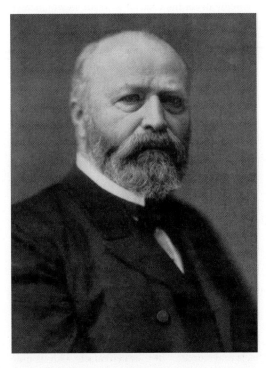

◘ Fig. 4.1. Bernhard von Gudden (1824–1886)

and as of 1869 professor of psychiatry at the University of Zurich. He was three years in Zurich when August von Solbrig died on May 31, 1872. Two weeks later Bernhard Gudden, then 48 years old, applied for the position as Solbrig's successor.

Gudden had started working in Zurich in 1869 and was director of the Cantonal Psychiatric Clinic »Burghoelzli«. »Burghoelzli« had been rebuilt and was not finished until 1870, during Gudden's term of office. The plans for the building, conceived by Wilhelm Griesinger, reflect the concept of a modern handling of psychiatric patients, which did not necessarily include locking them up and using coercive methods. Griesinger (1817–1868) was head of the chair for internal medicine in Zurich from 1860 to 1865 and was not only head of the Zurich Cantonal Hospital, but also head of the very old-fashioned and run-down Zurich »mental asylum«. Griesinger planned to replace the old mental asylum with a new building and energetically pursued his plan, although he accepted a position in Berlin before work was started on the new building. In Berlin, he was offered the chance to combine into **one** clinic the »department for the mentally ill« at the Charité with the newly formed »department for nervous diseases«, a completely innovative idea for the time. When Griesinger left Zurich, Gudden replaced him (after an almost four year vacancy) at the chair for psychiatry in Zurich.

From the outside it seemed as though Gudden was the successor of a great pioneer of German psychiatry and that as head of a completely newly built clinic he had achieved an ideal career break with exceptionally good working conditions. Apparently, however, this was not the case. Gudden's authority and competence were restricted by a very difficult and idiosyncratic head of administration; as a result, he was soon looking for the first opportunity to leave Zurich. For this reason and on hearing of A. von Solbrig's death, Gudden immediately applied for the job.

For various reasons the move was not an easy one. His motive for leaving a very good working atmosphere at Werneck was the connection to the university in Zurich. He had hoped for an cosmopolitan atmosphere in Zurich with pleasant contacts and stimuli. The Gudden family with its nine children between five and sixteen years of age had settled well in Zurich. There were good schools for the children and opportunities for further education. The living quarters and garden at Burghoelzli were spacious. The fees from private patients and the annual salary from the canton were considerable, but all the same Gudden applied for the position in Munich!

The Appointment to Munich

There was a particular reason leading to the decision to apply for the job in Munich. Already 13 years ago in 1859 Gudden had turned down the offer to take over the newly built Munich district mental hospital and with it the professorship for psychiatry at the Munich university. He had done so, because he did not want to turn his back on the construction work at the district mental hospital of Lower Franconia, Werneck.

When the situation in Zurich and the constant disagreements there became unbearable, Gudden applied in writing (13 years after turning down the position in Munich) to the Minister of the Interior, for Church and School Affairs of the Royal Bavarian Government. His application, as well as that of C. Westphal, Th. Meynert and others, was handled in depth, although in a rather controversial manner. The faculty decided finally in October 1872 to apply to the minister that not Gudden, but Max Hubrich (1837–1896), Gudden's successor at Werneck, should be offered the position of honorary professor for psychiatry. The faculty's proposal was obviously made with the intention that the ministry would make Hubrich director of the district mental hospital in Munich. However, this assumption was not correct and the ministry, also responsible for the district mental hospital, decided to give the management of the hospital to Gudden and not Hubrich! The faculty was informed and the ministry pointed out that it was prepared to negotiate with Gudden and to give him the title of full professor of psychiatry, just like in Zurich. With its comments the ministry pointed out that, considering the importance of psychiatry and the excellent reputation of Bernhard Gudden as doctor and scientist, it would refrain from reminding the faculty that when newly appointing positions the number of full professors should be kept to a minimum. (With hindsight it is understandable why the faculty had decided to give Hubrich an honorary or extraordinary professorship.) Gudden had made clear from the start that the would only come to Munich if he would be made »full professor«!

Bernhard von Gudden and the Wittelsbachs

Possibly, another point played an important role in the appointment of Gudden to Munich and it was a point concerning the royal family of Wittelsbach:

Gudden was supposed to take over the treatment of Prince Otto (1848–1916) (◘ Fig. 4.2), the younger brother of King Ludwig the Second (1845–1886) (◘ Fig. 4.3), who was ill.

Once the differing opinions between the medical faculty and the ministry in Munich were settled regarding the appointment of a successor for Solbrig. In November 1872 King Ludwig the Second let it be known (via his cabinet secretary Eisenhardt), that he, the King, had the »great desire« that Gudden similar to his predecessor Solbrig, would »periodically visit his Royal Highness, Prince Otto, who for a long time now had been suffering from nervousness as well as hallucinations«. (This assertion was based on an assessment of his condition made by Solbrig a couple of months prior to this death.) Gudden took on the task. Right from the beginning Gudden and some of his co-workers (known as the so-called »prince's doctors«) regularly visited the ailing Prince Otto at the Palace of Nymphenburg and later at the little castle of Fürstenried. Gudden wrote to the Queen Mother, Marie of Bavaria and mother of King Ludwig the Second, about these visits and their correspondence continued for the following 14 years. This contact also explains why Marie, widow of King Maximilian the Second (1811–1864), sent a letter of condolence, two weeks after the death of her son and Bernhard von Gudden, to Gudden's widow.

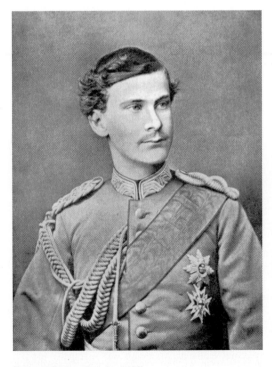

◘ **Fig. 4.2.** Prince Otto (ca. 1870)

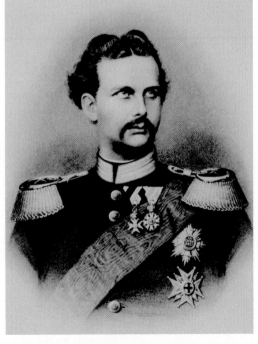

◘ **Fig. 4.3.** King Ludwig the Second (ca. 1870)

Before receiving the task of giving an expert opinion on the King in June of 1886, Gudden, together with Grashey, Hagen and Hubrich, had probably had no personal contact with the King. (Although during previous years they had probably met at an official reception.)

The expertise (□ Fig. 4.4) on Ludwig the Second, how he came to die and his and Bernhard von Gudden's death remain controversial today. The result is a flood of publications on the matter: Serious, scientific studies and daring speculations (e.g. about political motives), earnest attempts at literary commentaries and less tasteful accounts of the events, portrayed as comedies and comic strips, films and even series in the cheap newspapers.

The most absurd accounts are usually aimed at psychiatry, all of which contribute to the fact that the name of Bernhard von Gudden is only ever mentioned in connection with the death of Ludwig the Second.

Von Gudden, who from 1872 was responsible for taking care of the mentally disturbed Prince Otto, was first informed in March 1886 in a conversation with the Bavarian government about their concern that King Ludwig the Second was most likely ill as well and not in a position to take care of government business. It remains unclear whether von Gudden, based on his knowledge of the illness of the King's brother and its course, had already thought – prior to 1886 – that King Ludwig the Second had a similar illness. However, in March 1886 at the latest, von Gudden was confronted directly with the King's possible illness. In May 1886, in protracted meetings with the ministers of state, von Lutz and von Crailsheim, and based on the medical history and reports from people dealing with the King, von Gudden explained why he thought the King was possibly, psychiatrically ill. Consequently, he was given the task of making a professional report, as anchored in the Bavarian constitution, on the possibility that »for a long period of time His Majesty the King may be kept from carrying out his duties«. As proposed by von Gudden and due to the momentousness of such a task, a collegial expertise was made – together with Hubert Grashey (then full professor of psychiatry at the University of Wurzburg, ► Chapter 5), Friedrich Wilhelm Hagen (1814–1888; until 1887

extraordinary professor for psychiatry at the University of Erlangen and director of the district mental hospital in Erlangen) and Max Hubrich (then director of the district mental asylum Werneck). The collegial expertise was completed on June 8, 1886 and after a meeting of the four in Munich came to a unanimous conclusion that

1. »His Majesty is in a very advanced state of mental disorder and most probably suffering from what psychiatrists would refer to as paranoia (insanity);
2. With this type of illness, with its gradual, but advanced development and the fact that it has been noticed for quite some time His Majesty is to be declared irrevocably ill and it is possible that his mental condition will deteriorate;
3. Due to his illness, it is clear that His Majesty no longer has his own will and for this reason is most likely to be unable to govern, and that this situation will most likely last not only a year, but for the rest of his life.

Once the entire Ministry of State had been informed by von Gudden of the King's mental incapacity to govern the state, a stately commission travelled to Hohenschwangau on June 8, 1886, with the intention of visiting the Castle of Neuschwanstein the next day. On June 10, 1886, the regency of Prince Luitpold, the King's uncle, was proclaimed (□ Fig. 4.5). Von Gudden accompanied the commission to Hohenschwangau and suggested to take care of the King at Furstenried castle were his brother Otto stayed. First though, the Linderhof castle was considered a possibility until finally it was decided to confine him to Berg castle on the Lake of Starnberg.

On June 12 the King was brought to Berg castle by a commission, so that he could be cared for there by von Gudden's doctors and nurses. On June 13 von Gudden visited Berg castle and went for a walk with the King along the banks of the Lake of Starnberg. During the night King Ludwig the Second and Bernhard von Gudden were found dead in the lake, giving ground to many assumptions and often exaggerated speculations as to the cause of death. Although clear that their dear King was psychiatrically ill, his death was a tragedy for the Bavarians, and his doctor died with him.

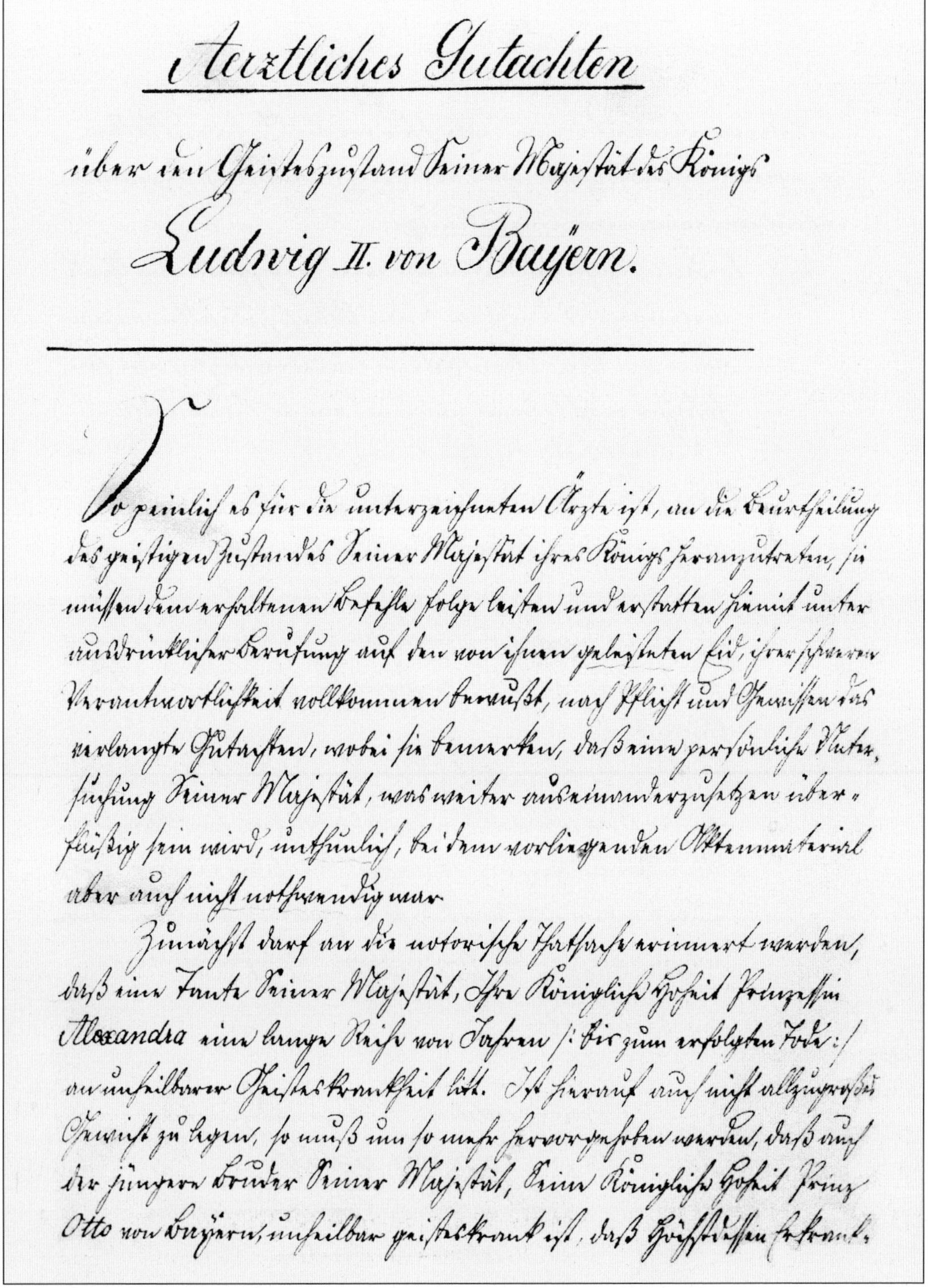

Aerztliches Gutachten

über den Geisteszustand Seiner Majestät des Königs

Ludwig II. von Bayern.

So peinlich es für die unterzeichneten Ärzte ist, an die Beurtheilung des geistigen Zustandes Seiner Majestät ihres Königs heranzutreten, sie müssen dem erhaltenen Befehle Folge leisten und erstatten hiemit unter ausdrücklicher Berufung auf den von ihnen geleisteten Eid, ihrer schweren Verantwortlichkeit vollkommen bewußt, nach Pflicht und Gewissen das verlangte Gutachten, wobei sie bemerken, daß eine persönliche Untersuchung Seiner Majestät, was weiter auseinanderzusetzen überflüssig sein wird, unthunlich, bei dem vorliegenden Aktenmaterial aber auch nicht nothwendig war.

Zunächst darf an die notorische Thatsache erinnert werden, daß eine Tante Seiner Majestät, Ihre Königliche Hoheit Prinzessin Alexandra eine lange Reihe von Jahren /: bis zum erfolgten Tode :/ an unheilbarer Geisteskrankheit litt. Ist hierauf auch nicht allzugroßes Gewicht zu legen, so muß um so mehr hervorgehoben werden, daß auch der jüngere Bruder Seiner Majestät, Seine Königliche Hoheit Prinz Otto von Bayern, unheilbar geisteskrank ist, daß Geschwister erkrankt,

Fig. 4.4. First and last page of the »Medical expertise on the mental condition of His Majesty the King, Ludwig the Second of Bavaria«, signed by the experts von Gudden, Hagen, Grashey and Hubrich, dated June 8, 1886

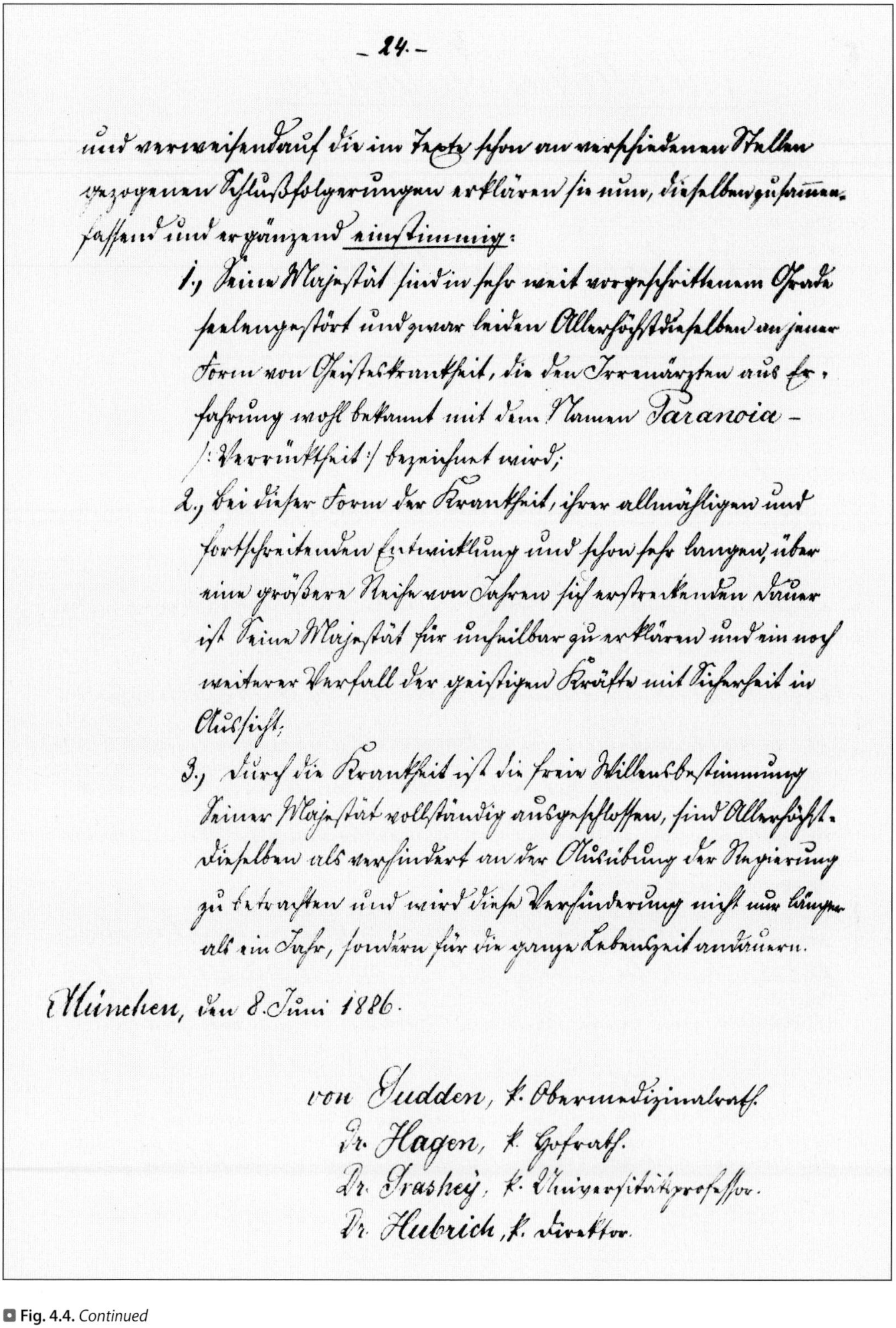

– 24. –

und verweisend auf die im Texte schon an verschiedenen Stellen gezogenen Schlußfolgerungen erklären sie nun, dieselben zusammenfassend und ergänzend einstimmig:

1.) Seine Majestät sind in sehr weit vorgeschrittenem Grade seelengestört und zwar leiden Allerhöchstdieselben an jener Form von Geisteskrankheit, die den Irrenärzten aus Erfahrung wohl bekannt mit dem Namen Paranoia – /:Verrücktheit:/ bezeichnet wird;

2.) bei dieser Form der Krankheit, ihrer allmähligen und fortschreitenden Entwicklung und schon sehr langen, über eine größere Reihe von Jahren sich erstreckenden Dauer ist Seine Majestät für unheilbar zu erklären und ein noch weiterer Verfall der geistigen Kräfte mit Sicherheit in Aussicht;

3.) durch die Krankheit ist die freie Willensbestimmung Seiner Majestät vollständig ausgeschlossen, sind Allerhöchstdieselben als verhindert an der Ausübung der Regierung zu betrachten und wird diese Verhinderung nicht nur länger als ein Jahr, sondern für die ganze Lebenszeit andauern.

München, den 8. Juni 1886.

von Gudden, k. Obermedizinalrath.
Dr. Hagen, k. Hofrath.
Dr. Grashey, k. Universitätsprofessor.
Dr. Hubrich, k. Direktor.

Fig. 4.4. *Continued*

»**Medical expertise on the mental condition of His Majesty the King, Ludwig the Second of Bavaria**

As embarrassing as it is for the undersigned doctors to make a judgement on the mental state of His Majesty the King, they must follow orders and report herewith under the oath they have sworn, realizing their serious responsibility, according to their duty and conscience, whereby it must be pointed out that a personal examination of His Majesty, which should not be further discussed here, was not necessary with the documentation available on the case.

It must be reminded that an aunt of His Majesty, Her Royal Highness Princess Alexandra, suffered for quite some years until her death from an untreatable mental disease. Should this not give the necessary emphasis, then it should be stressed that also the younger brother of His Majesty, His Royal Highness Prince Otto of Bavaria, is incurably mentally ill, so that exactly this disease, which originated already in his youth, automatically and clearly shows a relationship with certain aspects of His Majesty's disease.

His Royal Highness complained to the co-signing, senior medical officer, von Gudden, at a relatively symptom-free period that he had experienced awful attacks of anxiety and inner agitation every now and then during his youth, for example when he was lieutenant at the age of 17 years and had to stand guard for the first time at the »Residenz« palace. When the people of Munich gathered around him rejoicing and looking at him, he had a feeling that he was standing at the »stake of shame«; at the same time he had suffered from hallucinations and from the most repulsive feelings in his chest and lower body, from motoric excitement, which was expressed in various slinging and jumping movements of the arms and legs, was not seldom highly agitated and tended towards violent actions. Also, to the contrary and to a certain extent as counterbalance to some of his depressing sensations and associations, he reported often to be plagued by exceptionally high spirits and self-confidence, so that statements such as »no one can give me orders, not even the King« were often uttered and all efforts to influence His Royal Majesty with medical advice or the most gentle actions had no effect whatsoever.

The doctors herewith conclude their description and refer to their conclusions already made in various parts of the text and declare the following unanimously as summary and endorsement thereof:

1. His Majesty is in a progressive stage of mental illness and is suffering from a form of mental disease, which psychiatrists know from experience to be paranoia (madness);
2. With this form of disease, with its gradual and progressive development, which has been apparent for many years, His Majesty is to be declared as incurably ill and it is to be noted that a further deterioration of his mental faculties is to be expected with certainty;
3. Due to this disease, it is to be completely excluded that His Majesty is in charge of his own free will and he is therefore not capable of governing and that this incapacity will last not just for a year, but for the rest of his life.

Munich, June 8, 1886
Von Gudden, Senior Royal Medical Officer
Dr. Hagen, Royal Court Counsellor
Dr. Grashey, Royal University Professor
Dr. Hubrich, Royal Director«

◘ **Fig. 4.4.** *Continued*

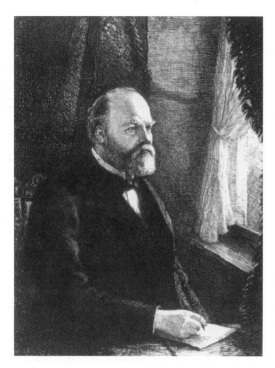

Fig. 4.5. Bernhard von Gudden at his desk (ca. 1880)

Bernhard von Gudden – a Progressive Doctor

Everything we know about Bernhard von Gudden as a doctor and his opinion on how to treat mentally ill patients, make it obvious for psychiatrists that the events on June 13, 1886, are the tragic death of a suicidal patient and his doctor. Von Gudden strongly believed in the (not generally accepted belief at that time) »no restraint principle« and most likely died whilst trying to stop a patient in his care from carrying out his suicide plan.

This interpretation is also supported by the publication of W. Wöbking on the 100th day of death of Ludwig the Second and Bernhard von Gudden entitled »The Death of King Ludwig the Second of Bavaria«. Wöbking at that time senior official at the Bavarian State Office of Criminal Investigation, evaluated many documents from the viewpoint of a lawyer and criminologist and drew his conclusions. All the information from the State

Archives of Bavaria as well as the secret archives of the House of Wittelsbach were put at his disposal.

As a result of events, the life work of von Gudden (◻ Fig. 4.5), as a significant doctor and scientist, has disappeared into the background and been almost completely forgotten. It has often been overlooked that Gudden made considerable contributions to the use of scientific methods in order to develop psychiatry as a medical discipline; he was the founder of modern neuo-anatomy. As a clinician, he was one of the first psychiatrists in Germany to almost completely forgo the use of methods of coercion in treatment and as such introduced the »no restraint« system in Werneck, as previously developed by the English psychiatrist Conolly, in Zurich. To introduce the system, he paid particular attention to changing the behaviour of the »psychiatric wardens« at Werneck and their attitude towards the patients. Von Gudden played a major part in converting the »psychiatric wardens« to »nursing staff«, which he had proved to be an urgent necessity following his studies on the origins of haematomas and broken ribs of psychiatric in-patients. When declaring these phenomena to be caused by patients being beaten by the wardens, he received much criticism. But he stood his point, entirely justified, and confirmed that haematomas and broken ribs were caused by wardens beating their patients.

In his clinic Gudden drafted directives for the nursing staff (◻ Fig. 4.6 and 4.7), forbidding any kind of rough treatment of patients by staff. He made a point of making sure that his directives were adhered to both in Werneck and later in Munich.

Bernhard von Gudden, the Scientist

At Werneck von Gudden had carried out more practical, clinical studies – in particular on the consequences of violence to asylum patients. To support his findings reliably, he conducted microscopic studies on traumatically battered ear cartilage and published the results. Due to the transition in to morphological studies, Gudden began his first neuro-anatomical studies at Werneck.

Comparative neuro-anatomical studies on 14 different species of animals and humans led to the

Dienstes-Anweisung

für das

Pflegepersonal

der

Kreisirrenanstalt München.

München.
Druck von Ludwig Mößl.
1884.

◨ **Fig. 4.6.** Instructions to the nursing staff by Bernhard von Gudden (1884)

Grundsätzliches.

1. Die Krankenpflege ist ein schwerer und verantwortlicher Beruf. Wer sich ihm widmen will, muß ein Herz für die Leiden seiner Mitmenschen haben und alle Vorurtheile ablegen, die noch gegen Geisteskranke bestehen.

2. Wie die meisten Krankheiten ohne Verschuldung sich einstellen, so kann auch die Geisteskrankheit den besten, ruhigsten und verständigsten Menschen befallen. Keiner ist unbedingt geschützt gegen dieselbe. Die Geisteskrankheit ist eine Gehirnkrankheit, und das Gehirn kann, wie jedes andere Organ durch die verschiedensten Ursachen in seiner Thätigkeit und in seinen Bestandtheilen beschädigt werden.

3. Geisteskrankheiten schließen die freie Selbstbestimmung mehr oder weniger aus. Keinem Geisteskranken ist das zuzurechnen, was er thut oder unterläßt. Selbst wenn er noch so bösartig erscheint und seine Umgebung noch so sehr und vielleicht sogar mit Ueberlegung und Absicht reizt und quält, so ist es der Zwang der Krankheit, dem er unterliegt, und nicht selten leiden gerade diejenigen Kranken, die am schwersten zu ertragen sind, am meisten und peinlichsten unter ihrer Krankheit.

4. Nicht große Muskelkräfte sind es, auf die es vorzugsweise bei der Pflege Geisteskranker ankommt. Eines einsichtsvollen, wohlwollenden und erfahrenen Pflegepersonals bedarf die Anstalt. Nur in seltenen Fällen wird es einem solchen nicht gelingen, aufgeregte Kranke durch geschickte Ablenkung zu beruhigen und Gewaltthätigkeiten fern zu halten.

5. Geduldig muß das Pflegepersonal sein, freundlich und gefällig gegen jeden Kranken ohne Unterschied, dabei die Rücksichten beobachten, die man dem Stande und der Bildung schuldig ist. Freundlich und geduldig gegen Kranke sich zu benehmen, die dafür empfänglich und dankbar sind, ist eine leicht zu erfüllende Aufgabe. Eine schwere Aufgabe aber ist es, freundlich und geduldig zu bleiben beispielsweise bei solchen Kranken, die gereizt und widerwärtig in ihrer Stimmung jeden Versuch, ihr Schicksal zu erleichtern, schnöde zurückweisen und sich

Fig. 4.7. First page of the instructions to the nursing staff of the District Hospital for Mental Diseases Munich

»In general:

1. Nursing is a difficult and responsible profession. Those who dedicate themselves to this profession, must be sympathetic towards the suffering of fellow human beings, and must rid themselves of all prejudice in respect of the mentally ill.

2. No one is to blame for becoming ill and similarly, even the best, quietest and most sensible people can become mentally ill. No one is immune to becoming mentally ill. Mental disease is a disease of the brain and the brain, like all other organs, can be damaged in its activity and capacity for the most varying reasons.

3. In most cases mental diseases eliminate one's self-control. No mentally ill person can be blamed for what he does or does not do. Even if he seems to be particularly malicious and annoys and tortures those who surround him in what seems to be an intentional manner, it is indeed the forces of disease steering him. It is not uncommon for those patients who are most difficult to put up with, to suffer the most from their own disease.

4. It is not physical strength that counts in the nursing care of the mentally ill. The institutions need understanding, kind and experienced nursing staff. In most cases it is possible to calm agitated patients with skilful diversion and it is not necessary to resort to violence.

5. The nursing staff must be patient, friendly and accommodating to each patient equally and make allowances according to status and education. It is an easy task to behave with kindness and patience towards patients, who are receptive and grateful for such treatment. However, it is difficult to remain friendly and patient towards those patients who are agitated and disagreeable, and who reject with disdain any attempts to improve their situation and ......«

◘ Fig. 4.7. *Continued*

discovery of what he called the »tractus penduncularis transverses«, the fibre bundle. In Zurich Gudden expanded on his animal-experimental studies to identify fibre bundles.

He studied the consequences of extirpation of sense organs and experimentally made lesions in certain brain regions of newly born animals. With this method of secondary atrophy after lesions he discovered a large number of fibre connections in the brain in many species of newly born animals. For his experiments he used the microtome which he had designed together with scientific assistants (e.g. A. Forel) and a builder of instruments. With the microtome it was possible to make a series of slides of the brain (◘ Fig. 4.8)

Von Gudden's method of retrograde degeneration and his microtome quickly ensured his scientific reputation and his methods and microtome were used by scientists world-wide. Gudden's reputation as a researcher from Werneck and his few years

in Zurich led to many young scientists wanting to work with him some of them becoming renowned psychiatrists and neuromorphologists.

The Students of Bernhard von Gudden

August Forel (1848–1931) (◘ Fig. 4.9), who later became professor of psychiatry in Zurich, followed von Gudden from Zurich to Munich. From 1873, Forel worked for almost six years with Gudden and qualified as professor under Gudden's auspices in Munich in 1877 with a study on brain anatomy and the tegmentum region. Forel's successor to the chair of psychiatry in Zurich, Eugen Bleuler (1857–1939), also worked for a couple of months with Gudden in Munich. Constantin von Monakow (1853–1930) visited von Gudden's clinic and laboratory – as did the student Friedrich von Müller (1858–1941), later ordinaries for internal medicine in Munich. According to his »memoires«, von Monakov had probably intended to work with Gudden for longer; but Gudden encouraged him to apply for a job with F. von Rinecker in Wurzburg, as the vacant positions at the district mental hospital in Munich were to be filled by Sigbert Ganser (1853–1931) and Anton Bumm (1849–1903).

Two of Gudden's students later became his successors at the Munich chair of psychiatry: Anton Bumm (► Chapter 5) and Emil Kraepelin (► Chapters 6 and 7).

The brain-anatomical laboratory was the centre of the clinic. All of Gudden's assistants were encouraged to do neuro-anatomical studies in addition to their clinical work. S. Ganser (◘ Fig. 4.10) qualified as professor under Gudden's guidance with an important study on the mole brain. Other assistants published studies on bird brains (A. Bumm)

XVI.

Ueber ein neues Microtom[1].

Der Apparat, um den es sich hier handelt, ist von sehr einfacher Construction und die Bezeichnung „neu" nur in relativem Sinne zulässig. Seine innere Verwandtschaft mit dem Welcker'schen erhellt aus der näheren Betrachtung beider.

Das Welcker'sche Microtom sucht seine Aufgabe folgendermassen zu lösen: durch Drehung einer Schraube führt es in genau messbaren minimalen Erhebungen das zu schneidende wohl fixirte Object dem Messer entgegen; dieses wird gestützt und getragen durch eine breite feste Unterlage und seine sonst freie Beweglichkeit erlaubt es, den für das Objekt schädlichen senkrechten Druck zu vermeiden; das Ausweichen der Schneide nach oben wird durch zwei kleine Vorsprünge verhütet, die den Rücken heben und die Adhäsion dadurch beseitigt, dass unter Wasser gearbeitet wird.

Aus eigener Erfahrung weiss ich, dass man mit dem Instrumente von Welcker sehr feine und schöne Schnitte anzufertigen im Stande ist. Dasselbe bestätigt als einer der competentesten Beurtheiler in Stricker's Handbuch der Lehre von den Geweben Cap. XXX. S. 678 der um die Anatomie des Rückenmarkes hochverdiente Gerlach. Auf seine kleinen Unvollkommenheiten, die jeder kennt, der mit ihm geschnitten hat, näher einzugehen, liegt nicht in meiner Absicht, aber geradezu unbrauchbar ist das Welcker'sche Microtom, sowie die Schnittmethode an die Zerlegung grösserer Objecte herantritt.

Das Ziel, welches mir vorschwebte, war, nicht blos feinste selbst für stärkste Vergrösserungen zugängliche Schnitte herzustellen, sondern auch solche zu Stande zu bringen, die sich über grössere, ja die sich über ganze menschliche Gehirne erstreckten.

Die Microtome von His und Rivatz sind beschrieben in Max Schultze's Archiv für mikroscopische Anatomie

Bd. VI und VII. Der Vorläufer des His'schen war das von Hensen (l. c. Bd. II). Sie genauer zu beschreiben, würde hier zu weit führen.

Grosses Aufsehen und zwar mit vollem Rechte erregten die Schnitte von Betz. Betz lieferte Querschnitte einer ganzen menschlichen Grosshirn-Hemisphäre. Das von ihm benutzte Instrument beschrieb er in Schultze's Archiv Bd. IX. Es besteht aus einem Cylinder mit schmalem Rande, in dem sich mittelst einer ziemlich groben Schraube ein Kolben bewegt. Instrumentenmacher Katsch in München fertigte nach der Betz'schen Zeichnung auf Veranlassung von Herrn Dr. Gierke ein Microtom, das ganz aus Metall gearbeitet, durch Anwendung einer Micrometerschraube, überhaupt durch äusserst sorgsame und präcise Arbeit imponirte und mich sehr bald über den Weg klar werden liess, auf dem das Ziel zu erreichen sei.

Nebenstehender Holzschnitt giebt eine klare Darstellung von dem neuen Apparate. a ist der im Metallcylinder sich bewegende Kolben. Der Cylinder hat einen Querdurchmesser im Lichten von 16 und einen Tiefendurchmesser von 22 Ctm. Zum Schneiden von nicht kleinen menschlichen Gehirnen in sagittaler Richtung sollte der Querdurchmesser allerdings etwas grösser sein, doch kann man sich durch Wegnahme der Spitzen von Stirn- und Hinterhauptshirn, auf die es weniger ankommt, einigermassen helfen. b ist der Rand des Cylinders, auf den das Messer zu liegen kommt. Derselbe ist 3 Ctm, d. h.

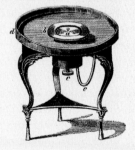

[1] Aus dem Archiv f. Psychiatrie, 5. Bd., 1875, pag. 229.
Gudden, Gesammelte Abhandlungen.   18

◘ **Fig. 4.8.** Picture of the »new microtome« – in »Bernhard von Gudden – collected and remaining essays«, edited by H. Grashey. J.F. Bergmann publishers, Wiesbaden 1889, page 137 (► Chapter 5, ◘ Fig. 5.4)

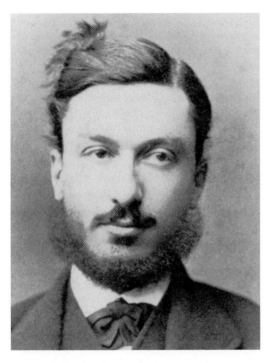

Fig. 4.9. August Forel (1843–1931)

and fish brains (P. Mayser); Kraepelin did anatomical studies on reptile brains.

In 1884, when von Gudden was dean, he had the right to choose a prize subject for the studies at the Munich faculty of medicine. As suggested by Ganser, the topic chosen was on methods for the histological ascertainment of pathological changes in nerve cells.

A 24-year old student presented a study on novel, specific nerve cell colorations, which the Munich anatomist, Karl Wilhelm Kupffer (1829–1902) did not consider worthy of a prize. Von Gudden, however, recognized the fundamental importance of the studies and ensured that the young student received the prize. The student was **Franz Nissl** (◧ Fig. 4.11). Nissl was von Gudden's last student (1885) prior to his death. Nissl quickly became one of the »prince's doctors« for the care of Prince Otto at Furstenried castle. Von Gudden had a small neuropathological laboratory installed at Furstenried, so that apart from his clinical duties, Nissl could also continue his scientific work.

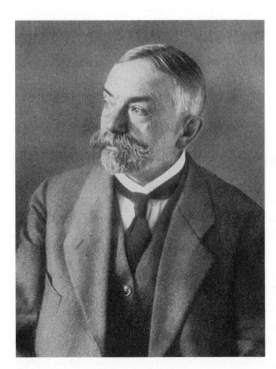

Fig. 4.10. Sigbert Ganser (1853–1931)

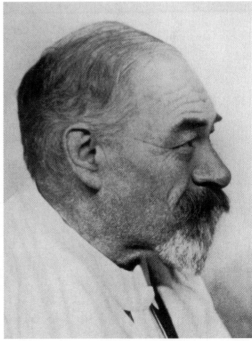

Fig. 4.11. Franz Nissl (1860–1919)

Von Gudden expected his co-workers to do research and deliver contributions to his research on comparative brain-anatomical studies. At the same time clinical work should not be neglected. Gudden himself only worked in the brain-anatomical laboratory during free time from his clinical duties; only during the holidays he found time to put his findings into writing.

For von Gudden and his circle of mainly scientifically interested young co-workers it was a great advantage that some of the assistants could dedicate almost all of their time to clinical work. In this context, **Melchior Josef Bandorf** (1845–1901) (◘ Fig. 4.12) played an important role by taking over the organizational tasks which automatically go side by side with clinical work.

Bandorf had already worked in various Bavarian district mental asylums (e.g. in Irsee and Kathaus-Prull) before joining Gudden in 1873 at the Munich hospital. He soon became senior consultant and von Gudden's deputy. For the assistants he was the »centre point« of the clinic next to Bernhard von Gudden and he gave them space for scientific research work. Emil Kraepelin, assistant at the Munich district mental hospital from 1878 to 1882 and then again from 1884 to 1885, characterized Bandorf in his »memoires« as an impressive

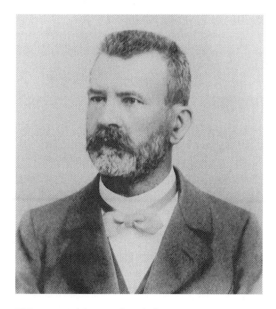

◘ **Fig. 4.12.** Melchior Josef Bandorf (1845–1901)

person: »He was superior due to the quiet and totally reliable implicitness with which he carried out his duties, knew about everything, anticipated everything and always had good advice. His friendly objectivity, also towards the youngest colleagues, meant that he was highly esteemed by all of us.«

With Melchior Josef Bandorf as senior consultant Bernhard von Gudden had started a tradition, which was noted at the 75-year anniversary of the clinic in the Nussbaumstrasse, that the Munich clinic was not only headed by »remarkable directors« – such as Bernhard von Gudden, Emil Kraepelin and Oswald Bumke – but also by the personalities of their senior clinical consultants.

Bandorf remained as senior consultant with von Gudden, until he became the first director of the newly built, second Upper Bavarian district mental hospital in Gabersee, near to Wasserburg.

Von Gudden had been involved decisively in the planning of Gabersee.

The constant over-occupancy of the Munich clinic had led to the creation of a care institution in Attel am Inn in 1873 (► Chapter 2); but this measure had not led to sustainable relief for the clinic in Munich and von Gudden saw the necessity to use his influence for the construction of a further district mental hospital in Upper Bavaria. The realization of the plan and the nomination of his senior consultant to be first director in Gabersee gave von Gudden great satisfaction, although von Gudden had no success – in spite of his initially very influential position in Munich – with his plans to build another clinic (see below).

In 1883 not only Bandorf, but also another older co-worker left the Munich clinic to take over one of the Bavarian district mental hospitals; a son of A. von Solbrig, August Solbrig jnr who was probably already assistant at the Munich clinic when von Gudden took over. As reported by Kraepelin, Solbrig jnr was also one of the »prince's doctors«.

On Solbrig's departure, Franz Carl Müller (1860–1913) joined the clinical in 1884 and soon became one of the »prince's doctors«. F. C. Müller's name is often remembered because he was on duty at Berg castle together with the nursing staff when von Gudden and Ludwig the Second died.

Not every assistant from the Munich district mental hospital was employed as a »prince's doctor« to take care of Prince Otto at Furstenried castle.

Although von Gudden could propose names of »prince's doctors«, he had to receive permission from the ministry and he did receive permission for one co-worker who is generally no longer remembered as psychiatrist: Oskar Panizza (1853–1923), (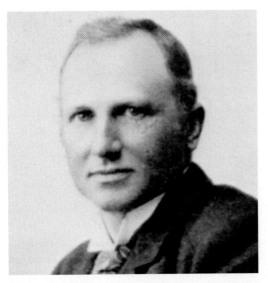 Fig. 4.13).

In 1895 Panizza, author of »Heaven's Tragedy: The Council of Love«, was condemned to prison for a year on charges of blasphemy. In this book, considered by Theodor Fontane to be »quite an important piece of literature«, Panizza described the »appearance of syphilis in Italy towards the end of the 15th century to have been caused by the depraved behaviour at the pope's court«. After serving his sentence, Panizza lived as a free-lance writer in Switzerland and France and composed a collection of poems »Parisana«, in which he denigrated the German Kaiser. As a result, he was a wanted man in Germany, but returned to Munich, where he was arrested and admitted to the district mental hospital for an expertise on his condition. This was the same clinic, where he had worked as assistant to von Gudden, but due to difficulties with the »boss«

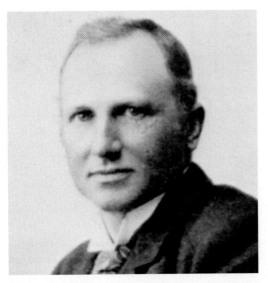

Fig. 4.13. Oskar Panizza (1853–1921)

and being scared of becoming mentally ill himself if he continued to work in a psychiatric clinic, he had left the clinic of his own accord. Several of Panizza's relatives were psychiatrically ill.

In 1901 an expertise confirmed that already before his first prison sentence in 1895 Panizza had been suffering from a chronically progressive paranoid and probably also hallucinatory psychosis. He was therefore placed under tutelage and not sentenced. From 1904 onwards until his death in 1921, and after his literary productivity had dried up, Panizza was a chronic patient at a sanatorium in Bayreuth.

The Development of Psychiatry in Munich during von Gudden's Last Years

After taking up office in Munich von Gudden quickly became an important person in the medical faculty. Already in 1872, he was nominated into the Medicinal Committee, whose task it was to advise the Ministry of the Interior in all medical issues for the entire Kingdom of Bavaria. In 1883 von Gudden was the second chairman of this committee which was otherwise headed by senior ministerial officials (J. v. Kerschensteiner). Further members of the committee at the time of von Gudden were B.M. von Pettenkofer and H. von Ziemssen.

The influential position and prestige occupied by von Gudden might suggest that his demands were always fulfilled. Immediately after his move to Munich Gudden took up A. von Solbrig's demand for a psychiatric university clinic independent of the district mental hospital and he was of the opinion that a full professorship and chair of psychiatry should also be separate from the management of the district mental hospital. The clinic should be located near to the other clinics of the medical faculty on the left bank of the river Isar. It was not until he was offered a position in Leipzig in 1874, the best position in Germany at the time, that his demands were suddenly taken seriously. On turning down the offer from Leipzig, he received a salary increase, was elevated into nobility and 200,000.- gilders were put aside for the construction of a new clinic (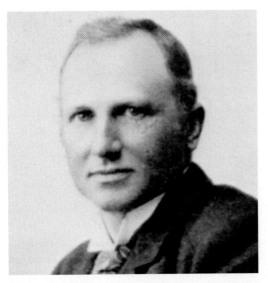 Fig. 4.14).

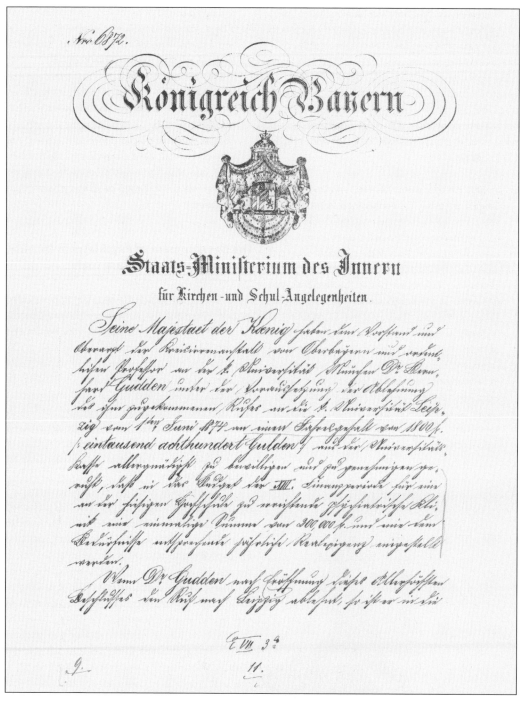

▣ Fig. 4.14. Certificate of May 31, 1874, memorandum from the Ministry of the Interior to the Senate of the University: **Kingdom of Bavaria State Ministry of the Interior for Church and School Matters. His Majesty the King has graciously agreed and proposes to the Head and Senior Consultant of the District Mental Asylum of Upper Bavaria and ordinary professor of the University of Munich, Dr. Bernhard von Gudden, assuming that he turns down the offer from the University of Leipzig of June 1, 1874, that he accepts an annual salary of 1,800 guilders from the University exchequer, and that a one-time sum of**

200,000 guilders be included in the budget for the 13ᵗʰ financial period for a psychiatric clinic to be established at the local university. If after publication of this highest resolution, Dr. Gudden turns down the offer from Leipzig, he will receive an additional sum of 600 guilders yearly and on the resolution by the presently assembled parliament the negotiations for the founding of a psychiatric clinic will begin immediately. In any case, after 8 days a report must be given on the status of the matter. Munich, May 31, 1874. By order of His Royal Majesty. Dr. v. Lutz (from the university arches Munich, signed: E-II-455)

However, after refusing Leipzig, his plans did not progress. In 1886, only a few months before his death, his application for the separation of the psychiatric professorship from the hospital management was turned down again on the grounds that the »psychiatric professorship as a complimentary additional office must suffice«.

At least von Gudden had initiated proceedings for the construction of the psychiatric clinic in the Nussbaumstrasse, which finally came to be 30 years after his move to Munich and 18 years after his tragic death.

Literature

Gudden, W. (1987): Bernhard von Gudden – Leben und Werk. Diss. Medical Faculty of the TU Munich

Gudden, W., Hippius, H., Steinberg, R. (in preparation): Bernhard von Gudden. Springer Verlag: Heidelberg

Wöbking, W. (1986): Der Tod Koenig Ludwigs II. Von Bayer – Eine Dokumentation. Rosenheimer Verlagshaus: Rosenheim

Planning and Construction of the Royal Psychiatric University Hospital in the Nussbaumstrasse

Hubert von Grashey and Anton Bumm

In many ways the death of Ludwig the Second and Bernhard von Gudden caused a serious incision in the development of psychiatry in Munich.

Since the beginning of 1886, the situation in the Kingdom of Bavaria and the tension between the King and the state ministries were mentioned more and more frequently in the press and abroad. In Bavaria the entire population was keenly interested in the events. The large expenditure by the King and his increasingly strange behaviour were criticised from all sides and not just in Bavaria, although allowances were made for him. The greater part of the Bavarians identified with their beloved King since his coronation in March 1864. The greater the quarrels about the King were in Bavaria in 1886, almost leading to a state crisis, the more unrest and discontent occurred.

In this atmosphere in March 1886, the members of the Bavarian government requested Bernhard von Gudden to give his professional opinion on the mental state of the King. As a consequence and as already mentioned (▶ Chapter 4), he met with the members of the state ministry to receive further information as to the King's conspicuousness and was handed files on the subject. By this time von Gudden was convinced that it was his duty to agree to this arduous task and on his proposal preparations were made for a collegial expertise. On June 8, 1886, von Gudden presented the colle-gial expertise to the entire ministry. In particular, it contained the explanation that from a professional point of view »the King was not expected to be able to govern the state for over a year« (▶ Chapter 4). The entire ministry then resolved to proclaim the King's uncle, Prince Luitpold, prince regent on June 10, 1886.

On communication of these developments at home and abroad the unrest in Bavaria grew; the beloved King had been forced to abdicate and a psychiatrist had helped to achieve this. Shortly afterwards sparce bits of news seeped out to the public about the events in Hohenschwangau and Neuschwanstein and how the King had been accompanied to Berg castle at the Lake of Starnberg by psychiatrists and nursing staff. The unrest increased further and not only von Gudden was blamed for the situation. And, finally the news of the death of Ludwig the Second and Bernhard von Gudden on June 13, 1886, was broken.

Still today Bavaria is suspicious of psychiatry and the roots of this suspicion no doubt originate from the events leading up to the death of Ludwig the Second.

In this context the situation for the Munich district mental hospital in June of 1886 was particularly difficult. With tremendous personal effort since his taking up office in 1872 von Gudden had managed to gain considerable appreciation for psychiatry and the Munich district mental hospital had a good reputation. All of a sudden this seemed no longer to apply and in many areas an anti-psychiatry mood was observed. The critical situation of the clinic was further aggravated during these days by staff problems which had already started prior to von Gudden's death.

From 1884 some particularly established and experienced co-workers (e.g. M.J. Bandorf, A. Bumm, S. Ganser, E. Kraepelin) had left the Munich district mental hospital to take on leading positions at other clinics. One senior consultant, who had been hired to fill the gap, was taken ill shortly after joining the clinic, was given sick leave for a year and finally had to resign at the end of April 1886.

All together, by the beginning of 1886, the situation at the clinic had become so precarious that von Gudden had to ask a former co-worker, Paul Mayser (1853–1922), to come and help out as senior consultant for a couple of months. Mayser had already worked in Munich for von Gudden, from 1876–1881, and then left to work for A. Forel in Zurich, where he habilitated. Forel agreed for Mayser to assist von Gudden, although he left Munich soon afterwards to take over a senior position at the institution in Saxony (Altscherbitz). He had already been offered the job whilst working for Forel in Zurich; Mayser had accepted and it was now requested that he go to Saxony, as the vacant position could no longer be kept vacant.

In spring 1886, Bernhard von Gudden had mainly young and inexperienced co-workers at his disposal. Only two of them had been at the clinic since 1884 and therefore had only two years of experience; F. C. Müller (1860–1913), (see page 42) and E. Rehm (1860–1913) (see page 41). Both assistants joined the clinic immediately after completing their medical studies and theses in 1884. F. Nissl (1860–1919) also worked at the clinic, although he did not join until 1885.

Due to the serious shortage of staff in spring 1886, von Gudden made E. Rehm his deputy as clinic director on June 1, 1886; F. C. Müller was to assist von Gudden with his plans for the care of the ill King in Berg castle. F. C. Müller had already worked as a »prince's doctor« in Fürstenried castle (▶ Chapter 4).

This was the situation at the Munich clinic, when suddenly, from one day to the next, the clinic was left without even a director!

Officially, the District Mental Hospital of Upper Bavaria had 550 beds, but until completion of the building in Gabersee and the end of the 1880's it had to admit 670–690 patients. E. Rehm, who had only just become deputy director two months previously, was faced with a difficult task: Following Ludwig the Second's death, F. C. Müller and F. Nissl were very busy taking care of his brother at Fürstenried castle. The entire job of running the clinic was left up to E. Rehm and three inexperienced young doctors who had only just started working there.

Obviously, E. Rehm mastered the task relatively well despite the difficult weeks and hostility towards psychiatry. In a letter from the end of June 1886 he wrote to A. Forel in Zurich, that »it had definitely been quite an effort to keep things going, but the situation is satisfactory or at least has to be satisfactory«.

Luckily the medical faculty made a quick decision on the successor for Bernhard von Gudden and the ministry nominated Hubert Grashey, who had been working in Wurzburg since 1884 as professor of psychiatry. On September 8, 1886, Prince Regent Luitpold wrote to the senate of the Munich University, informing them that as of September 1, 1886, Grashey was Full Professor of Psychiatry of the Munich University (▢ Fig. 5.1).

On September 20, 1886, Grashey became Professor of Psychiatry at the Medical Faculty of the University of Munich and at the same time director of the Upper Bavarian District Mental Hospital.

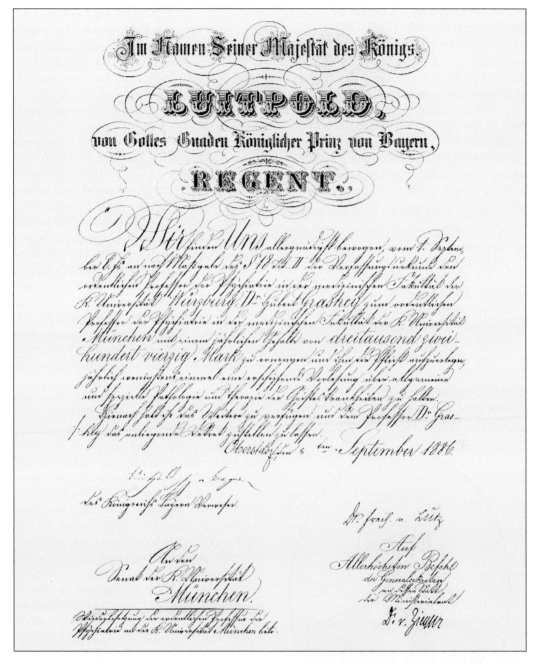

■ **Fig. 5.1.** Letter from the Prince Regent Luitpold to the Senate of the Munich University regarding the re-occupation of the ordinary chair for psychiatry: **In the name of His Majesty the King – Luitpold – by God's grace. Royal Prince of Bavaria – REGENT. We find ourselves disposed on September 1, according to para. 18, cit. II of the constitutional charter, to appoint the ordinary professor of psychiatry at the medical faculty of the Wurzburg University, Dr. Hubert Grashey, as ordinary professor of psychiatry at the medical faculty of the Munich University with an annual salary of three thousand two hundred and forty marks and to oblige him to give at least once a year a detailed lecture about general and special pathology and therapy of mental diseases. Hereby you are requested to carry out the necessary and to give the enclosed decree to Professor Dr. Grashey. Oberstdorf, September 8, 1886** (from the university archives, Munich, signed, E-II-1496)

Hubert von Grashey–Professor of Psychiatry in Munich (1886–1896)

Hubert Grashey (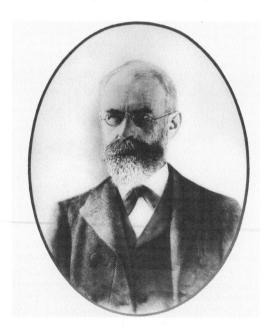 Fig. 5.2), son of a local judge, was born in Gronenbach/Allgau on October 31, 1839. He went to secondary school in Augsburg and then studied medicine in Wurzburg from 1859 to 1865. In Wurzburg he visited the lectures of Franz von Rinecker (1811–1883), one of the outstanding personalities at the Wurzburg medical faculty and an impressive academic teacher. Grashey became one of Rinecker's students.

> At the age of 25 F. Rinecker habilitated in 1836 in Wurzburg in internal medicine. In 1837 he became extraordinary professor and a year later full professor. He gave lectures on pharmacy, pediatrics and dermatology, later on physiology and microscopy; he founded the Institute of Physiology at Wurzburg. In 1863 Rinecker joined the Julius Hospital and took over the Department of Psychiatry; as of 1872 he was director of the Dermatological Clinic. As mentioned by Kraepelin in his memoires, Rinecker had many students who influenced sustainably the development of certain medical subjects, in particular psychiatry, and these included, F. Jolly, S. Ganser, K. Rieger, A. Bumm and E. Kraepelin.

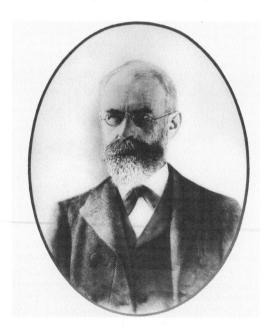

Fig. 5.2. Hubert von Grashey (1839–1914)

From 1864 until 1867 Grashey was assistant doctor at the Julius Hospital's department for the mentally ill, managed by Rinecker. Following that he went to the Lower Franconian district mental asylum, Werneck, whose director was Bernhard von Gudden. From Werneck Grashey visited the universities of Berlin and Vienna and their psychiatric clinics in 1868 and 1869.

It was also in Werneck that Grashey met Anna, Gudden's eldest daughter, who later became his wife. After the Gudden family moved to Zurich in 1872, Grashey remained for a further year as assistant to M. Hubrich (1837-1896), Gudden's successor until he was offered to take over the Lower Bavarian district mental asylum in Deggendorf. Shortly after moving to Deggendorf, he married Gudden's daughter. Grashey worked in Deggendorf for 11 years until he was offered a professorship for psychiatry at Wurzburg, following the death of his teacher, Rinecker. He managed the department for the mentally ill at the Julius Hospital until 1886, when he received an offer from Munich, following the death of his father-in-law (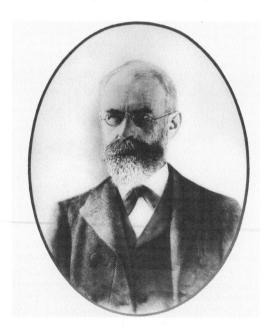 Fig. 5.3).

Under von Rinecker's influence Grashey, as a young scientist, had been working on the problem of using the method of sphygmorgraphy to study blood supply to the brain. To answer this question he developed physiological model trials (on elastic tubes) and clinical studies. He had wanted to re-visit these studies and continue them, but only ever managed to realize these plans in a limited scope for various reasons. According to contemporaries, Grashey was extremely thorough, precise and responsible; every aspect of each task had to be taken into consideration. On his move to Deggendorf, when he was 34 years' old, he dedicated himself to managing the clinic and scientific studies had only secondary value. Once the 11 years in Deggendorf were up, Grashey returned to Wurzburg intending to continue with his research, but he received an offer from Munich where he had little opportunity for undisturbed, scientific work.

In Munich Grashey considered it to be a matter of urgency to take over where von Gudden had left off and to stabilize the atmosphere in the clinic. He found a loyal supporter in E. Rehm.

Personal-Liste.

Familien- und Vorname.	Geburts- Ort.	Tag.	Monat.	Jahr.	Religion.	Familien-Stand	Kinder-Zahl Knaben	Mädchen	Graduirungen, erste Anstellung, Beförderungen.	Datum der Diplome, Rescripte etc. Tag.	Monat.	Jahr.	Titel und Ordens-Verleihungen etc.
Grashey Hubert	Grönenbach	30.	October	1839	katholisch	verheiratet	1	—	Zum Doktor der Medizin promoviert	17.	März	1866.	Inhaber des Verdienstordens vom hl. Michael IV. Klasse, k. Obermedizinalrat.
									Vom 1. Jänner 1869 an zum II. Hilfsarzt der Kreis-Irrenanstalt Werneck [illegible] ernannt.	22.	Feb.	1869.	
									Vom October 1869 bis März 1870 [illegible] Werneck aufgestellt	15.	Sept.	1869.	
									Vom 1. Mai 1870 an zum I. Hilfsarzt der Kreis-Irren-Anstalt Werneck ernannt.	29.	April	1870	
									Vom 1. Mai 1873 an zum Direktor der Kreis-Irrenanstalt Deggendorf ernannt	22.	April	1873	
									Zum ordentl. Professor der Psychiatrie [illegible] Würzburg vom 1. Aug. 1884 an ernannt.	9.	Juni	1884.	
									Vom 1. Sept. 1886 an zum Direktor der oberbayer. Kreis-Irrenanstalt in München ernannt.	31.	August	1886	
									Zum ordentl. Professor der Psychiatrie an der Universität München v. 1. Sept. 1886 an ernannt.	8.	Sept.	1886.	

München 24. October 1886 Prof. Grashey

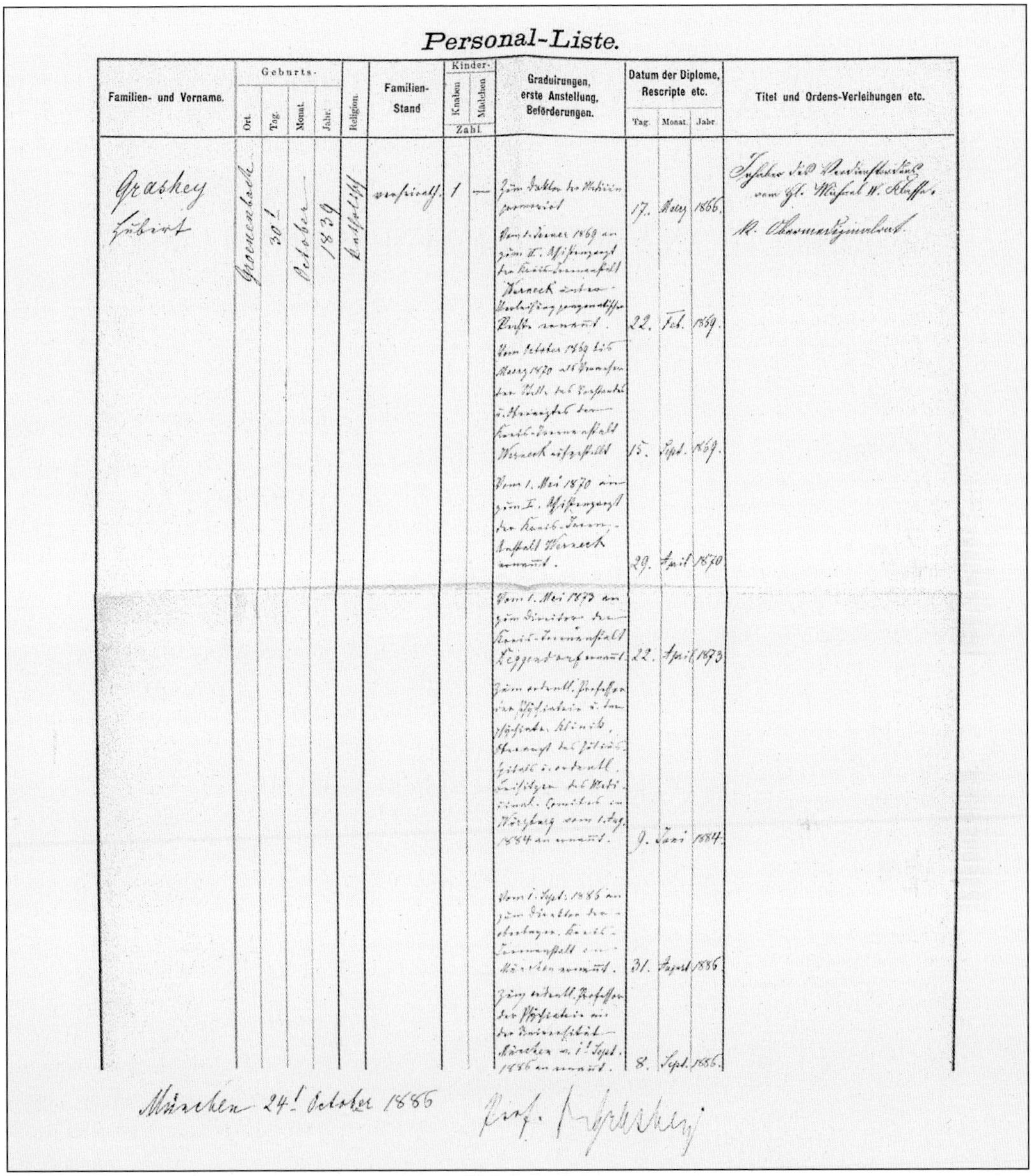

Fig. 5.3. Staff entry on Hubert Grashey, dated October 24, 1886 and signed by Grashey himself (from the University Archives, Munich, signed: E-II-1496)

E. Rehm had bridged the difficult time between von Gudden's death and Grashey's appointment. He remained at the clinic as senior consultant until 1892 and then became owner and director of the rehabilitation centre for nervous and mental diseases, called Neufriedheim, which had been built by two general practitioners from Munich. The clinic had capacity for 70, and later 90 male and female patients. F. Vocke, who had joined the clinic in 1890, became Rehm's successor as senior consultant with Grashey. Later Vocke worked for A. Bumm and then in 1901, he became the first director of the newly built district mental asylum in Eglfing (see below).

BERNHARD VON GUDDEN'S

GESAMMELTE UND HINTERLASSENE ABHANDLUNGEN.

HERAUSGEGEBEN

VON

DR. H. GRASHEY,

O. Ö. PROFESSOR DER UNIVERSITÄT UND DIRECTOR DER OBERBAYER. KREISIRRENANSTALT ZU MÜNCHEN.

MIT 41 IN KUPFER RADIRTEN TAFELN UND EINEM PORTRAIT.

WIESBADEN.

VERLAG VON J. F. BERGMANN.

1889.

◻ Fig. 5.4. Title page of the book »Bernhard von Gudden's collected and remaining essays«, 1889

When Grashey became von Gudden's successor it was inevitable that he would constantly be confronted with queries about the tragic events on June 13, 1886. He had to give an expertise, outlining his opinion on how both the King and his psychiatrist had died. After consideration of all the points he thought to be important, he composed a detailed obituary for his father-in-law. In the obituary he made his point of view clear: that Gudden had reacted without considering the consequences when he made a hand sign to the nursing staff accompanying him and the King on their evening stroll, sending him away. Grashey was of the opinion that the sign had been misinterpreted and that Gudden had not wanted to send the nurse away.

In the context of von Gudden's obituary, Grashey and F. C. Müller, a co-worker at Berg castle, were of differing opinions. F. C. Müller had been present at Berg castle on June 13, 1886, and had taken part in the search for the King and von Gudden. Grashey and Müller's disagreement became public and the situation further worsened the atmosphere at the clinic.

As assistant at the clinic Müller had a special position, being responsible for the care of Prince Otto, Ludwig's brother at Furstenried castle, even after Grashey had taken up office. At the beginning of 1887 Prince Regent Luitpold handed the task of taking care of King Otto to Grashey.

> F. C. Müller finally left the clinic in 1888 and took over the »Water Cure Institute« in Alexandersbad in the Fichtel mountains, but returned to Munich in 1896 and opened a practise as specialist for nervous diseases. In 1902, together with another psychiatrist, he founded an out-patient unit for the mentally ill.

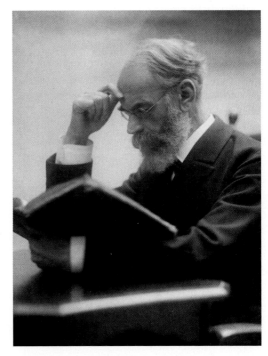

Fig. 5.5. Hubert von Grashey

In remembrance of von Gudden, in 1889 Grashey published a large volume entitled: »Bernhard von Gudden's Collected and Testated Works« (◘ Fig. 5.4). Grashey considered it his job to bring those matters that von Gudden could no longer work on, to a successful conclusion. Consequently, he emphatically committed himself to making sure that a psychiatric university clinic, separate from the district mental hospital, be set up. Grashey was a highly esteemed member of the medical faculty, had a good reputation at the Bavarian ministries and generally with the public health system of the Kingdom of Bavaria; he was a member of the Higher Medical Committee and became a member of the Medical Committee of the University of Munich in 1891. It was on his initiative in 1895 that the rule was laid down for psychiatric employees to become qualified as professional nursing staff. But however great his influence, Grashey did not manage to achieve much more than his predecessors, A. von Solbrig and B. von Gudden, when it came to the demand for an independent and new psychiatric university clinic!

It seems that this was the main reason for him to render his office as university professor and director of the district mental hospital in 1896. Prior to this he had been offered the job, at 57 years of age, to become consultant to the civil medical health system in the Kingdom of Bavaria. The specialist for internal medicine, J. von Kerschensteiner (1831–1896), had just resigned from this position. Presumably Grashey would have more influence as consultant in the Bavaria Ministry of the Interior with respect to the planning of the psychiatric clinic in Munich than he would have with a university job. In the Ministry of the Interior he made sure that in all areas of the Bavarian medical administration psychiatric training and studies in psychiatry be improved.

Grashey was gentrified in 1899 in Bavaria and became decorated for his services to the Bavarian Crown.

When Grashey (◘ Fig. 5.5) bade farewell to his university career, he was pleased to rid himself of his double roles which were increasingly becoming a burden. Soon he was given other tasks: 1897 he became extraordinary member of the Royal Public Health Department and in 1901 member of the Royal Imperial Health Council.

In 1904 von Grashey resigned from active duty for the Bavarian state. In 1909, almost 70 years of age, he finally retired, but still participated in some important matters and consequently was co-author of an expertise on the mental state of King Otto.

On August 24, 1914 at the age of almost 75 years von Grashey died in Munich.

Anton Bumm – Professor of Psychiatry in Munich (1896–1903)

Following Grashey's resignation as university professor and director of the district mental hospital, a successor had to be found as soon as possible. As proposed by the medical faculty Anton Bumm from Erlangen was offered the job.

Anton Bumm (■ Fig. 5.6) was born in Wurzburg on March 27, 1849.

> His father, Kasper Bumm, was teacher of the deaf and dumb. Bumm had an older sister and three younger brothers. All five children were exceptionally gifted. His sister, Franziska, managed to finish secondary school, which was something very unusual in the second half of the previous century; as the family could not afford to send her to university, she chose her father's profession and became teacher for the deaf and dumb. Two of A. Bumm's younger brothers became lawyers. Karl Bumm (note the index of names on pages 46 and 55) became an important official at the Bavarian Ministry of Culture, was gentrified and knighted. Franz Bumm became president of the Royal Imperial Health Council in Berlin and as such supported the research done by Robert Koch and Emil von Behring. Of all the brothers the most well known was Ernst Bumm. He became professor of gynaecology and obstetrics in Basle and Halle; in 1904 he became ordinarius for gynaecology at the Charité in Berlin and managed the University Clinic for Gynaecology there.

Anton Bumm began his medical studies in 1867 in Wurzburg and before finishing became assistant military doctor during the war against France in 1870/1871. He was given a medal for his services and later, for his commitment on behalf of the French prisoners, was decorated by the French.

His experiences as military doctor were the basis for his dissertation and in 1872 he graduated at the university of Wurzburg with a thesis »On Bullet Wounds«.

Like his brothers and sisters Anton Bumm was highly gifted. He was said to have spoken 14 languages, was universally educated and widely read. Amongst his colleagues and co-workers he was considered to have exceptional knowledge of the entire scientific psychiatric literature of the time.

Bumm began his psychiatric career in June 1873 at the Lower Franconian district mental asylum, Werneck which was managed after Gudden's resignation in 1872 by Max Hubrich. During his time at Werneck (1873–1877) Bumm received a travel grant from the State of Bavaria and Hubrich allowed him to take long research trips to Vienna (to Th. Meynert) and Paris (to J.M. Charcot at the Salpetrière).

In 1877 B. von Gudden invited A. Bumm to join the Munich districal mental hospital and to work on scientific research there. Bumm considered this proposition an honour. As he had already

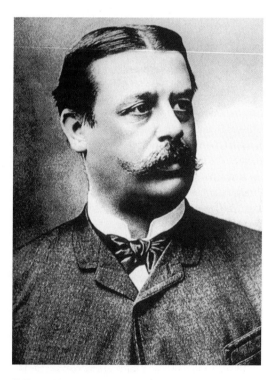

■ **Fig. 5.6.** Anton Bumm (1849–1903)

worked in Vienna with Meynert on neuro-anatomy, he fitted well into von Gudden's circle (along with A. Forel, S. Ganser and E. Kraepelin). Bumm did neuro-anatomical studies on bird brains and the retina of rabbits. After working with von Gudden's group for 6 six years, Bumm came to the conclusion he could not make a career by solely concentrating on neuro-anatomical topics and therefore, in the summer of 1883, applied for a job as »second assistant doctor« with F. W. Hagen (1814–1888) in Erlangen.

> F. W. Hagen had been managing the clinic in Erlangen since 1859 as successor to A. von Solbrig after his appointment to Munich.
> Hagen had studied theology, but then switched to medicine. At this time – similar to Solbrig – he visited the lectures of J.M. Leupoldt (see above); this was the period in which Hagen's interest in psychiatry was aroused. In 1836 and 1846 Hagen used the possibilities offered to him to work in various clinics at home and abroad. When the district mental hospital was opened in 1846 with Solbrig as director, Hagen returned to Erlangen and worked there for 3 years. In 1849 he was appointed as director of the newly opened district mental hospital, Irsee near to Kaufbeuren. When Solbrig was appointed to Munich in 1859, Hagen returned to Erlangen as Solbrig's successor after 10 years at Irsee.
> Hagen was – together with B. von Gudden, H. Grashey and M. Hubrich – one of the authors of the 1886 expertise on Ludwig the Second.

A. Bumm worked with Hagen in Erlangen for only a year; in 1884 he became – at 35 years of age being the youngest of all applicants – successor to H. Grashey as the head of the Lower Bavarian district mental asylum Deggendorf. In March 1888 Bumm was Hagen's successor in Erlangen as director of the clinic and professor of psychiatry at the university. Bumm successfully competed for the job against applicants such as S. Ganser and his previous boss, M. Hubrich.

When Bumm took over the professorship in Erlangen, an enormous amount of work was waiting for him: he had never taught at a university previously and had to prepare himself for these tasks in a very short period of time. During its 40 years' of existence the clinic in Erlangen became increas-

ingly overloaded with all kinds of new tasks and was constantly overcrowded. Consequently, Bumm soon proposed building a second clinic in Middle Franconia, but his suggestion was not accepted. As a result during his time in Erlangen, Bumm had to carry out small alterations and conversions to the building so that the situation there was not to become completely intolerable. Bumm ordered 8 large wards to be rebuilt; he also had work done on household and farming outbuildings, as well as quarters for the officials. Not one single year went past without Bumm having something done on some part of the building. In connection with the construction work Bumm studied the development of building for psychiatry in detail, in particular with the principle of the »panoptical mental asylum« (▶ Chapter 2; ◘ Fig. 2.1).

> The district mental asylum in Erlangen is the only psychiatric clinic in Germany which was built as a »panoptical institute«. This building principle, with buildings arranged like bicycle spokes, had been successful in England. For the custodial aspects of psychiatry it meant that in the »panoptical institute« the nursing staff could monitor centrally with a relatively small number of staff.

On his appointment to Munich in November 1896 as successor to Grashey (◘ Fig. 5.7), A. Bumm soon picked up where his predecessor had off in separating the job of head of the district mental asylum from the professorship for psychiatry at the medical faculty. In his first year of office, however, Bumm did not successed and the increasing burden caused by the double-function which had already caused Grashey to consider handing in his notice, grew even further for Bumm: exam duties increased because psychiatry had become an obligatory subject for a license in medicine; the load from forensic expertises became ever more extensive. To add to all this, the clinic was constantly overcrowded and subsequently the situation became unhealthy – facts leaked out to the public – leading finally to the decision of the Upper Bavarian diet (the body, which corresponds with today's district government) in 1899 to abandon the district mental hospital in the »Au«, near Munich, in order to construct a much larger new institution, but further away from the

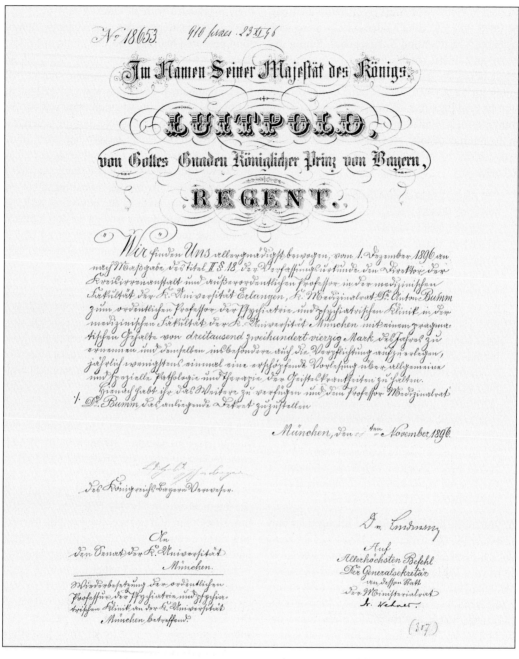

Fig. 5.7. Letter from the Prince Regent Luitpold to the Senate of the Munich University on November 21, 1896:
In the name of His Majesty the King – Luitpold – by God's grace. Royal Prince of Bavaria – REGENT. We find ourselves disposed as of December 1896, according to tit. II, para. 18 of the constitutional charter, to appoint the director of the District Mental Asylum and extraordinary professor of the medical faculty of the Erlangen University, Dr. Anton Bumm, as ordinary professor of psychiatry at the medical faculty of the Munich University with a pragmatic annual salary of three thousand two hundred and forty marks and in particular to oblige him to give at least once a year a detailed lecture about general and special pathology and therapy of mental diseases. Hereby you are requested to carry out the necessary and to give the enclosed decree to Professor and Medical Counsellor, Dr. Bumm. Munich, November 30, 1896 (from the university archives, signed: E-II-576)

city. This development fitted A. Bumm's plans perfectly and he could continue with his aim to have a independent university clinic near the city, situated close to the hospital on the left bank of the Isar (»Links der Isar«) together with the other university clinics.

Bumm's plans were supported by the Munich city authorities, since it had become increasingly difficult to cover the psychiatric needs of Munich's population. During Grashey's time in office all mentally ill Munich citizens could be admitted to the district mental asylum, but in the mid 90's this practise had been changed. After 1898 all psychiatric patients had to be first admitted to one of the city hospitals, examined and then transferred to the district mental asylum. Only after completion of these time-consuming formalities was it possible to transfer patients to the district mental asylum. Subsequently within a couple of years the number of psychiatric patients in Munich hospitals increased drastically (from approx. 150 to 700 per year).

As a result, Bumm could count on support from two sides – on one hand from the district authorities and on the other from the authorities of the city of Munich

Bumm prepared an expertise for the medical faculty in which he recommended the combination of a psychiatric university clinic with a »city asylum« (psychiatric hospital department for the citizens of Munich) with a total of 100 beds. The medical faculty and the senate of the Munich university agreed to his proposal and assigned a faculty commission, headed by Bumm, (and also including the internal specialist von Ziemssen) to make further suggestions for the actual realization of the concept. Bumm did the job with great dedication and completed it successfully!

In 1900 the commission's proposal was accepted and the building of a »Royal University Clinic for Psychiatry« on the site of the Hospital »Links der Isar« was agreed. The city of Munich offered a construction site on the corner of Nussbaum- and Goethestrasse, which belonged to the hospital foundation »Links der Isar«. In return, the university had to promise to admit the mentally ill of the city of Munich, at least temporarily, and to examine them there. Furthermore, the university should cover the construction costs, the furnishings and

the running of the clinic. Both the state government and the university agreed.

However, one further point had to be clarified: The intended building site belonged to the Sisters of Mercy of the Order of St. Vincent von Paul. The nuns used the land for agricultural purposes and there were doubts whether building a psychiatric clinic on this site would not lead to harassment. As compensation the nuns were offered a piece of land in Berg am Laim; also financial compensation was offered for the stable and agricultural buildings as well as the courtyard and garden. Negotiations with the nuns were successful and on top of it all the university and the order came to an agreement that the nuns would be responsible for the catering and nursing of the future psychiatry clinic (▶ Chapter 6).

Once the complicated negotiations had been completed, Bumm reduced his workload more and more; he delegated forensic-psychiatric expertises to his senior consultant F. Vocke.

Friedrich Vocke (1865–1927) (◨ Fig. 5.8) was already assistant doctor to Grashey in 1890. In 1892 he became senior consultant and was still in this position when Grashey resigned in 1896 and Bumm became his successor.

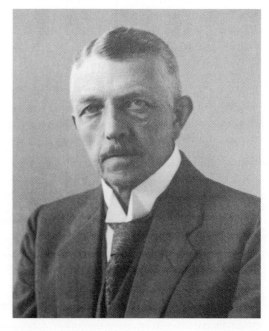

◨ **Fig. 5.8.** Friedrich Vocke (1865- 1927)

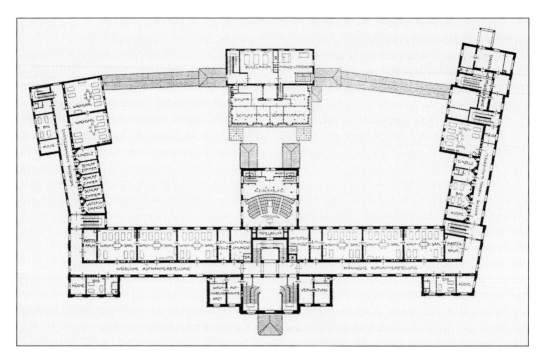

Fig. 5.9. From the building drafts: Floor plan for the 1st floor, signed Littmann (architect); dated 28.11.1901

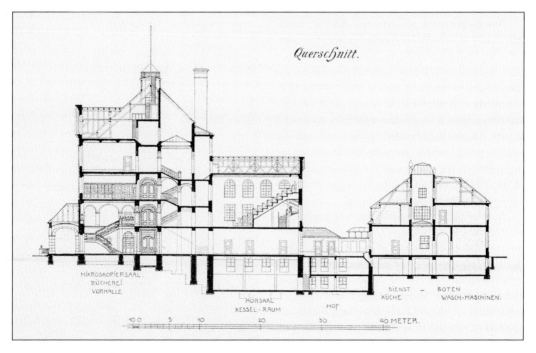

Fig. 5.10. From the building drafts: Section A–B of the middle tract – section through the ward building, auditorium and housekeeping building (builders: Heilmann and Littmann), signed by Littmann (architect); dated 28.11.1901

Vocke had achieved a special position not only through his forensic work, but also by assisting in the planning of the district mental asylum in Eglfing, for which Bumm remained responsible. With Vocke's support, Bumm had time to dedicate himself to the planning of the university clinic. Once the plans for Eglfing had been completed, Vocke was appointed director. Shortly after completion of Eglfing, Vocke pressed for a further building based on the expected overcrowding. His demands were accepted and a second asylum was built directly next to the Eglfing complex and opened in 1912: the asylum Haar (Haar and Eglfing were later – in 1931 – combined organizationally to make one large clinic).

Anton Bumm requested to be relieved from his duties in November 1900 in order to work solely on the planning and construction of the psychiatric clinic; he kept up his teaching activities as university professor. By resigning as director, a different and unexpected problem arose because the district authorities considered discontinuing the student lectures in the newly built asylum in Eglfing. Bumm managed to convince them to allow four-hour, weekly clinical training at Eglfing until the new clinic opened its doors.

In 1901 Bumm signed a contract which obliged him to become director of the new university clinic.

Another disagreement between Bumm and the Ministry of the Interior when Bumm demanded to increase the initially agreed 100 beds by a further 40 reserve beds. The reserve beds were intended for nursing staff, but in case of sudden overcrowding could be used for patients (e.g. when repair work was necessary or if new, special, closed wards were constructed, as could be the case for the examination of prisoners). In the opinion of the ministry Bumm's demand calling for a third floor in the west wing on the Goethestrasse, could not be fulfilled. However, the university senate was entirely on Bumm's side and in the end Bumm received the extra beds he had requested.

In every respect Bumm planned with foresight. For example, during the planning stages he made a request to the university senate to be generous when equipping the future clinic library (e.g. by acquiring the 56-volume edition of »Zeitschrift für klinische Psychiatrie und psychiatrisch-gerichtliche Medizin« (Journal of Clinical Psychiatry and Psychiatric-Forensic Medicine)).

The plans for the building of the psychiatric clinic were drawn up (◘ Fig. 5.9–5.10) by Professor Max Littmann, a very famous architect at the turn of the century; work began on the building in August 1902 by the construction company J. Heilmann. The clinic was to open its doors in 1904 (► Chapter 6).

The building work began, Bumm fell ill and had to postpone negotiations with the Sisters of Mercy on nursing and catering, since he wanted to travel to Carlsbad to recuperate. At the beginning of April 1903, Bumm thought he had recovered and wanted to leave for Carlsbad, but had to check into the Surgical University Clinic in the Nussbaumstrasse. On April 11, 1903, he was operated on the gall bladder and two days after surgery, at the age of 54, Anton Bumm died.

From his room at the Surgical Clinic Bumm could see the structural frame of the psychiatric clinic on the other side of the street.

The great life achievement of Anton Bumm was that by accomplishing his plans for the psychiatric clinic, he had set the prerequisites for all further developments in psychiatry at the university of Munich for the entire 20th century.

Literature

Bumm, A. (1896): Zur Geschichte der panoptischen Irrenanstalt. Festschrift zur Feier des fünfzigjährigen Bestehens der Kreisirrenanstalt für Mittelfranken in Erlangen. Erlangen: Junge u. Sohn

Grashey, H. (1886): Nekrolog auf Dr. B. v. Gudden. Arch Psychiat. Nervenkr. p. I – XXIX

Grashey, H. (1887): Nachtrag zum Nekrolog. Arch Psychiat. Nervenkr. 18: p. 898-910

Müller, N. (1997): Historische und aktuelle Bauprinzipien psychiatrischer Klinik. Nervenarzt 68: p. 184-195

Neupert (1903): Anton Bumm. Psychiatrisch-Neurologische Wochenschrift 14: p. 153-155

Schwarz, Th. (1982): Anton Bumm (1849-1903). Inaugural thesis. University Munich

Snell, O. (1917): Nachruf auf H. v. Grashey, Allg. Z. Psychiat. 73: p. 489-490

The Opening of the Psychiatric Hospital in 1904 by Emil Kraepelin

In April 1903 the »topping-out crown« was heaved up over the building of the Psychiatric Clinic on the Nussbaumstrasse, on which work had begun in August 1902. Work on the interior fittings was now begin and it was scheduled that a year and a half later the clinic should open its doors with the 54-year old Anton Bumm as its director. But Bumm had died unexpectedly on April 13, 1903.

Suddenly, the architect Max Littmann and the master builder, Jakob Heilmann, had no one with experienced, psychiatric knowledge to assist with the continuation of the job.

> At the turn of the century Professor Max Littmann (1862–1931; 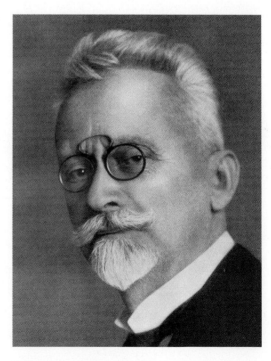 Fig. 6.1) was one of the most famous architects in Germany. In Munich the Schack-Gallerie (Schack Gallery), the Prinzregententheater (Prince Regent's Theatre), the new »Hofbräuhaus« at Platzl and the Anatomical Institute were built according to his designs. In other German cities many other, in particular public buildings were constructed according to his plans (e.g. in Stuttgart, the Königliches Hoftheater (the Theatre of the Royal Court), in Berlin the Schillertheater, in Weimar the Grossherzogliches Burgtheater (Theatre of the Grand-Duke).

Bumm had taken an active part in all the decisions on planning and building. His suggestions had been taken into account in the architect's concept for a long, four-storey main building on the Nussbaumstrasse with three low, comb-like, attached wing buildings. Bumm had also made proposals for the facade (◘ Fig. 6.2). He had laid down how the rooms should be set out and, together with the architect,

worked on the allocation of the rooms to different function areas. Bumm had also developed the first plans for the interior furnishings of the building.

In the early planning stage he had traveled to Berlin with Littmann and Heilmann to have a look at the psychiatric clinic of the Charité and in his discussions with the clinic director, F. Jolly (1844–1904), had acquired ideas for the new building in Munich. After this trip the plans which had

◘ **Fig. 6.1.** Max Littmann (1861–1931)

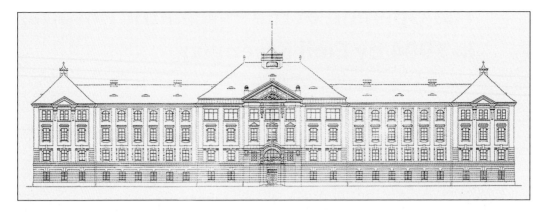

6

▫ **Fig. 6.2.** Facade of the clinic for nervous diseases: Draft from 1901 as proposed by Anton Bumm, but which was not the final design

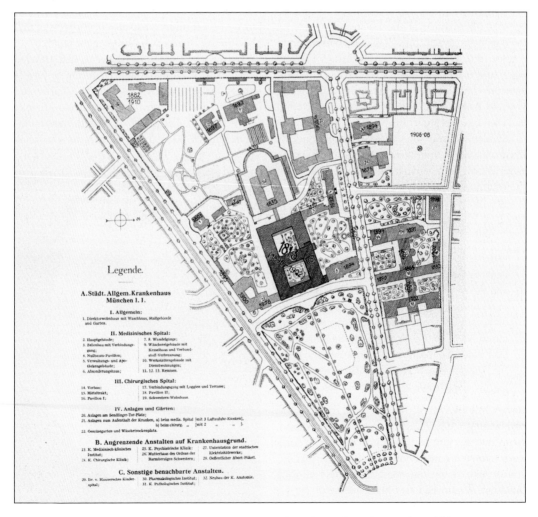

▫ **Fig. 6.3.** Site place of the Hospital »Links der Isar« (1903/1904) with psychiatric clinic (above, in the middle)

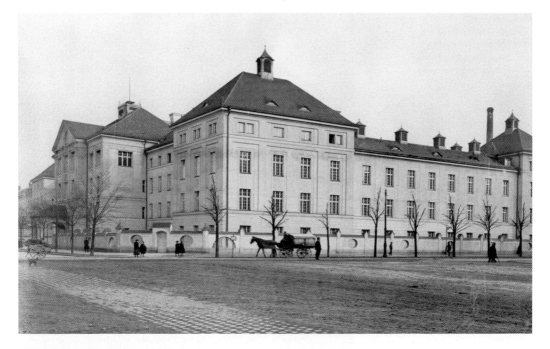

◻ **Fig. 6.4.** Psychiatric Clinic (ca. 1905)

been submitted to the city building authorities, were revised once again (◻ Fig. 6.3) and in 1902 the building work began (◻ Fig. 6.4).

On Bumm's death construction work ground to a halt.

In this situation the faculty and the university had to urgently look for a successor to Bumm in Munich. The decision was made within a few weeks during the summer term of 1903; In June 1903 Emil Kraepelin, at that time director of the Psychiatric Clinic of the University of Heidelberg, received an offer.

When Bumm died, and as a former pupil of von Gudden, Emil Kraepelin (◻ Fig. 6.5) expected an appointment in Munich. »Based on old memories and due to a love of Munich, it would have been a joy.« Whilst in his memoirs Kraepelin wrote that his »whole heart« was attached to the »beauty of Heidelberg« and what he particularly appreciated was the »quiet academic life« there.

During the first weeks after Bumm's death in April 1903, Kraepelin thought he would be spared having »to choose between the two«, when »finally in June 1903 the call came« after all. Kraepelin

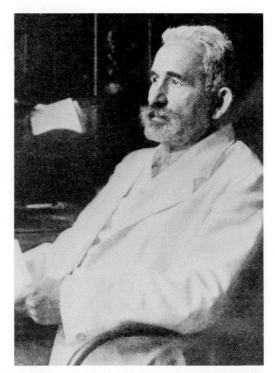

◻ **Fig. 6.5.** Emil Kraepelin (1910)

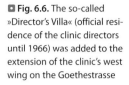
Fig. 6.6. The so-called »Director's Villa« (official residence of the clinic directors until 1966) was added to the extension of the clinic's west wing on the Goethestrasse

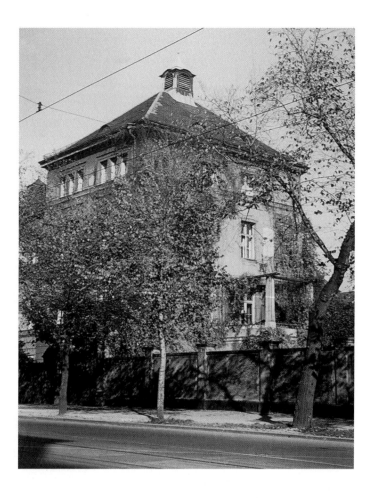

made up his mind quickly to go to Munich, probably because of the bad conditions at the Heidelberg clinic which were ignored in spite of his constant complaints. Kraepelin travelled to Munich that same month and together with the clinic consultant, the brother of the late Anton Bumm, inspected the structural works, shell and core of the building. Kraepelin was »downright amazed at the grandness of the building« and had to admit that there was »great potential for every kind of scientific work«. After a meeting with the dean of the medical faculty he made a couple of demands and offered to present a paper on the points he had mentioned. In this paper Kraepelin specified that on one hand the clinic had to be completely free to decide on patient admissions, on the other hand and under no circumstances should the clinic be forced to admit more patients than beds available. Kraepelin

also requested the erection of an official residence (**Fig. 6.6**) within the clinic's building and asked for permission to travel to south-east Asia for several month (**Fig. 6.7**). All requests were granted.

On Kraepelin's return to Heidelberg from his visit to Munich he received word from the Baden Ministry of Culture that they were at least prepared to support him in ridding the Heidelberg clinic of its »bad conditions«, but that the hindrances in the Baden Ministry of the Interior would probably not be overcome he then accepted the offer to go to Munich as of October 1, 1903 (**Fig. 6.8**) and subsequently moved there.

Construction work had been discontinued following Bumm's death and in order to get things going again and possibly make some suggestions for improvement, Kraepelin visited some of the newer clinics in Germany (Giessen, Kiel and Halle).

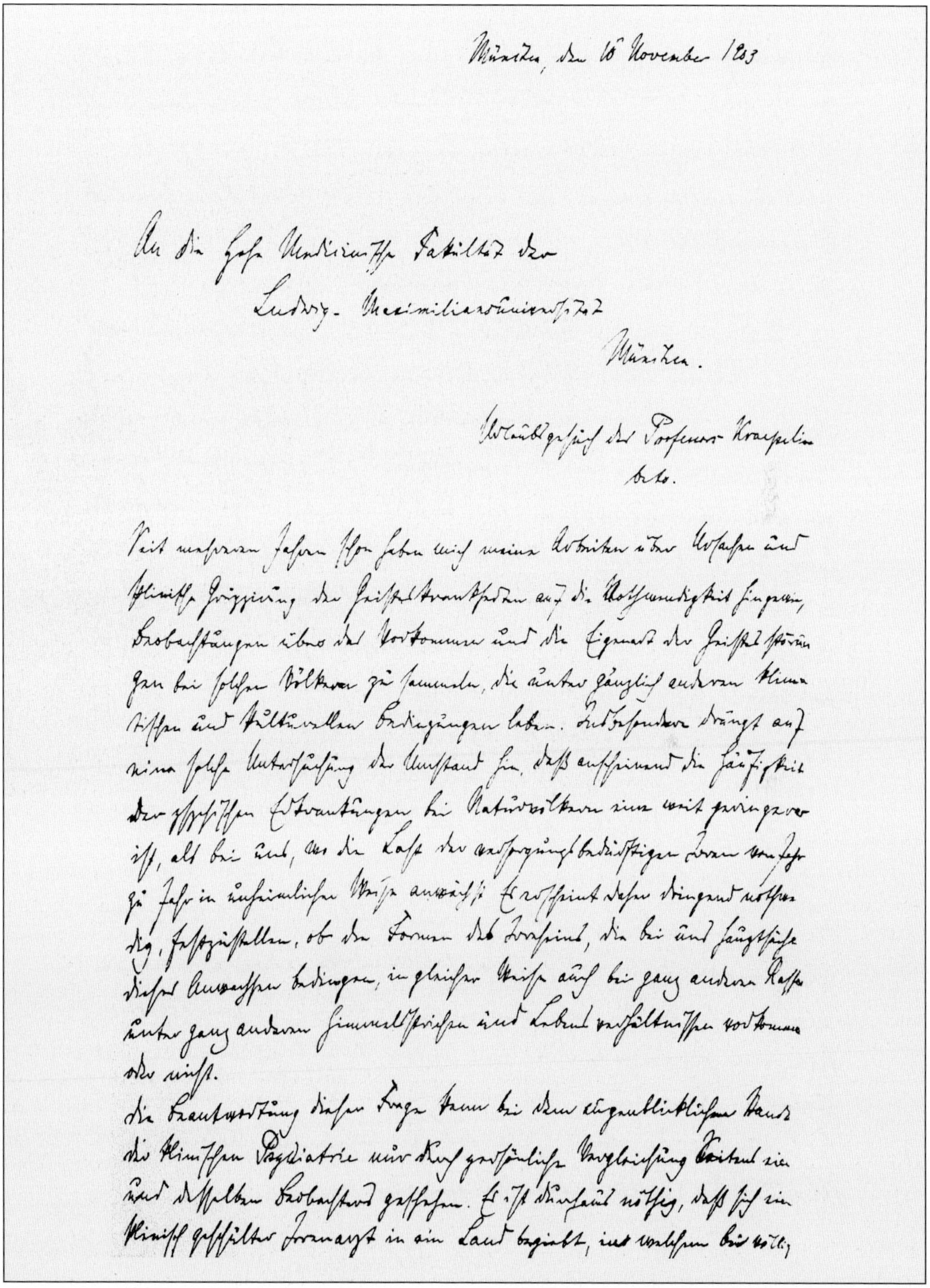

München, den 10 November 1903

An die hohe Medicinische Fakultät der
Ludwig-Maximiliansuniversität
München.

Urlaubsgesuch des Professor Kraepelin
betr.

Seit mehreren Jahren schon haben mich meine Arbeiten über Ursachen und klinische Gruppierung der Geisteskrankheiten auf die Notwendigkeit hingewiesen, Beobachtungen über das Vorkommen und die Eigenart der Geistesstörungen bei solchen Völkern zu sammeln, die unter gänzlich anderen klimatischen und kulturellen Bedingungen leben. Insbesondere drängt auf eine solche Untersuchung der Umstand hin, dass anscheinend die Häufigkeit der psychischen Erkrankungen bei Naturvölkern eine weit geringere ist, als bei uns, wo die Last der anstaltsbedürftigen Irren von Jahr zu Jahr in unheimlicher Weise anwächst. Es erscheint daher dringend notwendig, festzustellen, ob die Formen des Irreseins, die bei uns hauptsächlich diese Anwachsen bedingen, in gleicher Weise auch bei ganz anderen Rassen unter ganz anderen Himmelsstrichen und Lebensverhältnissen vorkommen oder nicht.
Die Beantwortung dieser Frage kann bei dem augenblicklichen Stande der klinischen Psychiatrie nur durch persönliche Vergleichung seitens eines und desselben Beobachters geschehen. Es ist durchaus nötig, dass sich ein klinisch geschulter Irrenarzt in ein Land begiebt, in welchem bis völlig

Fig. 6.7. Kraepelin's letter to the »High Medical Faculty of the Ludwig-Maximilians-University Munich« requesting permission to travel to Indonesia (»Dutch India«) from December 1903 until May 1904. Dated November 10, 1903 (from the archives of the Munich University, signed: E-II-621)

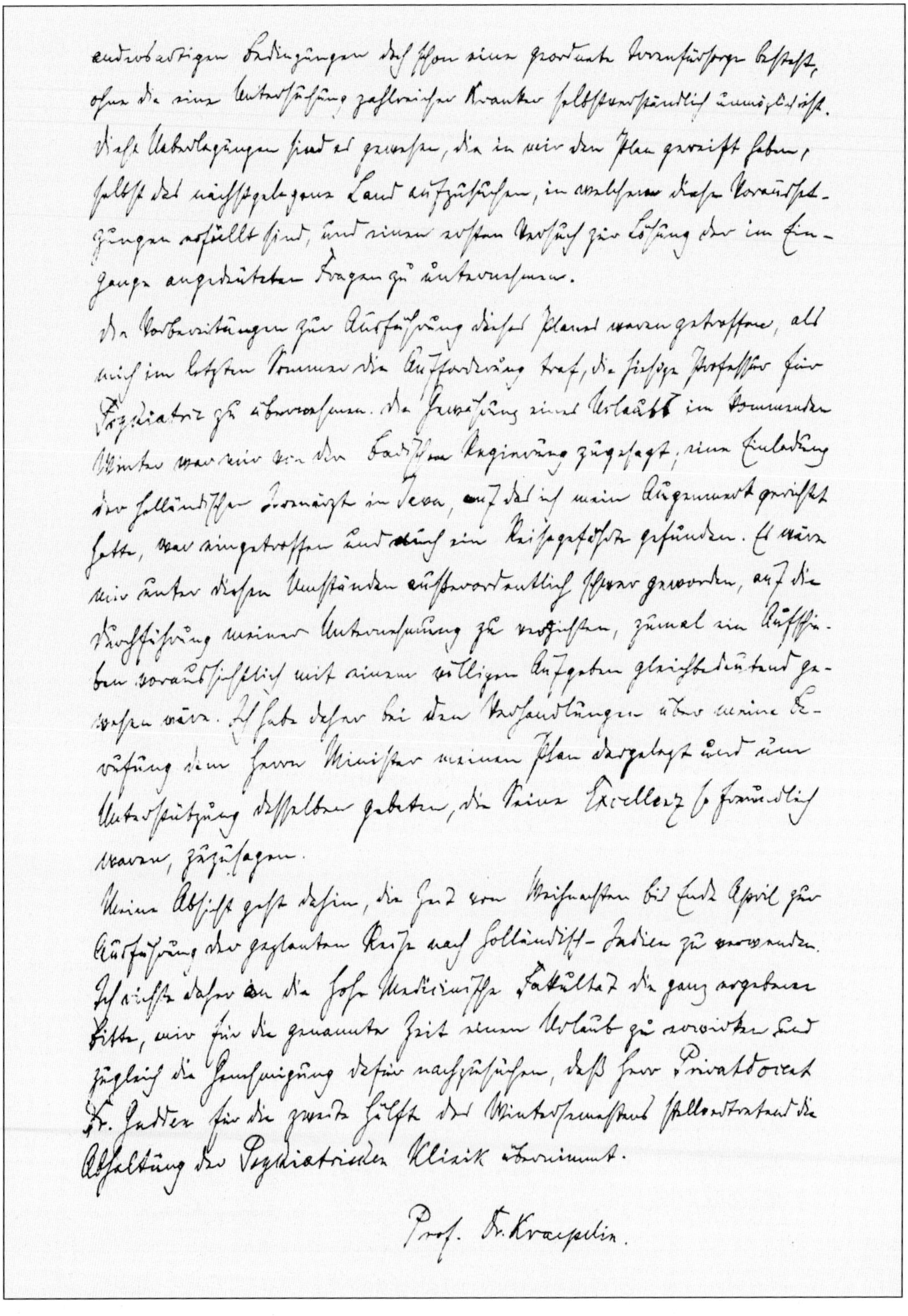
andersartigen Bedingungen doch schon eine geordnete Irrenfürsorge besteht, ohne die eine Untersuchung zahlreicher Kranker selbstverständlich unmöglich ist. Diese Ueberlegungen sind es gewesen, die in mir den Plan gereift haben, selbst das nächstgelegene Land aufzusuchen, in welchem diese Voraussetzungen erfüllt sind, und einen ersten Versuch zur Lösung der im Eingange angedeuteten Fragen zu unternehmen.

Die Vorbereitungen zur Ausführung dieses Planes waren getroffen, als mich im letzten Sommer die Aufforderung traf, die hiesige Professur für Psychiatrie zu übernehmen. Die Gewährung eines Urlaubs im kommenden Winter war mir von der Badischen Regierung zugesagt, eine Einladung der holländischen Irrenärzte in Java, auf das ich mein Augenmerk gerichtet hatte, war eingetroffen und auch ein Reisegefährte gefunden. Es wäre mir unter diesen Umständen außerordentlich schwer geworden, auf die Durchführung meiner Untersuchung zu verzichten, zumal ein Aufschieben voraussichtlich mit einem völligen Aufgeben gleichbedeutend gewesen wäre. Ich habe daher bei den Verhandlungen über meine Berufung dem Herrn Minister meinen Plan dargelegt und um Unterstützung desselben gebeten, die Seine Excellenz so freundlich waren, zuzusagen.

Meine Absicht geht dahin, die Zeit von Weihnachten bis Ende April zur Ausführung der geplanten Reise nach Holländisch-Indien zu verwenden. Ich richte daher an die hohe Medizinische Fakultät die ganz ergebene Bitte, mir für die genannte Zeit einen Urlaub zu erwirken und zugleich die Genehmigung dafür nachzusuchen, daß Herr Privatdocent Dr. Gaupp für die zweite Hälfte des Wintersemesters stellvertretend die Abhaltung der Psychiatrischen Klinik übernimmt.

Prof. Dr. Kraepelin.

Fig. 6.7. *Continued.*

»For several years now my studies on the causes and clinical grouping of mental diseases have made clear the necessity to collect observations on the types of mental diseases amongst those races, which live in totally different climatic and cultural conditions. In particular such study is advisable due to the fact that apparently the occurrence of mental diseases is much lower amongst the primitive peoples than with us, where the burden of the mentally ill in need of care increases year by year at an incredible rate. Therefore it seems urgent to find out whether the forms of mental disease, which cause this increase, occur similarly in completely different races, who live in totally different regions and conditions.

At the present level of clinical psychiatry, the answer to these questions can only be attained via personal comparison by one and the same observer. Therefore it is necessary that a clinically trained psychiatrist travels to a country, in which – although under totally different conditions – well-organized psychiatric care exists, so that numerous patients can be studied. These are the considerations, which have caused me to decide to visit the nearest possible country fulfilling these requirements and to make a first attempt at solving the previously mentioned questions.

The preparations to carry out this plan had been made, when I received the offer to take over the professorial chair for psychiatry in Munich. The Bavarian Government had given me permission to take leave during the upcoming winter; the invitation from Dutch psychiatrists in Java, which is the place I had chosen, had arrived and I had also found a travel companion. In this situation it had become extremely difficult to put off my trip, since to do such, or to postpone the trip, would probably have meant abandoning the entire plan. Therefore during negotiations on my transfer to Munich I explained the plan to the Minister and requested his support, which His Excellence was kind enough to agree to.

It is my intention to travel to Dutch India from Christmas until the end of April . I therefore request the High Medical Faculty with all my respect to grant my leave for the entire period and at the same time to agree that Dr. Gudden takes over the clinical psychiatry lectures during the second half of the winter term.«

◻ **Fig. 6.7.** *Continued.*

Little could be altered in the basic plan and the organization of the rooms; however the architect, Max Littmann, made every effort to fulfil Kraepelin's »additional wishes and to find a solution in cases of apparently impossible difficulties«. On approval by the Bavarian diet the construction plans were altered to include an official residence for Kraepelin in the so-called »male wing« (in the wing of the building on Goethestrasse). Also, Kraepelin's explicit request for »numerous and well equipped baths« (◻ Fig. 6.9) which he had used therapeutically in Heidelberg, was fulfilled. At that time warm baths, either for shorter or longer periods of time, were still considered one of the most effective methods of treatment for aroused and agitated patients and in order to fit in as many baths as possible, Kraepelin almost completely got rid of isolation rooms, which, according to his experiences in Heidelberg, were no longer necessary.

When Kraepelin arrived in Munich at the beginning of the winter term 1903/1904, his main task was »to inspect the building activities which had re-started«. He also gave a 4-hour lecture in the auditorium of the Clinic for Internal Medicine on »psychiatric clinic« and a 1-hour lecture on »general psychiatry«. During these lectures he presented patients from the admission department for psychiatric patients at the Hospital »Links der Isar«, which had been set up in 1898. **Hans Gudden** was head of this department and had taken over the job from Anton Bumm.

Hans Gudden (1866–1940, ◻ Fig. 6.10) was one of Bernhard von Gudden's sons and was born in Werneck in 1866. After graduating in Wurzburg (1891), he worked at the clinic for nervous disorders at the Charité in Berlin and then in Tubingen (1896). After habilitating in Tubingen in 1896, he took over the psychiatric department at the Hospital »Links der Isar«. The creation of such a department as a »city asylum« (roughly corresponding to an acute psychiatric clinic within a general hospital) had become necessary, once it had been realized that an independent, psychiatric clinic should be created and separated from the district mental asylum. Kraepelin deputized the lectures to Hans Gudden as of 1904; Kraepelin began his trip to Indonesia in December 1903 and was absent from Munich for five months.

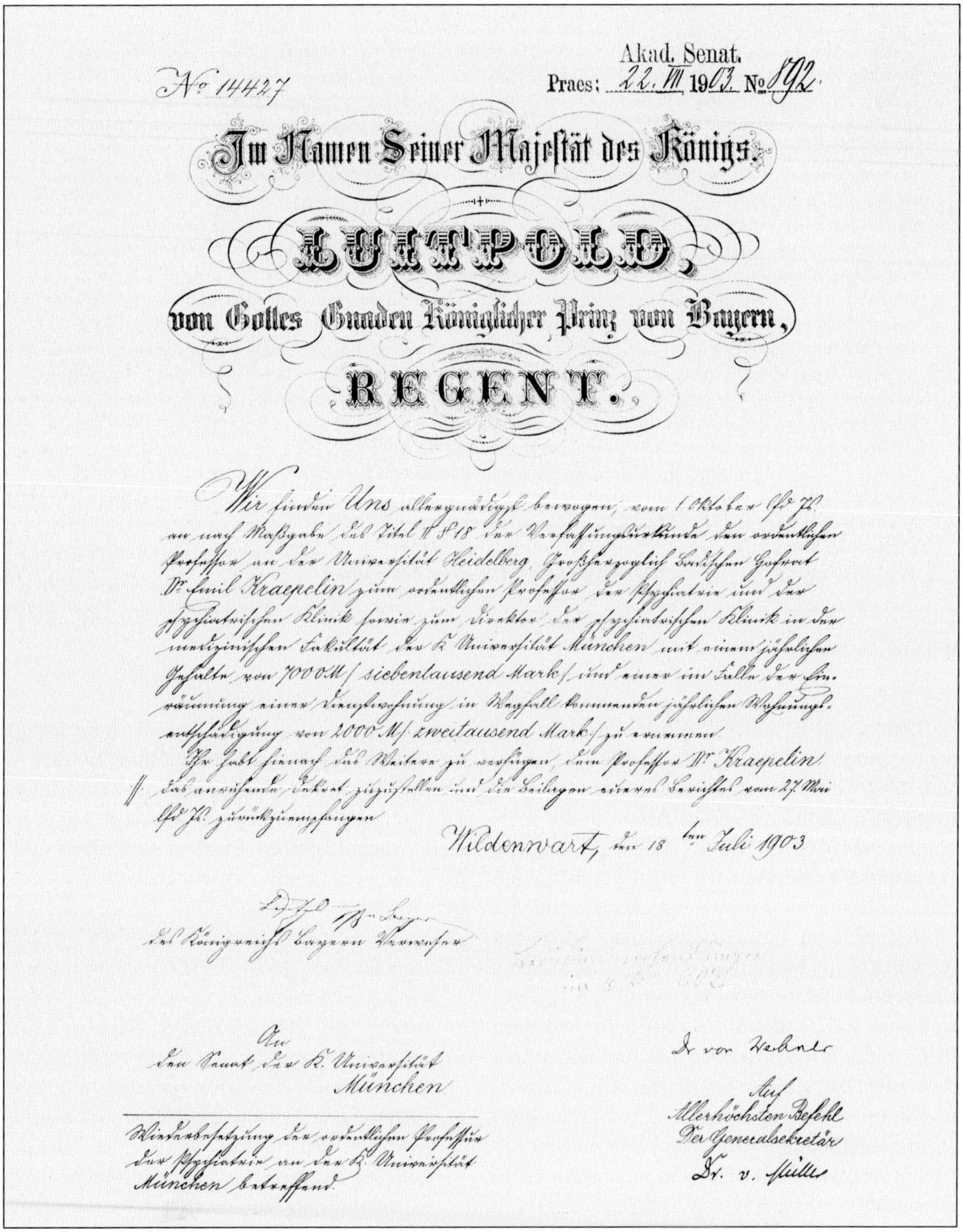

No 14427

Akad. Senat.
Praes: 22. VII 1903 No 892

Im Namen Seiner Majestät des Königs.

LUITPOLD,

von Gottes Gnaden Königlicher Prinz von Bayern,

REGENT.

Wir finden Uns allergnädigst bewogen, vom 1. Oktober lfd. Js. an nach Maßgabe des Titel II § 18 der Verfassungsurkunde den ordentlichen Professor an der Universität Heidelberg, Großherzoglich Badischen Hofrat Dr. Emil Kraepelin zum ordentlichen Professor der Psychiatrie und der psychiatrischen Klinik sowie zum Direktor der psychiatrischen Klinik in der medizinischen Fakultät der K. Universität München mit einem jährlichen Gehalte von 7000 M / siebentausend Mark / und einer im Falle der Einräumung einer Dienstwohnung in Wegfall kommenden jährlichen Wohnungsentschädigung von 2000 M / zweitausend Mark / zu ernennen.

Ihr habt hienach das Weitere zu verfügen, dem Professor Dr. Kraepelin das anliegende Dekret zuzustellen und die Beilagen eueres Berichtes vom 27. Mai lfd. Js. zurückzuempfangen.

Wildenwart, den 18ten Juli 1903

Luitpold Prinz von Bayern
des Königreichs Bayern Verweser

Dr. von Wehner

An
den Senat der K. Universität
München

Auf
Allerhöchsten Befehl
Der Generalsekretär
Dr. v. Müller

Wiederbesetzung der ordentlichen Professur der Psychiatrie an der K. Universität München betreffend.

Fig. 6.8. Letter from July 18, 1903 from the Prince Regent Luitpold to the Senate of the Munich University: *We find ourselves most graciously disposed as of October 1 of the present year, according to tit. II, para. 18 of the constitutional charter, to appoint the ordinary professor of the medical faculty of the Heidelberg University and counsellor to the Grand-Duchy of Baden, Dr. Emil Kraepelin, as ordinary professor of psychiatry at the medical faculty of the Munich University with a pragmatic annual salary of 7,000 marks, with 2,000 marks, should an official residence not be at his disposal. Hereby you are requested to carry out the necessary and to give the enclosed decree to Dr. Kraepelin and to receive the enclosures of your report of May 27 of this year.* (From the archives of the Munich university, signed: E-II-621)

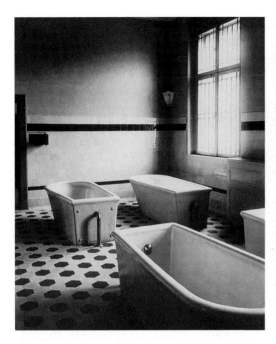

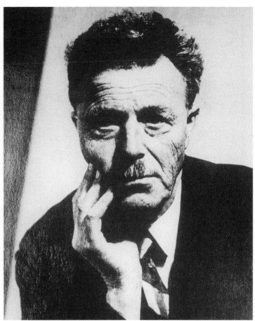

Fig. 6.9. One of Kraepelin's newly designed bathrooms for warm bath treatments

Fig. 6.10. Hans Gudden (1866–1940)

When the Psychiatric Clinic of the University was opened in autumn 1904, Hans Gudden moved to the new clinic and Kraepelin appointed him head of the Psychiatric Out-Patient Clinic. Gudden became extraordinary professor in 1904 and was head of the Out-Patient Clinic until 1922. He died in 1940.

During Kraepelin's journey to Indonesia Alois Alzheimer was primarily responsible for monitoring the building progress. Alzheimer (▶ Chapter 7) had joined Kraepelin in Heidelberg in 1903 from Frankfurt. A few months later, following Kraepelin's appointment to Munich, Alzheimer joined him in Munich.

During the year before the clinic's official opening, Alzheimer was able to exert considerable influence over the furnishing and equipping of the new clinic. In particular, this could be witnessed in the ample equipping of the hall for microscopic work which later became Alzheimer's famous place of work.

On his return from Indonesia in May 1904, Kraepelin also worked on the furnishing and equipping of the clinic. »To begin with I held back with respect to the acquisition of scientific equipment, in order to free myself from unnecessary or old-fashioned facilities, whilst it was necessary to take care of beds, all kinds of furniture, linen, kitchen and table crockery and cutlery, pictures, curtains, carpets and all other kinds of numerous details, which had to be available when the clinic opened.« Kraepelin was »involved in months of painstaking work to choose every single object according to type, size, number and price«. Alzheimer assisted Kraepelin in a »most thorough and constant manner«.

»Finally this difficult task was complete and on November 7, 1904, in the presence of the Minister of Culture and a large number of invited guests the festive opening of the clinic (▣ Fig. 6.11) took place.« In a celebratory speech Kraepelin gave a review of the almost 50-year history of clinical training in Munich and the »many plans for the building of a clinic«, which had luckily not been completed; »they would have all been in the way of the only perfect solution, which has now been accomplished«.

The celebratory speech of Kraepelin was later published together with a building description by the architect, Max Littmann.

Die Königliche
Psychiatrische Klinik
in München

I.

Festrede zur Eröffnung der Klinik
am 7. November 1904 von
Prof. Dr. **Emil Kraepelin**

II.

Baubeschreibung der Klinik
von **Heilmann** und **Littmann**

Mit 7 Ansichten und 5 Plänen

Leipzig 1905
VERLAG VON JOHANN AMBROSIUS BARTH

Fig. 6.11. Title page of the publication made on the occasion of the celebratory opening of the Royal Psychiatric University Clinic in Munich

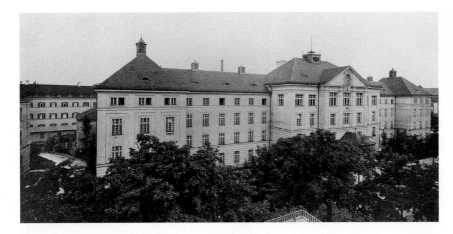

■ **Fig. 6.12.** The Psychiatric University Clinic on Nussbaumstrasse in 1907 (Photo from the municipal archives, Munich)

The Building

In the building description the ground plan, building and many details of the horse shoe-shaped building (■ Fig 5.9), (■ Fig. 6.12, 6.13):

- A long and stretched out main tract has three floors over the ground floor.
- From the main tract there are three wings in a comb-like shape (■ Fig 5.9) from which the east wing has one floor over the ground floor and the west wing three floors over the ground floor; there is access to the auditorium above the middle wing.
- The middle of the main tract is the entrance area of the clinic, with a spacious staircase leading from the ground floor to the first floor (■ Fig. 6.14).
- The middle construction of the main tract in front of the auditorium separates the male from the female wards.
- There are 100 beds (and 20 reserve beds) for patients, which are divided into 9 wards (2 private, 3 female and 4 male wards) (■ Fig. 6.15). For each ward the patients' rooms are on one side of the corridor (towards the clinic gardens). The wards' corridors have windows towards the street (■ Fig. 6.16).
- There is a small and a large auditorium for student training.
- In the middle of the main tract the library (■ Fig. 6.17), the microscopy laboratory (■ Fig. 6.18) and rooms for the director and senior consultants are located.

- The psychiatric out-patient department (with two large examining rooms, a room for a senior consultant, a waiting room for patients and a small auditorium) are located on the ground floor of the main building.

The building expenses for an area of 4,000 qm were 1,5 million marks; 200,000 marks were put aside for the furnishings.

A Selection of Clinic Patients

Since its opening 100 years ago, over 200,000 patients have been admitted as in-patients and treated, as far as possible with in the means at disposal.

In the archive of case histories the – almost complete – documents from these patients are filed.

As soon as he joined the clinic, Kraepelin introduced a standarized, systematic recording and presentation of the most important findings from each patient. He had already gained good experiences with this standardized method during his time in Heidelberg. Kraepelin used the documentation of each case as a basis for his scientific work and developed a »counting card system« for each trait or symptom. (The tradition of systematically registering the findings and course of the illness has generally been adhered to at the Munich clinic. Since 1971 all information on each clinic patient is registered with the AMDP system and documented in addition to the case history.)

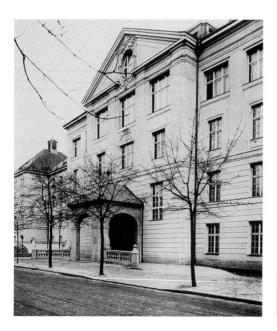

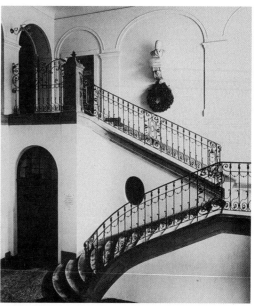

Fig. 6.13. View of the front of the clinic (1904)

Fig. 6.14. Staircase leading from the entry hall to the first floor (1904)

In the past 100 years many of the patients admitted to the clinic have been

- Contemporarily well-known persons (a)
- Representatives from cultural life (b)
- Patients, whose destinies have figured in important novels (c)
- Reference cases for the discovery or first-time description of a certain illness (d)
- Expertise cases which have been brought to public notice (e)

In the patient archives of the clinic there is some revealing information about the illness and destiny of patients, generally known to have been treated at the clinic at some time during their lives. However, there have also been famous patients treated at the clinic, totally unbeknown to the public.

Obviously, it would be particularly interesting to learn more about such patients, but for reasons of professional secrecy details cannot be given.

One of Kraepelin's patients (a) played a special role in the development of psychiatry: The very wealthy American, James Loeb (1867–1933) came to Munich in 1905 due to a relapsing, affective disorder, which had started 12 years previously,

to be treated by Kraepelin in case of recurrence. He resided in Munich and in Murnau on the Lake Staffel and was a generous patron of many cultural and scientific activities in the USA, England and particularly in Munich. Loeb played an important part in the founding of the Deutsche Forschungsanstalt für Psychiatrie (German Psychiatric Research Institute) in 1917 (▶ Chapter 8).

Towards the end of the 1st World War an important representative of literary expressionism was a patient at the clinic for a short period of time (b): Ernst Toller (1893–1939), who described his stay at the clinic in a book, published in 1933, »Eine Jugend in Deutschland« (An Adolescence in Germany). Toller broke off his law studies in Grenoble in 1914 in order to volunteer at the beginning of the war. After being badly wounded and treated at a military hospital he continued his studies in Munich. In the meantime, he changed into a militant pacifist and as a member and part-founder of the »Kulturpolitischer Bund der Jugend in Deutschland« (Cultural-Politcal Youth Alliance in Germany) had contact with many war opponents. In spring of 1918 he took part in a strike of the munition workers, was arrested and accused of treason. His mother

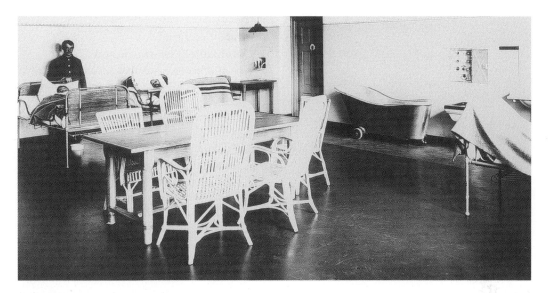

◘ Fig. 6.15. Lounge on the male ward

arranged for him to be admitted to the Psychiatric Clinic for examination and treatment, but he was discharged from the clinic a couple of days later and was enlisted again. During the last months of war he played a significant role in the November revolution and became a leading representative of the Munich council republic. On abatement of the revolution he was condemned to five years in prison. Toller emigrated in 1936, lived in New York in dreadful conditions and committed suicide there in 1939.

Liesl Karlstadt (1892–1960), known as the congenial partner of Karl Valentin and famous in Munich circles, was admitted to the clinic four times (b). The actress was admitted to the clinic for the first time in 1935 after trying to commit suicide by jumping into the river Isar. Apart from the usual case history there are also worried letters from Karl Valentin to the clinic director of that time, Oswald Bumke, regarding the condition of his partner. There is also a poem by the patient herself, in which she thanks the matron for the pleasant and good atmosphere created by the nuns during her stay.

From May 20 until August 4, 1910, the 25-year old patient, Alice Donath, was treated for a manic depressive disorder (c).

Alice D. is »Clarisse« in Robert Musil's »Mann ohne Eigenschaften« (Man Without Qualities). At the age of 22 Alice D. married the musician, librar-

ian and – less successful – composer Dr. Gustav Donath. Donath had been a friend of Musil's since their youth and is the role model »Walter« in Musil's novel.

Alice D. was already psychiatrically conspicuous as a young girl, was daughter of a Viennese artist and had become manic, aggressive and confused in Venice, during a journey from Vienna to Greece, to such an extent that she had to be admitted to hospital there. Her brother, a doctor from Vienna (»Siegmund« in Musil's novel) took her from Venice to Munich and to the clinic. Once discharged from the clinic, her condition improved for a while, but after giving birth to a child she became increasingly peculiar. She could no longer take care of household duties and retired to a house near Klagenfurt, avoiding all social contact. From 1926 until her death in 1939 she was a chronically ill patient of the Psychiatric Clinic of the City of Vienna at Steinhof.

The day labourer, Johann F. (1851–1907), was patient at the Munich clinic until a month before he died (d). The reason for admittance to the clinic was mentioned in the epicrisis as follows: The patient was forgetful, was disoriented and could no longer carry out simple tasks. The diagnosis in the case history was noted as organic brain disease (ateriosclerosis?).

The case of Johann F. became famous through a publication by Alois Alzheimer. In the publica-

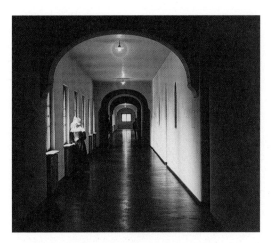

◘ Fig. 6.16. Ward corridor on the first floor (ca. 1905)

tion Alzheimer started that the case of J.F. must be a »special case« of dementia, as in the histology no fibrils could be found. According to present criteria this was the first documented reference case for »plaque only« cases.

Psychiatric **expertises** (e) by clinic doctors (E. Rüdin and E. Kahn) on members of the council republic caused sensation and protest, not only at the time. It is still worrying nowadays to think that in 1919, from a psychiatric point of view, one referred to »psychopaths as revolutionary leaders«, whilst the psychiatric opinion of Rüdin on the personality of Count Anton von Arco-Valley (1897–1945) made a definite contribution to his being condemned to death in 1920 for the murder of Kurt Eisner (February 21, 1919), the death penalty being converted into lifelong imprisonment and finally Arco being pardoned in 1924.

The Clinic Staff

At the opening of the clinic at the beginning of the 20th century there were mainly two groups of staff responsible for patient care; the doctors and the nursing staff and their work is the basis for the reputation of the clinic.

Doctors

In 1904 there were 4 paid doctors available for 100 patients:

1   Director
1   Senior Consultant
4   (as of 1906: 5) assistant doctors
2   (as of 1905: 3) »internal volunteer doctors« (unpaid, but with living and eating facilities in the clinic)
2   »external volunteer doctors« (unpaid)

In addition to the above there was also the senior consultant at the out-patient clinic; once the clinic had been opened and the existing (since 1898) psychiatric out-patient clinic at the Hospital »Links der Isar« had been closed, this position was taken over by the Psychiatric Clinic.

There were also 6 medical trainees and, as of 1905, the Bavarian Ministry of War placed a »military« doctor at the clinic for psychiatric training.

The staffing of the clinic was more than ample for that time, particularly when compared to the 7 doctors at the district mental asylum, responsible for 700 patients.

The 100 beds on the wards of the new clinic were soon filled: in 1905 1,600 patients were treated as in-patients (900 men; 610 women). In the following years the number of in-patients increased to 2,000 p.a.; the overbalance of male patients remained. As of 1905 about 500 patients were treated annually at the psychiatric out-patient clinic.

Nursing Staff

The plans for the nursing organisation at the new clinic had already been out lined at the time of A. Bumm. During negotiations with the Bavarian Ministry of Culture Kraepelin had been informed that the task »categorically had to be handed over to the Order of the Sisters of Mercy«. Kraepelin was »not entirely happy with this arrangement«. He soon realized that collaboration with the nuns went smoothly and according to his expectations; and he was satisfied that the agreement had advantages for him: »As the order was responsible for the entire catering and took care of it masterfully, this most difficult and trying part of administration was taken care of once and for all.«

On December 27 and 30, 1904 the contracts, prepared by the Bavarian Ministry of Culture, were signed by the university and the Order of the Sisters of Mercy, thus giving the order the entire

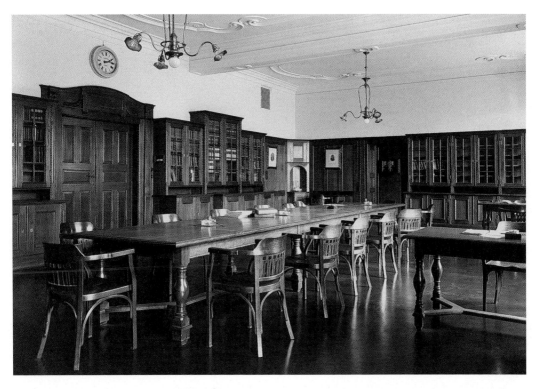

◻ Fig. 6.17. Library of the Psychiatric University Clinic

responsibility for the nursing, kitchen and laundry of the clinic. At the beginning of 1905, 23 nuns started work, »supported by 13 maids and 17 wardens«. Kraepelin soon acknowledged that the nuns were a »flock of reliable, experienced and devoted nurses«. This tradition, which started with Kraepelin, lasted for 85 years.

It was not until March 1991 that four of the last five nuns, some of whom had been working at the clinic for years, could no longer be replaced due to lack of younger successors, that the collaboration with the order had to be stopped, although they had particularly proved their worth in difficult times.

The »Sisters of Mercy of St. Vinzenz von Paul« came to Munich with their Matron, Ignatia Jorth von Strassburg, in March 1832 at the request of King Ludwig the First. First of all they took over nursing duties at the Medical Department of the General Hospital »Links der Isar«, now referred to as the Medical Clinic of the City Centre, then later during the 19th century,

they took over the nuring in the Hauner'schen Pediatric Hospital (1853) and the Surgical Department of the Hospital »Links der Isar« (1866).

The Psychiatric Clinic was the first **university clinic** to entrust the nursing to nuns when it opened.

In 1932 47 nuns were working at the clinic. Their convent with enclosure was located in the extension O. Bumke had built in 1926/1927. From 1933 until 1935 nursing staff with national socialistic tendencies tried to oust them from the clinic. O. Bumke intervened and in 1938 – when the congregation had reached an all-time high with approximately 2800 nuns – there were 50 nuns working at the clinic.

During both world wars the number of doctors and male nurses was reduced; the clinic was overcrowded with patients. In this situation the nuns had to take on many tasks and extensive responsibilities.

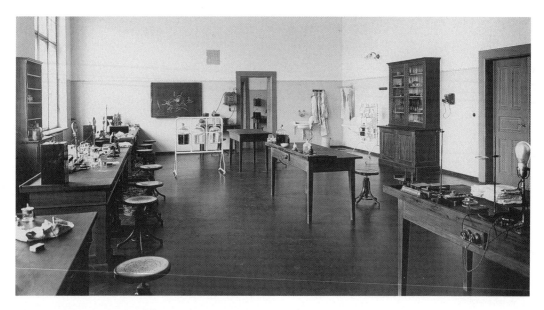

☐ **Fig. 6.18.** Alzheimer's microscopy laboratory on the clinic's third floor

During the air raids of the 2nd World War, the patients had to be evacuated either into bunkers in the vicinity or attended to in makeshift rooms in the clinic. The damage during the last years of the war had to be repaired over and over again (► Chapter 10). The daily work on the wards had to be seen to and the nuns were responsible for all these tasks: They lived in the clinic and hurried to »their« wards whenever help was needed.

For many patients of the Munich Clinic and their relations it has always been particularly important that the nuns could be counted on whenever necessary. It was especially important for those patients who repeatedly spent time in the clinic, that the same nuns would often work on the wards for a long time. Many nuns remained in the clinic for decades. One of the last matrons, Sister Clarella, worked at the clinic for 50 years (1926–1976; of which 32 years as matron).

The fact that the nuns did all the nursing at the clinic from the beginning until after the 2nd World War became problematic once their numbers began to dwindle. Somehow, well-trained male nursing staff and well trained, worldly nurses had to be found for the job.

The general aspects of psychiatric nursing had changed considerably since the opening of the clinic. The changes were based on the developments in psychiatry and the function itself of nurses in the psychiatric clinics.

When Kraepelin took over the clinic, jobs for 17 »wardens« had been created to support the nuns. »Wardens« had already existed in the oldest psychiatric institutions in the 19th century. The »wardens« (occasionally female »wardens« were employed) were supervising staff, who had to ensure peace and quiet and cleanliness. Both male and female wardens were subject to – if at all – a very lax medical supervision (► Chapter 1).

A job as »warden for the insane« did not have a particularly good reputation; the pay for such hard work was not good. The situation only changed minimally in the 19th century with the building of the care and nursing asylums: »Monitoring« of the patients remained their most important task. The »wardens« were scarcely supervised or instructed by the medical staff, but they had to follow strict regulations, which could include curfew and not being allowed to marry. It was not until the end of the 19th century that the state ministries of the German Reich were requested to improve the situation, as for example in Bavaria by H. von Grashey (► Chapter 4). During this period the »wardens« began to complain more clearly about their work-

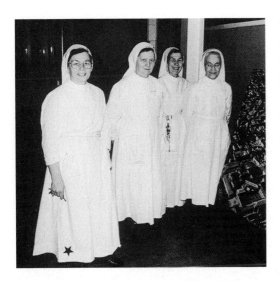

Fig. 6.19. Four of the last nuns working at the clinic (ca. 1990) (from left to right: Sister Belanda, Burgina, Frambalda, Imara)

ing conditions. In 1902 attempts were made to organize the »wardens« in a type of union. In certain states, as for example in Bavaria, plans were set up for a proper »job description« for the staff working in psychiatric asylums and clinic. The effect of these efforts led to changing the name for the female and male »wardens« into »nurse« and guidelines were set up to reflect the developments in general nursing of psychiatric patients.

Whilst Kraepelin was in office the situation for the male nursing staff did not improve considerably. Kraepelin set down strict rules of the house and other official regulations. Notice period was one month; »disobedience« could be grounds for immediate dismissal. If time-out was exceeded or the sleeping room for nursing staff was not left on time, the guilty party could be fined. On the wards there were time-punch machines, which were not abolished until 1971. The work day of a nurse lasted 15 hours (from 6 a.m. until 9 p.m.)

Obviously, under such working conditions and the increasing amount of work due to increasing numbers of in-patients misunderstandings between the clinic management and the nursing staff grew; towards the end of Kraepelin's time the threat of strikes loomed. The main demand from

the nursing staff was the creation of jobs for them as civil servants. However, Kraepelin wanted to reserve such jobs for some especially good nurses and for the »lecture nurse«. After the 1st World War Kraepelin fought the introduction of a three-shift working day, because he thought it would have a negative impact on the continuity of the nursing.

With the introduction of new legal and organizational regulations the situation for the male nurses gradually improved. The atmosphere between clinic management and the nursing staff calmed down. Even after the 2nd World War the nurses had a 60-hour week and the cleaning and maintenance of the wards still remained the responsibility of the nurses, as the clinic employed only a few cleaning staff.

The most important changes for the nurses came with the introduction of effective treatment methods into psychiatry. The collaboration with nurses was necessary for fever and insulin treatment and for electro-shock therapy. In particular the introduction of modern psychotropic drugs in the 20th century changed the general clinic atmosphere for the nursing staff – the nurses were increasingly included by the doctors in the monitoring and treatment of patients.

Until the seventies the nuns had the main responsibility for the nursing on the wards (Fig. 6.19). Once their numbers began to dwindle, more and more worldly sisters were employed; worldly sisters and male nurses were given jobs with personal responsibility.

After 1971 efforts were made to improve the training and further education of the entire nursing staff. On joining the clinic the nuns had already had a two-year training as nurse, whilst the other nursing staff – until after the 2nd World War – were only semi-skilled. After 1971 further education events were organized and finally in 1978 after negotiations with the Bavarian Ministry of Culture an »Institution for the Further Education of Psychiatric Nurses« was set up in cooperation with the Psychiatric Clinic, the Technical University and Max-Planck-Institute for Psychiatry and acknowledged by the German Hospital Association (Deutsche Krankenhausgesellschaft). By participating in the training events of the institution the nursing staff has the possibility to take part in a 2-year in-service training.

The changes in psychiatry since the beginning of the 20th century are not only reflected in the scientific development of the subject, the introduction of many new and efficacious methods of treatment and the broadening of medical perspectives in dealing with psychiatric patients: An especially important contribution is the strong development in the career and work profile of psychiatric nursing staff during the last 100 years.

Apart from the nursing staff there is other staff involved in the smooth running of the clinic:

Kitchen staff, medical secretaries, administrative staff, the porters and craftsmen. (Cleaning staff hardly existed initially, since the cleaning on the wards was taken care of by the nursing staff!) The doctors' work in the laboratories was assisted by a few workers.

The situation has changed significantly in the last 100 years. A psychiatric clinic can only offer the proper modern standards of care if it has not only the above mentioned staff, but also psychologists, medical-technical assistants, social-welfare workers, physiotherapists, work therapists, people for filing and registering, staff for special activities, such as art and music therapists.

The patient's impression of the clinic is not only based on the medical and nursing staff, as was the case at the opening of the clinic 100 years ago. Not just the number of staff employed by a clinic, but the »therapeutic atmosphere« is crucial.

It is interesting to take a look at how the staffing has changed over time.

When Kraepelin opened the clinic on November 7, 1904, with a celebratory speech nobody knew what changes would occur during the next 100 years.

Every development in psychiatry has been accommodated at the Munich clinic. It was an important milestone that the originally designed »Psychiatric Clinic« spent 50 years as a »Clinic for Nervous Disorders« (psychiatric and neurological clinic), before changing again into a »Psychiatric Clinic«, as Kraepelin had intended, in 1971.

As a matter of course, psychiatry became a clinical subject and is constantly developing fur-

ther. In this connection it will always be confronted with new challenges, e.g.

- With regard to the necessary changes in the building itself,
- With regard to
  - The necessary changes to the internal, organizational structure and
  - The improvement in the staffing (medical, nursing and other).

However one thing has remained unchanged since 1904: The aims of the Munich clinic with respect to

- Patient care,
- Presentation of the clinical training and in particular,
- Keeping research on a high level.

In 1904 Kraepelin thanked the Bavarian ministries, the medical faculty, the university authorities, the city of Munich, the architects, his predecessors and all those, who had been involved in the new clinic building, with the following words: »Many heads and many hands have worked together, to create all prerequisites for science, to encourage it to flourish, from the highest official to the last subworker. An unbelievable troop – all forces united to achieve one goal«. With this he rounded off his glimpse into the future, which has remained the same for the past 100 years: »May our energy and our success not lag too far behind our intentions!«

Literature

Hippius, H., Hoff, P. (1991): Psychiatrische Klinik der Ludwig-Maximilians Universität München: Dokumente zur Baugeschichte. Stelzl-Druck: Munich

Kraepelin, E. (1905): Die Königlich-Psychiatrische Klinik in München. J.A. Barth-Verlag: Munich

Mutterhaus der Barmherzigen Schwester vom hl. Vinzenz von Paul (Ed. 1982): Barmherzige Schwestern vom hl. Vinzenz von Paul – 150 Jahre in Bayern 1832–1982. Seitz Druck GmbH: Munich

The Munich Hospital Managed by Emil Kraepelin

With the opening of the clinic in 1904 and the appointment of Emil Kraepelin to the chair of psychiatry, Munich acquired world-standing in psychiatry at the beginning of the 20th century.

Kraepelin had already made a name for himself as a young assistant doctor (in Munich with B. von Gudden) with his first publication, a polemic paper about »Abolition of Penal Sentences« (◪ Fig. 7.1), had further received recognition in 1883 for his »Compendium of Psychiatry« (◪ Fig. 7.2) and had been appointed to chair of psychiatry (Dorpat 1886) at the age of 30. Due to his activities Kraepelin was one of the leading German psychiatrists of the 19th century. He further secured his reputation as an exceptional clinician and scientist with the rapid publication of the different editions of his **textbook »Psychiatry«** (◪ Fig. 7.3: 1887, 1889, 1893, 1896, 1899), which had emerged from the »Compendium«. The seventh, 2-volume edition of »Psychiatry« was published in 1903/1904 (◪ Fig. 7.4), after Kraepelin had worked for 12 years in Heidelberg and had decided to accept the chair in Munich. The last complete (4-volume) eighth edition (1909–1915) was written by Kraepelin in Munich. A ninth, 4-volume edition had been planned in collaboration with J. Lange (see below), but remained unfinished (◪ Fig. 7.5); two volumes were published by Johannes Lange after Kraepelin's death.

The nine editions of the textbook are the basis of Kraepelin's outstanding importance for psychiatry as a whole to date. The basics, developed from clinical view and observation, were tested empirically over and over again, taking new findings and knowledge into account, adapting Kraepelin's systemization of psychiatric clinical pictures, and remain valid today. The world-wide efforts to operationalize psychiatric diagnostics (in connection with the ICD classification (ICD-10)) of the WHO and American diagnosis classification DSM-III

Die

Abschaffung des Strafmaßes.

——

Ein Vorschlag

zur

Reform der heutigen Strafrechtspflege.

Pro humanitate!

Von

Dr. med. **Emil Kraepelin,**

Irrenarzt.

Stuttgart.

Verlag von Ferdinand Enke.

1880.

◪ **Fig. 7.1.** Kraepelin's pamphlet on »Abolition of Sentences« (1880)

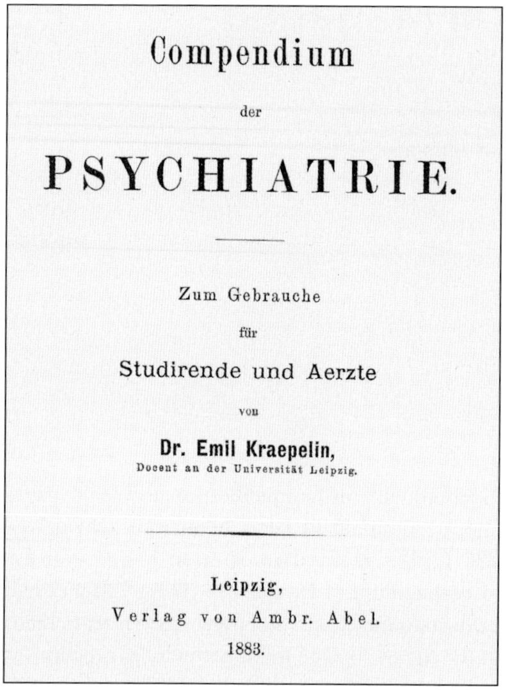

Compendium

der

PSYCHIATRIE.

Zum Gebrauche

für

Studirende und Aerzte

von

Dr. Emil Kraepelin,
Docent an der Universität Leipzig.

Leipzig,
Verlag von Ambr. Abel.
1883.

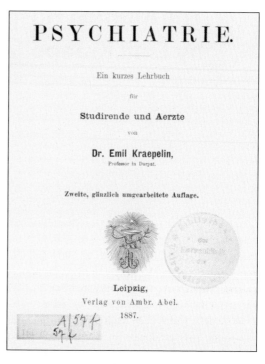

PSYCHIATRIE.

Ein kurzes Lehrbuch

für

Studirende und Aerzte

von

Dr. Emil Kraepelin,
Professor in Dorpat.

Zweite, gänzlich umgearbeitete Auflage.

Leipzig,
Verlag von Ambr. Abel.
1887.

■ **Fig. 7.2.** »Compendium of psychiatry« (1883), predecessor of Kraepelin's textbook, which was later published in 9 editions

■ **Fig. 7.3.** Second edition of E. Kraepelin's textbook in 1887: »Psychiatry – A Concise Textbook for Students and Doctors«

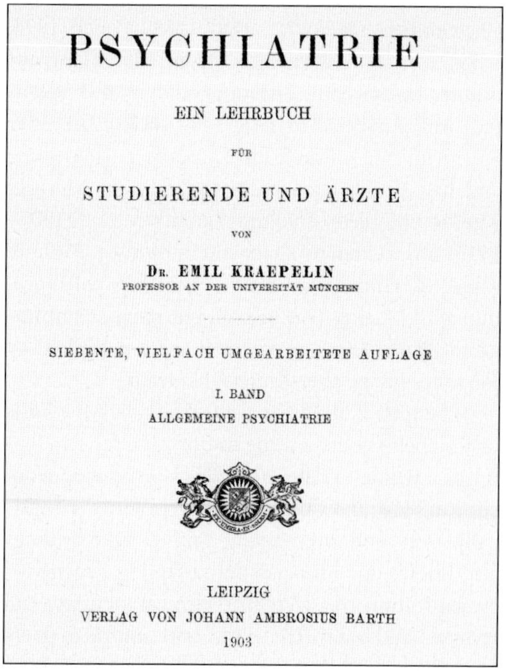

PSYCHIATRIE

EIN LEHRBUCH

FÜR

STUDIERENDE UND ÄRZTE

VON

Dr. EMIL KRAEPELIN
PROFESSOR AN DER UNIVERSITÄT MÜNCHEN

SIEBENTE, VIELFACH UMGEARBEITETE AUFLAGE

I. BAND
ALLGEMEINE PSYCHIATRIE

LEIPZIG
VERLAG VON JOHANN AMBROSIUS BARTH
1903

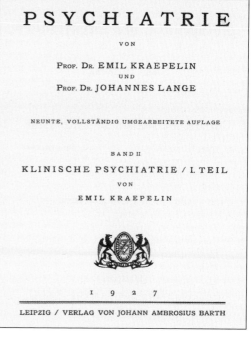

PSYCHIATRIE

VON

PROF. DR. EMIL KRAEPELIN
UND
PROF. DR. JOHANNES LANGE

NEUNTE, VOLLSTÄNDIG UMGEARBEITETE AUFLAGE

BAND II

KLINISCHE PSYCHIATRIE / I. TEIL

VON

EMIL KRAEPELIN

1 9 2 7

LEIPZIG / VERLAG VON JOHANN AMBROSIUS BARTH

■ **Fig. 7.4.** Seventh edition of E. Kraepelin's textbook of 1903, during his time in Munich

■ **Fig. 7.5.** Ninth, but incomplete edition of E. Kraepelin's textbook from 1927

and IV) reviewed Kraepelin's nosology and classification systems and regained importance during the past decades.

However, not only with his textbook »Psychiatry«, the core of his life work, did Kraepelin leave his mark on psychiatry as a clinical and scientific discipline. He also gave important, innovative impulses to many fields of research. Some budding scientific areas nowadays can be traced back to Kraepelin. He is one of the pioneers of experimental-psychological research in psychiatry and his work in this field set the trend to develop the methodology for clinical research in psychiatry. With his systematic method of recording and describing »types« and »courses« of psychiatric illnesses and by using statistical methods to evaluate the clinical data, he created a definite basis for modern clinical-psychiatric research. Some of Kraepelin's works were the starting point for modern pharmacopsychology and subsequently pharmacopsychiatry. Kraepelin also cultivated forensic psychiatry. The observations and experiences he made during one of his research journeys to south east Asia – described by Kraepelin as »comparative psychiatry« – became the starting point of transcultural psychiatry. Modern genetic research can also be traced back to the initiatives of Kraepelin and his co-workers; in this connection his work group was responsible for the evolution of psychiatric epidemiology.

Kraepelin considered methods of natural science to be the basis in order to progress in psychiatry and for this reason he particularly supported these branches of research, which are nowadays referred to as biological psychiatry. In spite of this preference for the biological-psychiatric approach, it is not justified to reduce his self-conception as doctor and scientist to a narrowed down and strictly materialistic position. Influenced by the Leipzig professor of psychology, Professor Wilhelm Wundt, who he considered to be his most important teacher (see below), he held a parallel view when dealing with the body and soul problem.

To do justice to Kraepelin and to illustrate his importance for psychiatry in the past 120 years, it is not sufficient to mention his classical textbook and the influence it had on psychiatric nosology and diagnosis classification, he also should be given credit for laying the foundation for new

branches of research; there are two other aspects of Kraepelin's life work illustrating his continuous influence:

- Kraepelin had a number of excellent students (see below).
- Kraepelin founded a research institute which became a world-wide model for the organization of psychiatric fundamental research (▶ Chapter 8).

The three founding pillars in Kraepelin's life work are linked directly to his own personal development – the textbook, the students, the research institute.

Emil Kraepelin Professor of Psychiatry in Munich (1903–1922)

Emil Kraepelin (□ Fig. 7.6) was born in Neustrelitz in Mecklenburg on February 15, 1856.

> Kraepelin's father, Karl (1817–1882) came from a family of teachers, had started to study theology, but then became actor and singer at the grand-duke's court theatre (Grossherzogliches Hoftheater) in Neustrelitz. When the theatre closed down (1848)

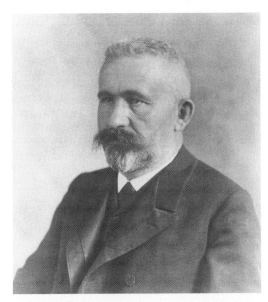

□ **Fig. 7.6.** Emil Kraepelin (1910)

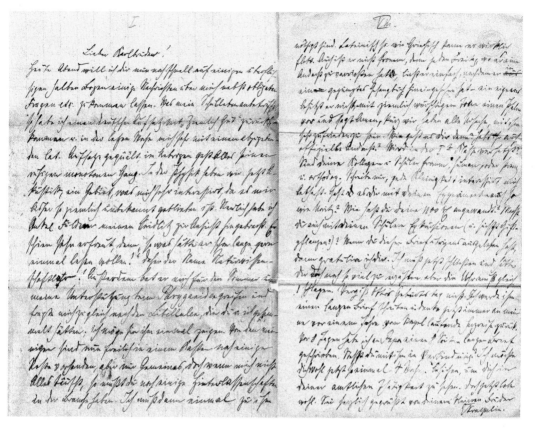

◘ Fig. 7.7. First and last page of an 8-page letter from E. Kraepelin to his brother Karl (not dated)

I.

My dear brother, Karl

This evening I want to send you some news about me on some spare sheets of paper as well as the usual obligatory questions. With regard to my student life my German essay has been returned to me with the mark »fairly good« and last week I tortured myself with a Latin essay, which had to be handed in; by the way everything is pretty monotonous as usual. In physics we are learning acoustics, a very interesting area, as I did not really know anything about it. Recently I showed my Seidlitz to uncle Julian (?). He was very pleased about it and said »he had wanted to read something like that for a long time!« Hence the name natural scientists!......

VIII.

…. I have to close now and would have lots more to tell you, but the clock is about to strike one. Don't forget Otto's birthday. I will write him a long letter and keep thinking of my short journey from Stapel (?) a year ago. Eight days ago, I wrote an 8-(?) page letter to papa. Are you in touch with him? I would like to visit you some time in H'bg and watch you at work. All the best! Best regards from your little brother

he became music teacher and later well-known »Reuter reader«, who made a great contribution to the tradition of the Low German dialect of Mecklenburg. Karl Kraepelin was a friend of Fritz Reuter.

Emil Kraepelin was the youngest of three brothers and sisters. His relationship to his elder brother by 9 years, Karl (1848–1915), was especially close. Emil Kraepelin was influenced in many ways by this brother, who later became director of the Museum for Natural History in Hamburg. His elder brother encouraged him to be interested in natural sciences, e.g. in botanical subjects and the identification of plants. The letters from Kraepelin, written during his youth, to his admired, big brother show the dominant and formative role that his brother played. One of his letters, describing how he had set up a herbarium for poisonous plants, is signed from »your little brother Emil« (◘ Fig. 7.7). The close contact between the two brothers remained until Karl's death in 1915 and shows the dominant role of the elder brother over and over again; for example when Kraepelin complains that Karl writes to him only seldom. The brothers went on many trips together, for example the 5-month long journey to Ceylon, South India, Singapore and Java (1903/1904) and a 2-month journey to North America (1908). Karl Kraepelin often chose the routes, as he wanted to follow his botanical interests en route. It is possible that Emil Kraepelin's tendency to classify and systematize in psychiatry comes from his brother's influence.

At school in Neustrelitz (1861–1874) Kraepelin was »quite a good pupil with a rather steady, but not particularly exceptional talent who did his work reliably, but without enthusiasm«. He remembered his time at school as being »coloured vividly by the regret to have lost much precious time of my youth with philological nothingness«.

Influenced by his father's friend, a doctor, Kraepelin decided at school to study medicine. On finishing school, he went to Leipzig for a year in the summer term 1874 and started studying there. In Leipzig he attended the lectures of **Wilhelm Wundt** (▶ Chapter 8).

Wilhelm Wundt (1832–1920) studied medicine, worked for a short period of time at a psychiatric clinic, following which he became pupil to the phys-

iologist H. Helmholtz (1821–1894). Wundt habilitated in Heidelberg on the subject of physiology. After publishing the 3-volume edition of »Basics of physiological psychology« (1873/1874), he was offered the chair of philosophy at the university of Zurich. He stayed there for a year and received a professorship for physiology in Leipzig in 1875. In Leipzig Wundt founded – as pioneer for other developments – an »Institute for Experimental Psychology« and continued teaching there until he retired honourably in 1915. After some years of retirement in Heidelberg, he returned to Saxony where he died at the age of 88 years near Leipzig.

Kraepelin had a good, even friendly contact to the 24-year older Wilhelm Wundt. They often wrote letters to each other. To begin with, Wundt addressed Kraepelin as »dear doctor« which he soon changed to »dear friend«. As Wundt had difficulties seeing and his writing was almost illegible, he started using a typewriter before the turn of the century. Much of the letters' content was professional and scientific, where Kraepelin was looking for Wundt's advice. They also talked about meeting each other and made appointments sending each other invitations.

In the commemorative address on Kraepelin's death, held at the annual meeting of the German Research Institution for Psychiatry in Munich, W. Spielmeyer (▶ Chapter 13/14) emphasized the strong influence Wundt had on Kraepelin and that Kraepelin had once said that his work with psychology had proved to be the »starting point for (his) choice of career«. Kraepelin's professional career and his scientific studies were moulded by Wundt's approach. He tried to use the methods he had learnt from Wundt in his scientific work in psychiatry. These formed the origins for his first »mental measurement of time under the influence of various substances such as alcohol, caffeine and tea« and the setting up of a »working curve«.

From the beginning of the summer term 1875 Kraepelin studied in Wurzburg and visited the lectures of Hermann Emminghaus.

After studying and graduating in Jena, Hermann Emminghaus (1845–1904), whose name has recently been mentioned more frequently in connection with one of he earlier works on bulimia, worked for two years at a psychiatric clinic, a clinic for internal medicine and at a physiological institute. In 1873 he opened a practise in Wurzburg and habilitated in the same year for psychiatry. He gave lectures on psychiatry and internal medicine and one of the students attending these lectures was Emil Kraepelin. In 1879 Emminghaus gave up his practise and the lectures at the university of Wurzburg. He worked for a year at the psychiatric institution in Heppenheim (Hessen) and in 1880 became ordinary professor for psychiatric at the newly founded Psychiatric Clinic of the Baltic University in Dorpat. In 1886 he was appointed to the chair of psychiatry in Freiburg. Due to a cerebal-organic disease after 10 years in Freiburg Emminghaus was given temporary leave in 1890; in 1902 he officially retired and died in Freiburg in 1904.

Kraepelin did his preliminary medical examination in Wurzburg and, with encouragement from Emminghaus, as a student at the Wurzburg university began working for a prize on the topic »About the influence of acute diseases on the onset of mental diseases«. Kraepelin won the prize, although he had to admit that no one else had entered the competition. A few years later in 1881/1882 Kraepelin published the work in the form of five bulletins for the »Archive of Psychiatry » (Archiv für Psychiatrie). After spending one term in Leipzig, Kraepelin returned to Wurzburg for the winter term 1877/1878, where F. von Rinecker offered him a job as assistant doctor. He took the job at the end of 1877, although he did not take his final exams until 1878 and used a revised version of his prize topic as his thesis for graduation. Whilst von Rinecker was absent from the clinic for a few weeks, Emminghaus became his deputy; in this manner Kraepelin, the student, came into contact with him again and referred to him as his »old teacher«. The relationship they had begun in Wurzburg continued and subsequently Emminghaus proposed Kraepelin to be his successor in Dorpat in 1886.

Von Rinecker made B. von Gudden aware of Kraepelin; he offered him a job at the district mental hospital in Munich starting August 1, 1878. It seems Kraepelin's first contact with psychiatry had been rather »discouraging«. In particular, a certain »powerlessness of medical treatment« is noted and

he was worried by the sheer number of psychiatric diseases which he considered only a »confusing mass«, a pure »confusion of observations«.

With his scientific interests Kraepelin soon made contacts at the Munich clinic with some of the co-workers at the clinic, who were having success with neuro-anatomy as patronized by B. von Gudden (▶ Chapter 4).

Kraepelin was very impressed by B. von Gudden as doctor and researcher, but was apparently not so enthusiastic about the kind of research he was doing. He had been given the task of studying reptile brains from a neuro-anatomical point of view. It is not clear how intensively he worked on this area, but during his four years with von Gudden (1878–1882) he did not publish any scientific work on this topic.

During his time with von Gudden, Kraepelin had to do the second part of his military service in Neustrelitz (October 1879 – May 1880). He used the time to write, in three weeks, a scientific paper, which made him famous: He wrote a polemic pamphlet on a publication by the lawyer Mittelstaedt (1834–1899) in which he vehemently criticized Mittelstadt's retaliation theory from a »psychiatrist's point of view«. Kraepelin demanded that the sentences be served in a similar manner to treatment in a mental asylum (◘ Fig. 7.1).

When he started working again in Munich, he found that, although he was very proud of the scientific reputation of the Munich clinic and personally admired B. von Gudden, he could not follow his own scientific plans and intentions. In the summer of 1882 he accepted Paul Flechsig's offer and became assistant doctor at the Psychiatric Clinic of the University of Leipzig. Flechsig assured Kraepelin that he would be able to habilitate on the subject of psychiatry in Leipzig with his support.

Paul Flechsig (1847–1929) had been professor of psychiatry in Leipzig since 1877 and paved the way for the construction of a psychiatric clinic at the Leipzig medical faculty. When Kraepelin arrived in Leipzig in February 1882, the clinic was planned to be opened on May 1, 1882. Flechsig gave Kraepelin orders to set up a psychological laboratory in time for the clinic opening. Kraepelin welcomed the task as an opportunity to work with Wilhelm Wundt (who he had admired since his student days in Leipzig as philosopher and psychologist) in his laboratory.

Five weeks after the opening of the clinic Flechsig dismissed Kraepelin! (There is no clear evidence about the cause of disagreement between Flechsig and Kraepelin. It is presumed that Kraepelin spent more time in Wilhelm Wundt's institute than at the Leipzig clinic.) Two weeks after the dismissal Kraepelin had to leave the clinic; furthermore, Flechsig withdrew his offer of habilitation.

With the help of Wilhelm Wundt and Wilhelm Erb (1840–1921), doctor for internal medicine and neurology in Leipzig, Kraepelin did manage to habilitate in Leipzig.

Kraepelin used the following months to intensify scientific work in Wundt's Psychological Laboratory, but he no longer had a secure income. To earn some money and at Wundt's suggestion he wrote the »Compendium of Psychiatry« during the Easter holidays in 1883 (◘ Fig. 7.2), although he would have preferred publishing something on criminal psychology. Due to his uncertain financial situation Kraepelin considered going to Gorlitz at the beginning of 1883 to work as assistant to K.L. Kahlbaum (1828–1899). Gorlitz did not work at the university, but had an excellent scientific reputation. Wundt dissuaded Kraepelin from this idea.

Following these difficulties, Kraepelin considered resigning from the medical faculty to join the philosophical faculty as Wundt's pupil for »experimental psychology« and to habilitate there. However, Wundt discouraged him from this step too, since the chances of a career as university lecturer for experimental psychology at the philosophical faculty were particularly bad. In autumn 1883 Kraepelin asked B. von Gudden for his advice which path to choose. Gudden offered him to return to Munich and Kraepelin left Leipzig. In autumn 1883 he started work again in Munich for von Gudden and very soon habilitated under the deanship of M. von Pettenkofer (1818–1901) at the Munich medical faculty giving his trial lecture on the »Psychological Point of View in Psychiatry«.

As B. von Gudden had allowed S. Ganser (► Chapter 4), a befriended colleague of Kraepelin's to give the lectures on »Psychiatry«, Kraepelin gave his first lectures as private lecturer on »Criminal Psychology« and »Experimental Psychology«.

By taking on the job as assistant with B. von Gudden and being able to earn some money, Kraepelin was finally in the situation to be able to marry at the age of 28 and start a family. Since 1871 he had been engaged to Ina Schwabe from Neustrelitz,

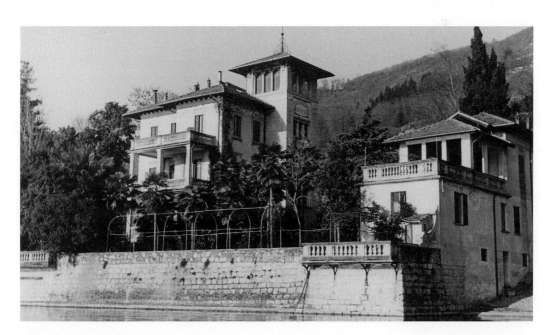

◘ **Fig. 7.8.** The house in Pallanza on Lago Maggiore

who was 7 months older than him. He still waited before getting married.

On his return to B. von Gudden Kraepelin had completely lost all interest in brain-anatomical studies. Whilst with Wundt he had decided to work scientifically on experimental psychology and not – as many psychiatrists at the time – to work clinically and scientifically on anatomy of the brain. Kraepelin felt himself to be a »pure psychiatrist with psychological tendencies«. During 1884 which was filled with much doubt and deliberation for Kraepelin, he (yet again as in 1883) decided »to give up an academic career and marry«. He became senior consultant at the Silesian institution, Leubus, and married on October 4, 1884. A few months later he was offered the post of head doctor at the department for mental disorders at the General Hospital of Dresden; he accepted the offer and began to work there in spring 1884. In November 1885 in Dresden, his first daughter was born but died a few hours after birth.

After being in Dresden for a year and on recommendation of his Wurzburg friend, H. Emminghaus, he was offered the chair of psychiatry at the Baltic University of Dorpat.

From 1886 until 1891 Kraepelin was professor of Psychiatry in Dorpat. He managed to improve the conditions at the Dorpat clinic significantly. And, supported by younger assistants and students, he began to work scientifically: With simple means he built up a laboratory for experimental psychology (▶ Chapter 8).

In 1891 Kraepelin was offered the chair of psychiatry in Heidelberg as successor to Carl Fürstner (1848–1906). He received the offer on November 9, 1890, on the day his first son was born.

For the Kraepelin family the years spent in Dorpat had been fairly tragic ones. After their first daughter had died in 1885, a second daughter was born in 1887 and a third in 1888. The third daughter died two years later in Dorpat; and before the family moved to Heidelberg, their son also died. Consequently only Kraepelin, his wife and daughter, born in 1887, moved to Heidelberg.

The years in Heidelberg (1891–1903) were a happy time for the Kraepelin family: Another four daughters were born.

As a member of the highly esteemed Heidelberg medical faculty, Kraepelin's reputation as an academic teacher and scientist grew. In spite of a huge amount of work he continued to work scientifically and revised three editions of his well-known textbook »Psychiatry«.

In Heidelberg Kraepelin managed to attract younger scientists with special research projects to the clinic. Amongst this group was G. Aschaffenburg, R. Gaupp, E. Rüdin, P. Schröder, A. Weygandt and in particular F. Nissl who joined the clinic in 1895. Aschaffenburg, Weygandt and Rüdin, who

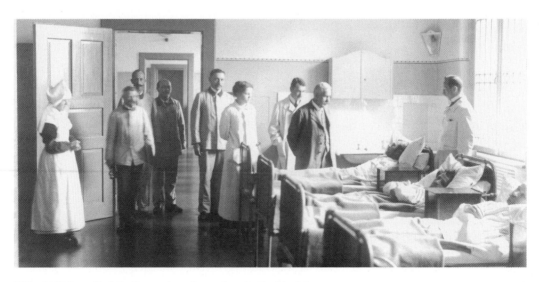

◨ **Fig. 7.9.** E. Kraepelin doing his rounds on the wards at the Munich clinic

joined in 1900, left the clinic whilst Kraepelin was still there.

Following the sudden death of Anton Bumm (► Chapters 5 and 6), Kraepelin assumed that the chances of receiving an offer to Munich were good. He decided to apply for the job, since he was disappointed that during his 12 years in Heidelberg he had not managed to improve the conditions at the clinic. The ministries in Baden had only ever reacted inertly to his demands. Kraepelin's application to Munich was accepted. Various co-workers followed him to Munich in 1903 to continue their work with him, as was the case for R. Gaupp, A. Alzheimer and P. Nitsche (see below). Some followed at a later date (e.g. F. Lotmar, E. Reiss and E. Rohdc). Rohde, highly esteemed by Kraepelin, built the first chemical laboratory in Munich which was later run by F. Lotmar and then R. Allers (see below), when Rohde returned to Heidelberg.

Although Kraepelin thought that his move to Munich meant he was »sacrificing his personal happiness for the sake of science«, he later admitted that his »second period in Munich« (1903–1926) scientifically, professionally as well as privately the most important time of his life. Kraepelin's relations with most members of the medical faculty were not particularly close and he found it »showed signs of a final-stage university, as no one tended to leave the Munich university«, but he did have many contacts to the outside world, maintained old relationships and made new contacts to a great number of his professional colleagues.

Not only for Kraepelin himself, but also for his family, the change from Heidelberg to Munich was a very pleasant one. On his appointment Kraepelin had negotiated that a large, official residence (the »villa«), annexed to the new clinic, would be put at his disposal. In 1906 Kraepelin purchased a large piece of land between Hoellriegelskreuth and Baierbrunn where he later wanted to live with his family in the pleasant Isar valley to the south of Munich. However, Kraepelin soon changed his mind and reverted to the plans he had already made in Heidelberg. Kraepelin's financial situation in Munich had improved to such an extent that he now considered seriously constructing a house in Pallanza, on the shores of Lago Maggiore (◘ Fig. 7.8), land he had bought in 1902 whilst in Heidelberg. Kraepelin and

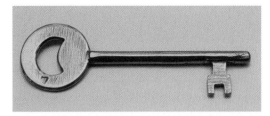

◘ **Fig. 7.10.** Key which worked on the locks of his official residence in Munich and his house in Pallanza

his wife kept these plans secret and it was not until they moved into the house with its large garden, located right on the banks of the lake, that he surprised his family; from then on the house was used for holidays and Christmas celebrations. Kraepelin also used the house regularly during the term holidays, escaping many obligations he had in Munich in order, to concentrate on his scientific work. For the entire family »a period of blessed work and great enjoyment of life gradually developed in our Italian house«.

Large parts of Kraepelin's scientific works were compiled in Munich and written in Pallanza. Regularly, Kraepelin left Munich immediately after term time with a couple of boxes of records and clinical notes which were to be scientifically evaluated and possibly included in the next edition of his textbook (◘ Fig. 7.9). To a certain extent Pallanza became a »scientific outpost« of the Munich clinic and a symbol of this attitude was that he had a key prepared not only as »passpartout« for all the clinic's locks and for his official residence, but also opening the doors of his house at Pallanza! (This also explains why he pointed out what otherwise would have seemed a trivial matter: He placed »particular importance on the practical solution as far as the key problem was concerned.«) (◘ Fig. 7.10)

After original scepticism Kraepelin and his family enjoyed the pleasant living and general life in Munich. He was able to go on many of the trips he had planned which he always considered an »escape« from his professional obligations. Soon after taking up office in Munich, he wrote to his brother Karl (letter of January 27, 1905): »At the moment my main aim is to earn enough money to travel wherever I want without any problem« (◘ Fig. 7.11). Kraepelin had already been travelling

München,den 27.Januar 1905.

Lieber Korl !

Es hat mir sehr leid gethan,dass die Sache mit den Diapositiven so
missglückt ist,aber Ina wird Dir wohl schon geschildert haben;dass ich
mir alle Mühe gegeben hatte,alles in die Reihe zu bringen.Ich bin natürlich bereit;die Bilder,wenn Du sie nicht brauchen kannst,auf meine Ko-
sten zu übernehmen.Wir können das ja später bei unserer Abrechnung be-
rücksichtigen.Ich werde mir ohnedies wohl noch eine grössere Zahl von
Diapositiven anfertigen oder anfertigen lassen.Dass Dein Vortrag so gut
ausgefallen ist,hat mich sehr gefreut;es war ja bei dem reichen Stoffe
nicht anders zu erwarten.Vor kurzem habe ich übrigens noch einige Bilder aus Johore und Colombo hier gefunden,die Du noch nicht gesehen hast;
ich schicke sie Dir gelegentlich zu,wenn sie copirt sind.

Aus Deinem Briefe an Willerts habe ich leider ersehen,dass Deine
Neigung,im Herbst mit uns zu reisen,sehr gering ist.Willerts möchten auf
begreiflichen Gründen einmal den Orient kennen lernen und haben dazu
keine andere Jahreszeit zur Verfügung,als den Herbst.Ich halte zwar Deine Schilderung der Fährlichkeiten des Südens nach unseren Erfahrungen
in Süditalien für viel zu schwarz,aber ich bin gern bereit,auf irgend
einen anderen Plan einzugehen,der besser ist,da ich ja Tunis;das mich
interessiren würde,jederzeit besuchen kann.Darum habe ich Willerts zunächst Constantinopel vorgeschlagen,das wegen seiner landschaftlichen
Umgebung im August ganz gut zu besuchen ist.Man könnte den Hinweg durch
die Balkanstaaten,etwa durch Rumänien nehmen,ein paar Tage in Wien bleiben,die Donau ein Stück entlang fahren und über das schwarze Meer in den
Bosporus einlaufen;um zurück durch das Mittelmeer nach Triest oder Venedig zu fahren.Hier wären ernsthafte klimatische Bedenken gewiss nicht,
nachdem wir vor einigen Jahren um dieselbe Zeit in Neapel und Rom wa-
ren.Oder weisst Du einen anderen Plan,der Willerts Wunsch erfüllen könnte?Es liesse sich ja etwa an Algier denken,aber Constantinopel ist ohne

■ **Fig 7.11.** Letter of 27.01.1905 from Kraepelin to his brother Karl Munich, January 27, 1905

Zweifel weit lohnender.Wie lange dauern Deine Ferien?Vier Wochen wirst
Du Dich doch frei machen können?Da könnten ja Willerts zunächst einige
Zeit hier,in Salzburg und Wien verbringen,und wir könnten dort gegen
den 15.mit Dir zusammentreffen,um über Budapest,Belgrad,Bukarest,Varna
weiterzufahren.Für Konstantinopel würde ich etwa 10 Tage rechnen;ich habe dort gute Beziehungen.Ein Abstecher nach Brussa wäre mit dabei,dann
vielleidht noch Smyrna mit Ausflug nach Ephesus.Jetzt zu Ostern werde
ich mit Ina wohl über Graz und Triest nach Abbazia und weiter nach Fiume,Gravosa,Ragusa,Antivari gehen,zurück über Venedig und Pallanza nach
Heidelberg,um dort noch etwas zu arbeiten.Mitte März gehen wir fort und
sind Mitte April in H.Das Semester beginnt mich stark mitzunehmen;ich
habe jetzt schon 6 Unterrichtsstunden und bekomme im nächsten Monate
noch 3 dazu in einem Curse für Oberstabsärzte.Mit meinem Buche bin ich
daher immer noch nicht ganz fertig und komme fast gar nicht aus dem Hau-
se.In Folge dessen werde ich dick und schwerfällig,so dass es höchste
Zeit wird,die Glieder wieder mehr zu regen.Der Geist in der Klinik wird
allmählich ein besserer;es beginnt sich eine Tradition herauszubilden,
was ich allerdings nur durch volles Aufgebot meiner Person erreicht ha-
be.Wöchentlich findet ein wissenschaftlicher Nachmittag,alle zwei Wochen ein Referirabend statt,so dass mein Einfluss nach und nach die bun-
te Masse der Neulinge zusammenschweissen kann.Zu den Abenden kommen auch
die Fachgenossen aus den Anstalten;ausserdem haben wir schon wieder einen ganzen Schwarm von Mitläufern und Arbeitern.An die grosse Reise den-
ke ich tagtäglich mit Wehmuth zurück;und ich schwöre mir zu,dass sie
noch viele Nachfolger haben soll.Money,travelling spent,is well spent.
Heute vor einem Jahre trafen wir von Nuwara Eliya in Colombo ein und
sassen Abends am Strande;übermorgen geht es nach Südindien.Ich habe zur
Zeit nur das Hauptziel vor Augen,soviel Geld zu verdienen;dass ich un-
bedenklich reisen kann,wohin ich mag.Unsere Kinder gehen Ostern auch
nach Heidelberg.Bei Euch ist hoffentlich die Krankheit endlich vorüber;
solche Dinge sind oft schrecklich hartnäckig.Toni schreibt bald einen
Dankesbrief;sie ist sehr angestrengt.Viele Grüsse!

Emil.

■ Fig 7.11. *Continued*

Dear Karl

I am sorry that it went so wrong with the slides, but Ina will have explained to you that I did all I could to sort it out. Of course I am prepared to pay for the pictures, if they are of no use to you. We can consider that when we draw up an account later. I want to prepare or at least have a number of slides prepared for me. I am glad to hear that your lecture was so successful; but with such interesting material it is hardly surprising. By the way, I recently found some pictures from Jahore and Colombo which you have not yet seen and I will send them to you, once they have been copied.

From your letter to Willerts I see that you are not so keen on travelling with us in autumn. For obvious reasons Willerts would like to see the Orient and only has the autumn months free to do it. In our experience I consider your description of the dangers of south Italy to be far too negative, but am more than prepared to hear any better plans, since I would be interested in Tunis, but can visit it anytime I want. That is why I have suggested Constantinopel and its surroundings to Willerts, as August should be a good time to visit. We could go there via the Baltic States, for example Rumania, spend a couple of days in Vienna, travel down the Danube and go to the Black Sea via the Bosphorus returning via the Mediterranean to Triest or Venice. We would not have any serious climatic worries in this area, since we were in Naples and Rome at the same time a couple of years ago. Or do you have another plan matching Willerts wishes? For example Algiers, but Constantinopel is definitely more worthwhile. How long are your holidays? You will be able to take 4 weeks off, I imagine? Willerts could spend some time here, in Salzburg and Vienna and we could meet you there around the 15th and travel together via Budapest, Bucharest and Varna. I would estimate about 10 days for Constantinopel; I have some good contacts there. We could visit Brussa and then maybe Smyrna with a trip to Ephesus. Over Easter I will travel with Ina to Fiume, Gravosa, Ragusa, Antivari and then back via Venice and Pallanza to Heidelberg to do some work. We will leave mid March and be in H. mid April. The term has become very busy and I already have 6 hours of tuition and will have another 5-hour course for senior major surgeons. I still have not finished my book and cannot get out of the house. As a result, I am becoming fat and slow and it is time to move my joints a bit. The spirit in the clinic is gradually improving; a tradition seems to be growing, but only really due to my personal commitment. Every week we have a scientific afternoon and every second week some kind of evening presentation; with my influence drawing together the colourful mass of newcomers. We invite colleagues from other psychiatric institutes to the evening presentations and have quite a number of followers now. I think longingly of the big trip we made and swear that it will not be the last. Money spent travelling is money spent well. Exactly a year ago today, we arrived in Nuwara Eliya in Colombo and sat on the beach in the evening; the day after tomorrow we are off to south India. I only have one main aim at present, to earn enough money so that I can travel whenever I want. Our children will be going to Heidelberg at Easter. I hope that you have finally recovered from your illness; such things are often extremely difficult to get rid of. Toni will soon write a thank-you letter; she is working hard. Many greetings! Emil.

◻ **Fig 7.11.** *Continued*

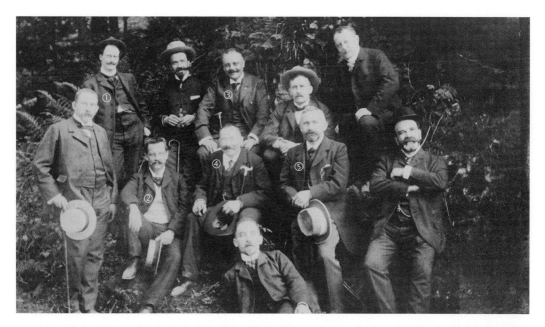

◻ Fig. 7.12. Meeting of the South German psychiatrists in Baden-Baden (»Wanderversammlung der Sueddeutschen Psychiater«): 1. Albrecht Bethe, 2. Robert Gaupp, 3. Alois Alzheimer, 4. Franz Nissl, 5. Emil Kraepelin

from Dorpat and from Heidelberg, and he continued in this fashion from Munich. Apart from the regular trips to Italy, his journeys to South-East Asia (1903/1904) and his visits to America (1908 and 1922) are the most well known. He made a journey by ship to Madeira, to the North African coast and to Portugal. In 1915/1916 a 9-month trip he had planned via Russia to Siberia and then from China via Burma to Singapore had to be abandoned due to the First World War.

Neither did the India trip during the winter months of 1926/1927 materialize, which Kraepelin had planned with J. Lange during the work on the 9ᵗʰ edition of the textbook »Psychiatry«, because Kraepelin died in Munich shortly after falling ill with pneumonia on October 7, 1926.

Although Kraepelin particularly enjoyed long distance journeys, he also considered his trips within Europe to be important and often combined them with visits to psychiatric clinics. Usually together with his wife or daughters, he explored the near and far regions of Munich on long bicycle trips or by foot. »As long as my professional life allowed, I fled into the fresh air.« He spent holidays in Berchtesgaden with his wife or on the »Frauen-

insel« in Chiemsee (Lake Chiem). He spent one longer working holiday with his daughter Toni at the house of James Loeb in Murnau on Lake Staffel (► Chapter 8) and got to know the foothills of the Alps in Garmisch. In his memoires Kraepelin mentioned his »alpine crossing« (from Munich to Pallanza) by bicycle; Pallanza was often used as the starting point for »10 to 15-hour hikes«.

Some tiring mountain hikes with colleagues are jokingly referred to as »Catatonic walks« (◻ Fig. 7.12). Once travelling became restricted during the First World War, Kraepelin and his daughters went on a long bicycle trip from Munich via central Germany to his home in Mecklenburg to explore his ancestry.

From contemporaries' reports it can be concluded that the fulfilment of duties was Kraepelin's main principle in life; but he found many of his duties to be something he had to put up with and did so with little joy and enthusiasm. As son of a Prussian teacher »Zeitgeist«, education and character no doubt contributed to his personal qualities. Fears, worries and his somewhat obsessive personality traits lead him to his crusade against alcohol at the end of the 19ᵗʰ century: »Worry about the German people, his clinic and his scientific authority were expressed here and shaped his actions«. The effect of substances of abuse on performance was something that had been preoccupying Kraepelin since 1881; in the following years he made a number of studies on the subject (»On the effect of some medicinal substances on the duration of simple mental processes, 1881). Having studied alcohol experimentally (altogether he wrote 19 publications on the subject of alcohol) and having seen the detrimental effects of acute and long-term intake, his conclusions led to his complete abstinence intending to set an example for others. Alcohol was strictly forbidden at the Munich clinic, although he had originally praised alcohol as a calming substance for aroused patients. Instead of alcohol, the patients were given his own recipe, a type of lemonade, the so-called »Kraepelin sparkling wine«. He also demanded sanatoriums for alcoholics which was turned down by the Ministry of the Interior. The Munich breweries protested and criticized Kraepelin's ideas expressing themselves vehemently, both personally and via the daily press.

> Coming from a middle-class family, Kraepelin remained conservative and bourgeois for his entire life. He was also a zealous autocrat who was austere, but treated his co-workers with fairness. Apart from psychiatry he was also interested in the arts, such as music, theatre and painting, although he was by no means convivial but the older he got, the less time he had for these interests.

Emil Kraepelin's Co-Workers and Pupils at the Munich Hospital

During the first four years as assistant to von Gudden Kraepelin belonged to a circle of young scientists who, under the auspices of von Gudden, all worked on one scientific area: Studies on comparative neuro-anatomy of the brain of different species of animal. For this reason, and rightly so, the Munich study group was often referred to as von Gudden's school, as the »first Munich school«. Kraepelin is also generally referred to as Gudden's scientific student, although no neuro-anatomical studies by him exist.

Without question von Gudden was Kraepelin's clinical teacher, although Kraepelin considered Wilhlem Wundt to be his main teacher despite the fact that Kraepelin had only spent a short time with him as student and later assistant.

As soon as Kraepelin occupied positions in the eighties giving him the opportunity to instruct young scientists, he entrusted them with certain research projects. To begin with, his co-workers dealt with questions of experimental psychology, in particular with regard to pharmaco-psychology. Kraepelin motivated his students and younger assistant doctors to participate in scientific studies. It became apparent that Kraepelin would one day found a »school« with the central topic »experimental psychology« in psychiatry. One of Kraepelin's first doctoral candidates in Dorpat, H. Dehio, graduated with a thesis on »Studies on the effect of caffeine and tea on the duration of simple psychological processes«, a topic, which had interested Kraepelin some years previously with W. Wundt and which he later summarized in a book in 1892 »On the influence of drugs on simple psychic processes«.

However, contrary to B. von Gudden, Kraepelin did not found a »school«, in which the co-workers had to study a certain subject of particular importance to the »boss«. Kraepelin took pains to make sure that as many »auxiliary sciences« as possible were included in clinical-psychiatric research and in order to achieve this he allowed his co-workers to deal with problems from completely different research areas. This was the reason that in Heidelberg and even more so after his move to Munich, he added researchers to his work groups, who worked successfully in other areas than his own (e.g. on physiological chemistry, serology, genealogy or neuropathology). He expected to make the most progress in experimental psychology, but wanted to create an atmosphere where the »auxiliary sciences« could contribute to psychiatric research. Kraepelin was convinced that progress could only be made by taking as many »auxiliary sciences« into consideration as possible and by using its methodological diversity to the advantage of clinical psychiatry.

As such Kraepelin did not found a »school« like the »school« of von Gudden, which could be compared with the »Berlin school« of C. Westphal or the »schools« of the later centuries (e.g. the Tubingen school of R. Gaupp and E. Kretschmer or the Heidelberg school of K. Wilmanns and K. Schneider). But with his students at the Munich clinic, and later with co-workers of the »German Psychiatric Research Institute«, he did have a large number of pupils and co-workers, who influenced psychiatry world-wide sustainably for generations without coming from a particular school of thought.

In a summary of Kraepelin's most important co-workers at the Munich clinic from 1904 to 1992 54 names can be mentioned. The list would be even longer if the numerous guests, who worked in the clinic or in one of the laboratories (e.g. Alzheimer's microscopy laboratory), were included as well.

The list of names to be mentioned is long and it is only possible to give the details of a few (e.g. the senior consultants), and most of them only cursorily.

F. Nissl (▶ Chapter 4) and K. Brodmann (▶ Chapter 8) should also be mentioned here; in 1918 they were not appointed as clinic co-workers, but went straight to the German Psychiatric Research Institute. Together with co-workers from the clinic they built up the German Psychiatric Research Institute (▶ Chapter 8): E. Rüdin, F. Plaut and W. Spielmeyer resigned formally (1917/1918) from the clinic and became members of the Research Institute; however, their ties to the clinic remained to a certain degree, as the Research Institute was accommodated completely in rooms within the clinic up until 1924, and up until 1928 it had some of its departments at the clinic.

In a complete list of Kraepelin's co-workers there are names of some scientists most of whom have been forgotten.

For example; U. Ebbecke (1883–1960) worked with Kraepelin and the neurologist, G. Schaltenbrand, (1897–1979) who was one of his doctoral candidates in Munich.

Many of Kraepelin's co-workers would hold important positions in psychiatry, but not until they had left the clinic and worked in other clinics: For example

A. Serko (1879–1938): 1909 until 1912 assistant in Munich; 1912–1914 assistant to Wagner von Jauregg in Vienna; postdoctoral lecture qualification in Prague 1919; from 1919 ordinary professor for psychiatry in Laibach (Ljubljana).

F. Meggendorfer (1880–1953): 1911–1913 Graduation and first assistant with Kraepelin; later with Rüdin at the German Psychiatric Research Institute; 1934–1945 ordinary professor for psychiatry and director of the Psychiatric Clinic in Erlangen.

Some directors of large psychiatric institutions, who played important roles in the development of psychiatry, came from Kraepelin's clinic.

There are also names hardly ever connected with the Munich clinic, like O. Gross and M.H. Göring.

Otto Gross (1877–1920) has recently been rediscovered as an »expressionist of the Schwabing cultural revolution«.

Gross habilitated at his home town of Graz, Austria, with G. Anton (1858–1933) in the field of psychopathology. He was assistant at the Munich clinic from 1906 until 1910. During this period he worked scientifically on the problems of disintegration of the conscience, with the differential diagnostics of negativistic phenomena, and he published a book »On Psychopathic Inferiorities«. He was also very interested in psychoanalysis; he had done psychoanalysis with C. G. Jung and was well respected by S. Freud. In 1908 Freud referred to him as a most original person, but soon judged him as being »dangerous for the psychoanalytical movement«.

In Munich Gross joined the art circles of Schwabing with their revolutionary ideas. He became addicted to drugs; Freud asked C. G. Jung to treat him. After moving to Switzerland and also later in Austria he encountered problems with the authorities due to his »revolutionary activities«. During the First World War in Prague Gross belonged to the circle of M. Brod, F. Werfel and F. Kafka. He was treated on several occasions in psychiatric clinics, most likely not only due to his dependence on drugs, but also because he was psychotically ill. He died in Berlin in 1920.

Another of Kraepelin's assistants was Matthias Heinrich Göring. He worked at the Munich clinic from 1908 until 1910, then changed to psychoanalysis, habilitated in psychiatry in Giessen and from 1936 onwards managed the »Reich's Institute for Psychological Research and Psychotherapy«, which was tolerated by the national socialists. This somewhat bizarre constellation could occur because

M.H. Göring was a cousin of Hermann Göring and therefore enjoyed special treatment.

> One of Kraepelin's assistants, P. Nitsche (1876–1947) played a disastrous role in national socialism. Nitsche had already worked with Kraepelin in Heidelberg as assistant doctor and in a letter to his brother Karl Kraepelin referred to him as one of his best assistants. For this reason Kraepelin took Nitsche, as well as Gaupp and Alzheimer to Munich; he hoped that »he would help to further a harmonious and purposeful working atmosphere with colleagues from very different institutions«. Nitsche worked at the Munich clinic until 1907.
>
> After his time in Munich, Nitsche held managing positions at various other psychiatric clinics and asylums in Saxony (Dresden, Leipzig, Sonnenstein near Pirna). Together with E. Rüdin and C. Schneider he wrote a paper in 1943 about the »Reorganization of Psychiatry in the German Reich«.
>
> As senior expert Nitsche became one of the main people responsible for the national socialist plan to exterminate the mentally ill (euthanasia program). In 1947 he was condemned to death by a jury court in Dresden and hanged.

It would be an important task to follow the lives and developments of all psychiatrists, who worked at the Munich clinic at the beginning of the century. No doubt many unknown connections would show up and probably the one or other claim could be put down as unproven speculation. However, there are gaps in some of the stories, but one person, E. Rüdin, has been studied in detail; he was senior consultant in Munich with Kraepelin and later, during the Third Reich, headed the German Psychiatric Research Institute (► Chapter 8).

Recently, Emil Kraepelin has been reproached for his national-conservative attitude, but the sweeping statement that Kraepelin was a precursor of national socialism and a militant anti-Semite is not justified.

Obviously, it would be important to take these aspects into account, considering the interest in Kraepelin's scientific work, which has grown during the past few years. Overhasty accusations and judgement should be avoided, neither should worldly or political statements by Kraepelin be considered harmless. A careful analysis of these aspects of Kraepelin's work should not be limited to a single, select publication (e.g. to the »Psychiatric Side Comments to Contemporary History« from 1919), but should be looked at in its contemporary, historical context.

It is to be assumed that the publication of all available material about Kraepelin, currently being processed by M. Weber from the Max-Planck-Institute for Psychiatry (together with W. Burgmair and J.E. Engstrom) will shed ample light on this problem. (Four volumes of the planned eight volumes entitled »Emil Kraepelin« were already published in 2000 by »Belleville« publishers – Munich).

Kraepelin's co-workers at the Munich clinic were his **senior consultants**:

R. Gaupp (1904–1906)
A. Alzheimer (1906–1909)
E. Rüdin (1909–1917)
G. Stertz (1919–1921)
E. Kahn (1921–1922; then – after Kraepelin's retirement – provisional director of the clinic: 1922–1924)

Robert Gaupp (1870–1953) (◻ Fig. 7.13) was the first senior consultant at the clinic when it opened; he had already worked with Kraepelin in Heidelberg.

From 1894 until 1898 Gaupp was assistant to C. Wernicke in Breslau, before going for a couple of months to a psychiatric asylum in his Swabian home town, Zwiefalten, as senior consultant. Because he did not enjoy the work there, he returned to the clinic in Breslau. He worked for a further year for Bonhoeffer, but then left the Breslau clinic and set up a practise for psychiatry in Breslau in 1899. When Kraepelin heard what Gaupp was doing, he invited him to Heidelberg. Gaupp agreed, habilitated in Heidelberg in 1901 and followed Kraepelin to Munich in 1904. In 1906 Gaupp left for Tubingen where he became full professor and clinic director. He managed the clinic in Tubingen until his retirement in 1936.

Wernicke trained Gaupp to record symptoms and analyse them thoroughly. After working for Kraepelin in Heidelberg and Munich, he realized that with Wernicke he was »only seeing one side of psychiatric science« and that progress could only be made with Kraepelin's clinical concepts (e.g. with

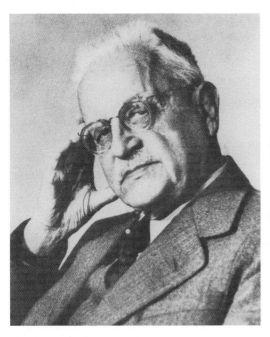

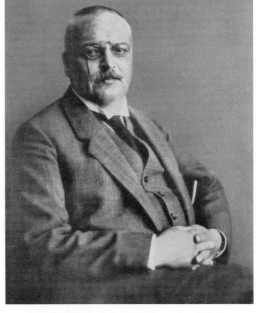

the »dichotomy« of endogenous psychoses). Gaupp agreed with Kraepelin's opinion that it was not sufficient to define differences between various psychiatric diseases based purely on clinical observation of the short-term findings. Already in Heidelberg and later in Munich, Gaupp developed his own ideas on the fundamentals of clinical psychiatry. He criticised that psychiatry at the turn of the century had been too restricted by natural sciences; as a consequence the psychological aspects of mental illness had been neglected. Gaupp expected psychiatrists to know their patients »inside out« and to follow up on the »mental legality of their statements on life«.

Whilst working for Kraepelin, the scientific topics Gaupp had been studying with Wernicke took a back seat. During his short stay in Munich he published works »On the Limits of Psychiatric Knowledge«, on »Depressive Disorders in Old Age«, »On Suicide« and about »The Clinical Anomalies of Our City Population«.

Kraepelin admired Gaupp and regretted that he left the Munich clinic in 1906. The good contact between the two did not diminish once Gaupp left for Tubingen. Even scientific differences of opinion (e.g. on the question of paranoia) had no influence

on their good personal relations and Kraepelin would have liked Gaupp to be his successor in Munich.

Alois Alzheimer (1864–1915) (◼ Fig. 7.14) was R. Gaupp's successor as senior consultant in 1906.

Alzheimer was born in Marktbreit am Main in Lower Franconia on June 14, 1864, as son of a notary. He studied in Berlin, Tubingen and Wurzburg. In 1888 he became assistant to E. Sioli (1852–1922) at the Municipal Mental Asylum in Frankfurt am Main. He worked there for 15 years and was influenced decisively by Sioli, who was particularly progressive for his time. One year after Alzheimer joined the Frankfurt clinic, F. Nissl started working with Sioli in 1889 as »Second Doctor« at the Frankfurter Clinic, due to his several years of working experience with B. von Gudden in Munich and with von Grashey.

Alzheimer and Nissl who was four years older, soon became good friends. Nissl showed Alzheimer his staining techniques and »with his test material and experimental results convinced him of the accuracy and the importance of neuro-histopathological methods for research into psychiatric diseases, which was not necessarily generally accepted

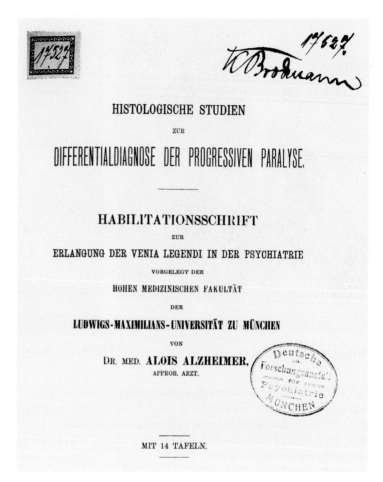

HISTOLOGISCHE STUDIEN

ZUR

DIFFERENTIALDIAGNOSE DER PROGRESSIVEN PARALYSE.

HABILITATIONSSCHRIFT

ZUR

ERLANGUNG DER VENIA LEGENDI IN DER PSYCHIATRIE

VORGELEGT DER

HOHEN MEDIZINISCHEN FAKULTÄT

DER

LUDWIGS-MAXIMILIANS-UNIVERSITÄT ZU MÜNCHEN

VON

DR. MED. ALOIS ALZHEIMER,

APPROB. ARZT.

MIT 14 TAFELN.

◻ **Fig. 7.15.** Thesis for the postdoctural lecturer qualification by Alois Alzheimer on »Differential diagnosis of progressive paralysis« (1904)

at the time«. Influenced by Nissl, Alzheimer started in Frankfurt with his neuropathological studies, which later brought him worldwide fame. Nissl and Alzheimer had the same »precise target: To record the fundamentals of the pathological process in mental illness«.

When Nissl left Frankfurt in 1895 to join Kraepelin at the clinic in Heidelberg, Alzheimer became Nissl's successor in Frankfurt as »Second Doctor«.

During his time at the clinic in Frankfurt it had not been Alzheimer's intention to have a scientific career, but to become director of a psychiatric institution. This was probably connected to the fact that Alzheimer's wife and mother of their three children died in 1901, when Alzheimer was 37 years old. As a result, Alzheimer turned down Kraepelin's offer to join him in Heidelberg and instead he applied for the job as director of a cure and care institu-

tion in Hessen. When Nissl informed Kraepelin of Alzheimer's plans, he urged him not to take this step, but to start an academic career. »Unfortunately this advice was not heeded at first. It was not until his plans to become asylum director had failed, that he came to me (Kraepelin) and I managed to convince him to join our circle.«

Alzheimer was in Heidelberg for less than a year, when his plans to habilitate had to be postponed. Kraepelin received an offer to go to Munich and moved there in October the same year. Alzheimer also moved to Munich in October 1903, as Kraepelin had given him the job to supervise the completion and equipping of the clinic.

In 1904 Alzheimer habilitated at the Munich faculty with a thesis »On histological studies on the differential diagnosis of progressive paralysis« (◻ Fig. 7.15).

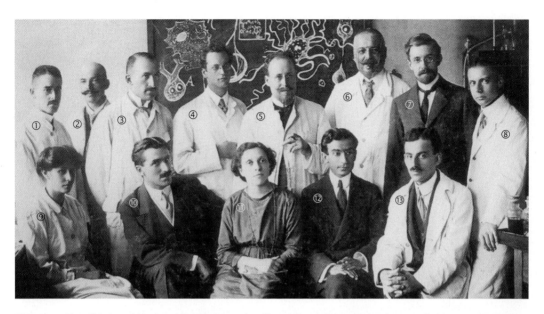

Fig. 7.16. Alois Alzheimer (6) in the midst of his co-workers (from left to right, upper then lower row): 1) Lotmar, 2) ?, 3) Rosental, 4) Allers(?), 5) ?, 7) Achucarro, 8) Levy, 9) Grombach, 10) Cerletti, 11) ?, 12) Bonfiglio, 13) Perusini

Whilst working as senior consultant in Frankfurt at the end of 1901, Alzheimer had examined a female patient (»Auguste D.«). She had been admitted to the Frankfurt clinic in 1901 because after showing ideas of jealousy she had developed a quickly progressing loss of memory, helplessness and finally complete confusion with distinct motor agitation. Alzheimer observed the course of illness until he left for Heidelberg in 1903 and then for Munich. However, he remained in contact with the Frankfurt clinic due to the course of Auguste D.'s illness. The patient died having been ill for 4 ½ years, at the age of 56. Sioli gave the file and the brain of the patient to Alzheimer for scientific examination and Alzheimer's work on this case became the starting point for the first description of Alzheimer's form of dementia!

Alzheimer gave his first report of the case findings with a »strange and serious disease process of the cerebral cortex« at a psychiatric symposium in Tubingen in 1907. He presented his meticulous clinical, pathological-anatomical and microscopic histological findings in detail; however his exemplary presentation of the case found no resonance at the meeting: Neither the chairman of the meeting nor the audience deemed it necessary to discuss the case! Kraepelin realized the principal importance of the case of Auguste D. He included Alzheimer's observations in his textbook and named it »Alzheimer's disease«.

In Munich, to begin with Alzheimer was employed – like E. Rüdin, F. Plaut and M. Isserlin later – as »scientific assistant«: He was unpaid, but could use his time freely for research.

Before the opening of the clinic Alzheimer was Kraepelin's deputy and as such responsible for the final touches to the building and furnishings. Once the clinic had been opened he wanted to dedicate his time to research. Alzheimer's own working area was the large microscopy laboratory, equipped with 13 workspaces and a room for microphotography. It did not take long for researchers from all over the world to join Alzheimer in his work. Within a few years Alzheimer's microscopy laboratory had developed into a centre for neurohistological research. Some co-workers and pupils of Alzheimer were U. Cerletti (1877–1963), G. Perusini (1879–1907?) and F. Lotmar (1878–?), (■ Fig. 7.16). H.G. Creutzfeldt (1885–1964) (■ Fig. 7.17) and A.M. Jakob (1884–1931) (■ Fig. 7.18) worked for Alzheimer and later – separately – described the Jakob-Creutzfeldt disease bearing their name.

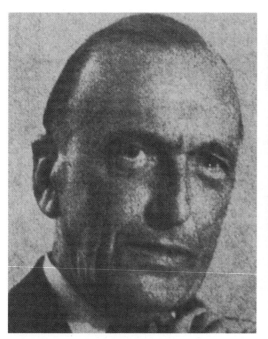

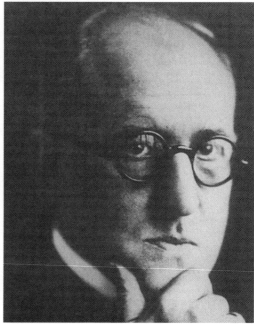

■ **Fig. 7.17.** H.G. Creutzfeld (1885–1964)   ■ **Fig. 7.18.** A.M. Jakob (1884–1931)

Once the clinic had been completed and officially opened, Alzheimer had to take on a vast number of tasks, which stopped him from working scientifically. After habilitating in 1904 and with the start of the summer term in 1905 (until leaving the clinic after the winter term 1912/1913), he had extensive lecture duties. After Gaupp's appointment to Tubingen (1906), Alzheimer became a paid doctor and Kraepelin's deputy. During the following three years he had a particularly large workload to tackle and due to Kraepelin's absences during the summer holidays he was never able to go on holiday.

At Alzheimer's urgent request Kraepelin handed over the duties of senior consultant to E. Rüdin in April 1909 and once again Alzheimer had the status of an unpaid »scientific assistant« with more time for scientific work; on one occasion he was given free time (during the summer term of 1909) for a study trip.

In 1912 Alzheimer became Bonhoeffer's successor at the psychiatric chair in Breslau. He left Munich only reluctantly.

Alzheimer managed the clinic in Breslau for only three years. On leaving Munich he soon became ill.

It is possible that he was suffering from endocarditis and later also from a kidney disease. Alois Alzheimer died aged 51 on December 19, 1915 in Breslau.

Ernst Rüdin (1874–1952) (■ Fig. 7.19) had already once worked for Kraepelin (1900 until 1901 in Heidelberg) before becoming Kraepelin's co-worker for a second time in 1907.

Ernst Rüdin was born in St. Gallen (Switzerland) as son of a teacher who later worked as a textile salesman. Rüdin grew up with his three elder sisters. The second eldest sister influenced him strongly and in many different ways. She was eight years older than him, was extremely assertive and was one of the first women in Switzerland to graduate in medicine. During her studies she met Alfred Julius Ploetz (1860–1940), who came from Silesia, was economist and founder of the racial hygiene movement in Germany. With his social-Darwinist views on »racial hygiene« Ploetz made a lasting impression on the young Ernst Rüdin. Even after Ploetz and Rüdin's sister divorced, Ploetz and Ernst Rüdin kept in contact. Apart from being influenced by Ploetz's initially utopian ideas, which later turned into the actual reality of racial

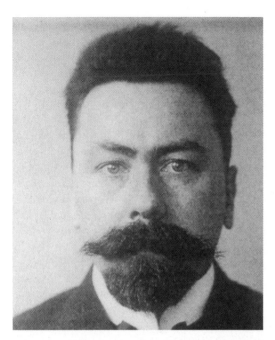

Fig. 7.19. Ernst Rüdin (1874–1952) during his time as senior consultant at the Munich Clinic

hygiene, Rüdin was also influenced as a young man by the works of A. Forel (► Chapter 4). Forel had been Professor for Psychiatry in Zurich since 1879, managed the Psychiatric Clinic Burgholzli in Zurich and was a committed member of the Swiss abstinence movement. Already during his school days, Rüdin combined Ploetz' social reforming postulate and concept of racial hygiene with the efforts of Forel enforcing the ideas of the abstinence movement.

Influenced by these ideas Rüdin began his medical studies in 1893, which took him to Switzerland, Italy, Germany and Ireland. After graduation in Zurich in 1898 he worked for a year at the Psychiatric Clinic for Forel's successor E. Bleuler (1857–1939), before leaving to join Kraepelin in Heidelberg. His graduation in Zurich was entitled »About the clinical forms of prison psychoses«. After working in Heidelberg for a short time, Rüdin's career took him back to Bleuler in Zurich and then finally to Berlin where he – after working in neurology for H. Oppenheim (1858–1919) – worked at the observation department of the prison Berlin-Moabit. During this time Rüdin was

again in close contact with A. Ploetz; plans to publish a new journal – »Archive of Biological Hygiene for Race and Society« – were established. The editor and co-publisher of this journal was Rüdin and he was co-founder of an »Association for Racial Hygiene«. The »Archive of Biological Hygiene for Race and Society« followed up on the »degeneration doctrine« developed by French psychiatrists during the second half of the 19th century and set down procedures for »prophylaxes of madness«.

From 1905 until 1907 Rüdin worked mainly as editor of the »Archive of Biological Hygiene for Race and Society«. Then he returned to psychiatry: He became assistant to Kraepelin at the Munich clinic. At this time, Kraepelin was preoccupied with work on the hereditary aspects of mental diseases and was critically analyzing the degeneration doctrine which he found to be conceptually inaccurate. Rüdin stayed with Kraepelin for 18 years, having studied at 6 or 7 different universities, after working for 6 years at many different clinics and finally having spent two and a half years as publisher and editor of a journal. He worked at the Munich clinic for 10 years and then at the German Psychiatric Research Institute, which Kraepelin had founded. During his entire time with Kraepelin Rüdin remained a dedicated advocate of »racial hygiene«.

Two years after joining the Munich clinic, Rüdin habilitated in 1909 at the medical faculty with a thesis »About the clinical research of mental disorders in prisoners sentenced to life-long imprisonment« and in doing so, followed up on his graduation topic in Zurich. Forensic-psychiatric problems were always of interest to Rüdin; he lectured on forensic psychiatry. From 1911 onwards he lectured on »Facts, Problem and Prophylaxis of Degeneration«.

After habilitating, Rüdin began his work on the »Empirical hereditary prognosis«. With his study on dementia praecox he became a founder of modern psychiatric-genetic research.

In 1909 Kraepelin made Rüdin clinical senior consultant in place of Alzheimer who wanted to dedicate himself to scientific work. Consequently, Rüdin was responsible for the Psychiatric Out-Patient Clinic and met Ida Senger, a co-worker of Hans Gudden. Rüdin married Ida Senger in 1920.

Kraepelin had hesitated for a while before making Rüdin clinical senior consultant. Following Gaupp's appointment to Tubingen (1906), Alzheimer took over the job of senior consultant on an interim basis. Kraepelin tried to convince Alzheimer to keep the job as long as possible, but Alzheimer constantly urged to be freed from his duties and Kraepelin finally decided to give Rüdin the job in 1909.

Kraepelin was very critical of many of Rüdin's ideas.

When Rüdin left the clinic in 1917, he took over the genealogical-demographic department of the Research Institute and continued to collaborate with the clinic doctors. This situation was possible because the Research Institute occupied rooms at the clinic for quite some time.

During the last months of the war and the first years following the First World War, Rüdin made some important forensic-psychiatric expertises. For example, together with E. Kahn (see below), he gave his expert opion on some of the members of the revolutionary unrest which had played a role in the founding of the Munich council republic. The »revolutionary leaders« were judged according to psychopathological criteria as »ethically defective, seriously psychopathic personalities«. These expert opinions were in considerable contrast to the forensic-psychiatric expertise Rüdin made on Count von Arco-Valley, who had shot the Bavarian Minister President Eisner in 1919: In Arco-Valley »no grounds for mental disease« could be found, but »only an immature personality tending towards impulsive acts« (this expertise by Rüdin from 1918/1919 is nowadays an unsettling example – and justifiably so – of how a psychiatric evaluation can unfortunately be defined by the personal conviction of a single expert).

Rüdin remained head of the genealogical-demographic department of the Research Institute until 1925; he then was offered the chair for psychiatry in Basle. He managed the Basle clinic for three years and after Kraepelin's death returned to the Research Institute in Munich in 1928. In Basle he was not able to carry out his plans for psychiatric-genetics studies as wished. In Munich, with the building of the Research Institute sponsored by the Rockefeller Foundation, he received the research

opportunity he had been looking for. In 1931 he became manager of the Research Institute and in 1933 was given the title and academic rights of an ordinary professor of psychiatry of the University of Munich.

In the following years he extended his department with considerable organizational talent. After 1933 he profited from the fact that his genetic-psychiatric research and ideas of racial hygiene were exactly what the new potentates were looking for. As early as 1933, Rüdin became head of the »Working Group for Racial Hygiene and Racial Politics« for the advisory council for »Racial and Population Politics« to the Reichs-Minister of the Interior, became assessor at the Court for Genetic Health and thus became more and more involved in the calamitous developments of the national-socialistic regime. The genealogical-demographic department of the German Psychiatric Research Institute was subsidized directly by funds from the Reich's Chancellor.

Immediately after the end of the Second World War the Swiss authorities withdrew Rüdin's citizenship. In autumn 1945 he was dismissed from office by the American Military Government and interned. Within the denazification project he was considered to be amongst the »less guilty« and after probation he was classified as »follower«. Rüdin died in Munich on October 22, 1952.

The opening of the German Research Institute had been so much work for Kraepelin in 1917/1918 that the problems at the clinic had second priority. When Rüdin left the clinic in 1917 to take over the genealogical-demographic department at the Research Institute, the job of senior consultant remained unoccupied for the time being. In 1919 G. Stertz became senior consultant at the clinic (▶ Chapter 10); and when Stertz was appointed to Marburg two years later, E. Kahn took his place. Kahn managed the clinic after Kraepelin's retirement and did so provisionally until O. Bumke took over (▶ Chapter 8).

Eugen Kahn (1887–1973) (◻ Fig. 7.20) has quite wrongly been forgotten in Germany; even in America only a few remember him, although he played an outstanding role during the thirties when he became Chairman of the Department of Psychiatry at Yale (1930).

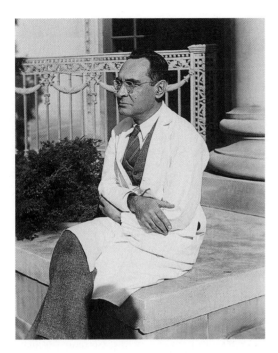

Fig. 7.20. Eugen Kahn (1887–1973) (ca. 1937)

Eugen Kahn was born on May 20, 1887, in Stuttgart, where he went to school. He studied medicine in Heidelberg, Berlin and Munich. After graduating in 1911, he worked as a medical trainee at the Psychiatric Clinic in Munich and in 1912 he became assistant to Kraepelin. He remained at the clinic as co-worker for 18 years until he was appointed to Yale.

Kahn became senior consultant in 1921 and was provisional director from 1922 until 1924 on Kraepelin's retirement. Kahn's work to become qualified as a postdoctoral lecturer was supervised by Kraepelin (and Rüdin); he habilitated with a thesis on the topic »Contribution to the genetics of schizophrenics and schizoid personalities with particular consideration of the children of married schizophrenic couples«. When Bumke took over the clinic in 1924 and brought his senior consultant with him from Leipzig, A. Bostroem (1886–1944), Kahn remained senior consultant together with Boestroem and Bumke. In 1927 he was appointed extraordinary professor.

Kraepelin entrusted Kahn with difficult tasks – for example with the forensic expertise on the leader of the Munich council republic, i.e. of Ernst Toller, Erich Mühsam and Rudolf Eglhofer, who became known in Munich as commander of the »Red Army«. Kraepelin and Rüdin worked together with Kahn on these expertises. This work formed the beginning of Kahn's interest in problems of psychopathy. Although the starting point of Kahn's work is problematic nowadays, his contribution to the teaching of psychopathy in Bumke's »Handbook of Mental Diseases« shows Kahn to be a profound scientist who 70 years ago worked on an otherwise neglected psychiatric problem in a trend-setting manner.

In 1930 Kahn joined Yale University and as clinician laid down the foundations for its fame in the field of »Social Psychiatry«.

Through his appointment to Yale, Kahn, son of a Jewish mother, avoided having to emigrate.

In 1946 Kahn left his position as Professor and Chairman of the »Department of Psychiatry and Mental Hygiene« at Yale, New Haven, and remained in America, never to return to Germany. He worked at the »New Haven Hospital«; from 1949–1951 he travelled in Europe, staying mainly in Switzerland. He then returned to America and became Professor of Psychiatry at the »Baylor University College of Medicine« in Houston, Texas. At the age of 74 he was still working as a psychiatric consultant at the »Veterans Administration Hospital« in Houston.

Eugen Kahn died at the age of 85 in Houston in January 1973.

Eugen Kahn was a very productive and original scientist; in particular, he was interested in the psychopathological form of psychoses and personality disorders. During his time in Munich, together with Rüdin, he developed a remarkable concept on the genetics of schizophrenic psychoses. Kahn differentiated between the schizoid reaction type as a trait, which he considered to be dominantly inheritable, and a recessively inheritable disposition to litigious psychoses. In his opinion, schizophrenic psychoses were manifested when the two genetic dispositions met.

Kahn had an especially good reputation as academic teacher. He gave lectures with topics far beyond the usual psychiatric ones, often dealing with philosophical and phenomenological problems.

Eugen Kahn's special service to the Munich clinic was that he managed it with great commitment and responsibility toward the clinic staff during difficult times after Kraepelin's retirement. The clinic staff considered him to be a particularly caring and conscientious »clinic boss«.

Apart from Kraepelin, his senior consultants (Alzheimer, Rüdin, Stertz and Kahn) and the department heads (see below), the scientific assistants also made their contribution to the clinic's good reputation. The unpaid scientific assistants, who could research freely, were not only Alzheimer and Rüdin, but later also F. Plaut and M. Isserlin.

Felix Plaut (1877–1940) was born in Kassel (◘ Fig. 7.21) and is rightfully known nowadays as one of the pioneers of modern neuroimmunology. Plaut joined Kraepelin at the Munich clinic in 1904. He studied medicine in Geneva, Berlin and Munich. In Munich he passed the medical exams and graduated in 1902 with a thesis »On cryptogenetic septic-uraemia«. He was assistant at the Berlin hospital »Am Urban« and co-worker at the Robert-Koch-Institute, headed by P. Ehrlich. In Berlin, together with A. Wassermann, he began serological studies of liquor cerebrospinalis from

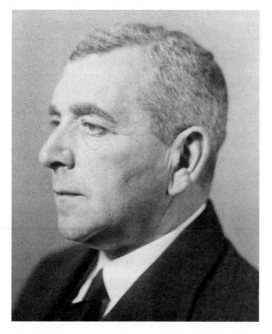

◘ **Fig. 7.21.** Felix Plaut (1877–1940)

patients with neurosyphilis. In 1904 he moved to Munich. To begin with, he worked on subjects Kraepelin had pointed out to him, e.g. experimental studies of the effect of long, warm baths; psychological studies of accident victims. But he soon returned to his serological studies on neurosyphilis and supplemented them with clinical studies. As scientific assistant Plaut was granted holidays to research in Wassermann's laboratory in Berlin. Later, Plaut and his co-workers carried out animal experiments on the pathogenesis and therapy of neurosyphilis.

For over 30 years the immunology of neurosyphilis remained Plaut's main research topic. He published almost 100 scientific papers on the subject and became internationally known. He was the first person to use animal experiments and clinical studies to prove, that an autochthon production of antibodies takes place in the brain. In 1909 he became postdoctoral lecturer.

With the founding of the German Psychiatric Research Institute Plaut became head of the serological laboratory; his serological department remained at the clinic until the building of the Research Institute was complete.

In 1925 Plaut accompanied Kraepelin on a trip to America, which had been organized by James Loeb (▶ Chapter 8), for Kraepelin to present his plans for a psychiatric research institute to the Rockefeller Foundation in New York. It was hoped that the Rockefeller Foundation would financially support Kraepelin's plans. The aim was achieved and the Rockefeller Foundation enabled the construction of the Research Institute's own building. Plaut's studies were also generously supported by the Rockefeller Foundation. After Kraepelin's death both F. Plaut and W. Spielmeyer managed the German Research Institute.

Being Jewish, it became difficult for Plaut to live in Germany after 1933. In 1933 Max Planck stepped in personally to avert Plaut's dismissal, but in October 1935 Plaut received a letter from Rüdin, who had become director of the Research Institute in the meantime, suspending him from duty.

Plaut knew England from his teaching and research sojourns there; he also had numerous personal and profession acquaintants there and in 1936 he emigrated to Epsom. He received further support from the Rockefeller Foundation for his research work and continued his studies on neurosyphilis and malaria therapy. Personally, he never got over his forced emigration and the loss of his prominent position at the German Research Institute. Plaut was embittered and disappointed and his impending internment as a German emigrant led him to commit suicide on June 27, 1940.

As well as Alzheimer, Plaut and Rüdin, Max Isserlin was also a member of the small group of »scientific assistants« gathered around Kraepelin, who were unpaid, but free from clinical routine work to do their own research.

Max Isserlin (1879–1941) (■ Fig. 7.22) came from a Jewish, East Prussian family and studied in Koenigsberg. As a young student of medicine he had been particularly interested in philosophy; aged 21, he wrote an essay on »Helmholtz as philosopher«. After the medical exams and graduation in Koenigsberg he turned to psychiatry. He worked at the university clinics of Giessen and Heidelberg for a short time, and on recovering from tuberculosis he joined the Munich clinic in 1906. As Isserlin had already worked on association tests in Giessen and Heidelberg, he became a member of

the psychological department and thus belonged to Kraepelin's inner circle of workers. Kraepelin suggested that he should work in the field of work psychology, of tiredness and experimental studies on simple voluntary movements. Isserlin soon became one of Kraepelin's most important co-workers. In 1910 he received his postdoctoral lecturer qualification for an experimental study on the »Analysis of simple movement processes (finger movements) in the mentally ill«.

Isserlin was professionally an all-rounder and was always open for new ideas. Following up on his own studies on association tests, he was intensely involved with the work of C.G. Jung. In this manner he came into contact with psychoanalysis. Through the publications of S. Freud, C.G. Jung and other psychoanalysts he received impulses for his own ideas and studies. Although Isserlin initially considered psychoanalysis to be plausible and inspiring, he soon became critical of the speculative nature of psychoanalytical theories. He criticized the psychoanalytical »art of interpretation« and complained about the – in his opinion – unscientific basis of psychoanalysis. Isserlin always tried to be fair to psychoanalysis since it had given him »numerous psychological stimuli«. Finally Isserlin decided that psychoanalysis was a »philosophy of life«, which has led to a »confusion of facts« and which wrongfully maintains to have solved psychological problems scientifically and empirically. Isserlin referred to C. G. Jung's opinions as »complex mythology«.

It was obvious that the situation would lead to conflicts between both sides acrimoniously. Jung complained to Freud that an assistant of Kraepelin had »killed« him with his arguments. Freud was initially more conciliatory, but soon regarded Isserlin's comments to be »shots from the enemy camp« and arguments from a man »from the blackest clique in Munich«. The climax of the conflict came in 1910 when C.G. Jung had Isserlin officially expelled from the Congress of the Psychoanalytical Association in Nuremberg.

Isserlin continued with experimental psychological studies after habilitating in 1910. He picked up on Kraepelin's old studies on the effects of small doses of alcohol. He also edited »omnibus reports« on experimental psychological and psychopathol-

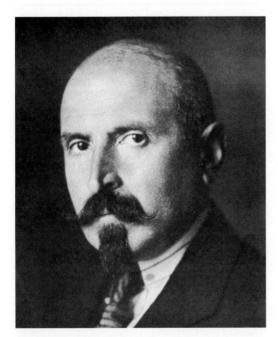

■ Fig. 7.22. Max Isserlin (1879–1941)

ogy. As postdoctoral lecturer Isserlin was entrusted by Kraepelin with the lectures on »Experimental Psychology«, which had been Kraepelin's own special, personal concern since his time in Dorpat.

Hans Gudden got Isserlin involved in psychiatric juvenile care; problems of medical pedagogy and the psychopathology of infancy later became areas of particular interest to Isserlin (see below).

At the outbreak of the First World War Isserlin's professional career turned into another new direction. In 1915 Isserlin was drafted and became staff doctor of the »department for nervous disorders« at a military hospital in Munich. In 1916 the department was turned into a department for brain injuries. In this situation during and after the First World War Isserlin was committed to the treatment of »mentally and nervously ill soldiers«. He turned the military hospital's ward into a model ward for the treatment and rehabilitation of patients with brain injuries and set up a school for teachers, doctors and later psychologists dealing with soldiers suffering from brain injuries.

Although Isserlin's clinical-practical duties during the war were manifold, he continued his scientific work during this period. He followed up on his research into apraxia and apthasia with which he had started his scientific career and introduced systematic examination method for patients with brain injuries. At the end of the war Isserlin did not return to the Psychiatric Clinic, but continued to dedicate his work to former war soldiers with brain injuries.

At the end of the First World War the military hospital was dissolved and consequently Isserlin's work was endangered. Isserlin managed to ensure that the department for brain injuries was kept, integrated into the hospital in Schwabing (Schwabinger Krankenhaus) and known as the »Supply Hospital For War Victims With Brain Injuries«. Isserlin became head of this department.

Apart from Isserlin's efforts to keep the Schwabing hospital as a supply hospital for patients with brain injuries during the years following the war, there were various initiatives in Munich to improve the situation of war victims. The American industrialist, A. Heckscher, launched a foundation for nervously ill war victims. In 1922 on Heckscher's initiative a further clinical department (Heckscher's Research Institute for Nervous Diseases) was set up at the Hospital Rechts der Isar (on the right bank of the river Isar) and the neurologist, G. von Malaisé (1875–1923), became director. In the same year with support from the pension office Isserlin bought a building in Schwabing, at Parzivalplatz to house the association he had founded, »Association for the Care of Seriously Injured War Veterans«. When von Malaisé suddenly died in 1923, Isserlin tried to coordinate all efforts in Munich to improve the care of brain injured patients and through this work came into contact with A. Heckscher. With support from Heckscher Isserlin's proposal in 1925 to set up the »Heckscher Research Institute for Nervous Diseases and War Victims with Brain Injuries« in Schwabing on Tristan-Street (Tristanstrasse) came to be. Isserlin became director of the institute and set up a clinical treatment institution for patients with brain injuries as well as an annexed home and workshops.

When Heckscher first visited Munich in 1927, Isserlin persuaded him to set up a similar institution for children. Heckscher established a similar foundation, which supported the new building of the »Children's Department of the Heckscher Research Institute for Nervous Diseases« in 1929. As of 1930 the institution also had its own »Orthopedagogy Outreach Clinic«, which was run together with the Pediatric Clinic of the University at Hauner's Pediatric Hospital.

During the twenties Isserlin's work was pioneering in two areas: Based on his initiatives, the clinics for brain injuries and the Clinic for Child Psychiatry were established in Munich!

After the national socialists came to power, Isserlin was dismissed from the position of director of the clinic for brain injuries in the summer of 1933. Being of Jewish origin, he had to hand over his responsibility for the Heckscher Clinic in 1938, and also for for the connecting school. In 1938 Isserlin and his family emigrated to England; on February 4, 1941 he died in Sheffield.

In 1904 Kraepelin had set up several **laboratories** (departments) for the »auxiliary sciences«. The idea was for young assistants to be schooled by advanced researchers on scientific subjects.

When Kraepelin and Alzheimer asked themselves prior to the opening of the clinic which laboratories should be established, they decided that

- A **Laboratory for Experimental Psychology**
- A **Laboratory for Neuropathology** (the »microscopy laboratory«) and
- A **Laboratory for Chemistry**
  were necessary.

Later, they added

- A **Serological Laboratory**
- A **Genealogical Demographic Laboratory** and
- A large **archive** for case histories

The **Laboratory for Experimental Psychology** was Kraepelin's own working area. Many young clinic assistants (incl. M. Isserlin) worked here. Kraepelin published the results of his studies in the Laboratory for Psychology in the eight-volume »Psychological Studies« (1896–1914) (◘ Fig. 7.23).

Under the guidance of Alzheimer many scientists from home and abroad, who later made a name for themselves (see above), worked in the **Laboratory for Neuropathology**. When it seemed as though the leading role of neuropathological research at the Munich clinic would be endangered by Alzheimer's resignation in 1912, Kraepelin, supported by Alzheimer, employed a young neuropathologist: Walter Spielmeyer came to Munich in 1912 and took over management of the laboratory in 1913 (◘ Fig. 7.24), before Alzheimer left Munich to take over the hospital in Breslau.

Walter Spielmeyer (1879–1935) had been interested in neuropathology since his student days in Greifswald and Halle. During his last years of study he worked in the neuro-anatomical laboratory of the Clinic for Nervous Diseases in Halle, headed by E. Hitzig (1838–1907); in 1902 he graduated with Hitzig's guidance with a »Contribution to the knowledge on encephalitis«. He then spent 10 years in Freiburg as assistant to Alfred E. Hoche (1865–1943), Kraepelin's great opponent. Spielmeyer became known during his Freiburg days due to his numerous, informative studies on neuro-histopathology. In 1906 he habilitated with a study on the topic »Clinical and anatomical studies on a special type of familial amaurotic idiocy«. Because

Spielmeyer was mainly interested in neuro-histology, once he had received his doctoral lecturer qualifications, he considered leaving Freiburg for Munich to work with Alzheimer. In 1912 Kraepelin summoned him to Munich! Spielmeyer was only able to work with Alzheimer for a couple of months. When Alzheimer left Munich in 1913, Kraepelin gave Spielmeyer responsibility for the laboratory, which continued to enjoy an excellent reputation. Scientists from all over the world came to Munich to work with Spielmeyer.

During the First World War Spielmeyer was responsible for the department for nervous diseases at the Munich military hospital. This gave him the opportunity to prove himself as an excellent clinician and consequently in 1917 the Heidelberg medical faculty offered him to take over the chair for psychiatry from F. Nissl, as well as the psychiatric clinic! (Nissl had decided to give up the chair for psychiatry in Heidelberg and to move to Munich to the newly founded« German Psychiatric Research Institute and to take over the histopathological department there.) Kraepelin was worried that his long time plan »to bring Nissl and Spielmeyer together to work« would be thwarted by these developments. Spielmeyer was supposed to take over a second histopathological department at the Research Institute in Munich.

Kraepelin was relieved when Spielmeyer turned down the offer from Heidelberg and was prepared to stay in Munich for the time being. Hence the future of neuro-morphology at the Research Institute finally seems to be secured.

However, two deaths overcast these promising developments: In August 1918 Korbinian Brodmann (born 1868) died. He had joined the Research Institute as head of the topographic-anatomical department. A year later, in August 1919 Franz Nissl died all of a sudden. At Kraepelin's suggestion the three originally planned neuro-morphological departments were combined into one and headed by Spielmeyer. Spielmeyer bore the entire responsibility (after having formally left the Munich clinic in 1917 on the founding of the Research Institute) and also headed the neuropathological laboratory at the clinic with combined staff. This ruling remained until Bumke came into office in 1924 (► Chapter 9).

7

PSYCHOLOGISCHE ARBEITEN

HERAUSGEGEBEN

VON

EMIL KRAEPELIN
PROFESSOR IN MÜNCHEN

FÜNFTER BAND

MIT 51 FIGUREN IM TEXT UND 4 TAFELN

LEIPZIG
VERLAG VON WILHELM ENGELMANN
1910

◻ Fig. 7.23. Fifth volume of the eight-volume series of E. Kraepelin's psychological study results: »Psychological Studies«

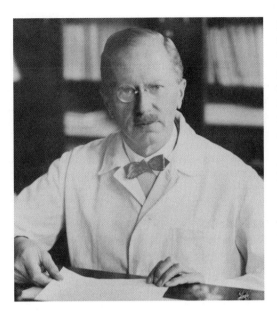

■ **Fig. 7.24.** Walter Spielmeyer (1879–1935)

At this point Spielmeyer gave up his double function, although he remained with his staff in rooms at the clinic until 1928 (► Chapter 9).

After Kraepelin's death in 1926, together with Plaut, he became director of the German Research Institute and kept this office until 1931, when E. Rüdin became his successor.

W. Spielmeyer died in Munich on February 6, 1935.

The **Laboratory for Chemistry** was headed by **Erwin Rohde** during the first year after the clinic's opening. Rohde had already worked in Heidelberg with Kraepelin. In 1908 he left the Munich clinic, returned to Heidelberg and habilitated in pharmacology. Following Rohde's departure, one of Alzheimer's co-workers headed the Laboratory for Chemistry, a Swiss, **Fritz Lotmar**, for a short period of time (1908/09); then Rudolf Allers took over.

The Austrian, Rudolf Allers (1883–1963), worked at a research laboratory in Vienna following his studies and then for Alfred Pick (1851–1924) at the Psychiatric Clinic of the German University in Prague. Allers' publications on »Metabolic pathological studies of psychoses« and »Contributions on the chemistry of the senile brain«, which he published at the Munich clinic as of 1909, proved to be pioneering studies in the field of biochemical

psychiatry developing since the beginning of the century. In 1910 Kraepelin offered him a position at the Munich hospital. In 1912 Allers was given a grant by the Bavarian Academy of Sciences for his metabolic studies on the mentally ill. In 1913 he received his doctoral lecturer qualification with a »Study on the metabolism of progressive paralysis«.

The many-facetted Allers was a particularly productive scientist. As assistant lecturer he lectured on »General Psychopathology«. As member of the Austrian army he was drafted during the First World War. After the war Kraepelin offered him to return to Munich to take over the Chemical Laboratory, not at the clinic, but at the German Research Institute. Allers accepted, but returned to Vienna a year later in 1919. In Vienna he worked for a short period at the Physiological Institute, but then left the university. He opened a practise in Vienna, but in order to belong to the university once again, he went through a second doctoral lecturer process in 1927 and held lectures. In 1938 he emigrated to America, lived in Washington and was professor for philosophy and psychology at the Georgetown University. Allers visited Austria again after the war, although he did not return to Europe for good and remained in America. He died near Washington aged 80 years.

The Chemical Laboratory of the clinic had been headed by Otto Wuth (1885–1945) before Allers moved to the Research Institute to head the Chemical Laboratory

Wuth studied and graduated in Munich before the war and was assistant to Friedrich von Müller for 4 years at the Clinic for Internal Medicine. When Wuth took over the Chemical Laboratory of the Psychiatric Clinic after the war, he followed up on research topics which Allers had been working on at the clinic until the outbreak of war. Wuth habilitated in 1921 with »Studies on physical disorders of the mentally ill«.

After Kraepelin's retirement Wuth remained with Bumke as head of the Chemical Laboratory until 1925, then went to the John Hopkins Hospital in Baltimore, USA, for 3 years. He returned in 1928 and worked in Switzerland at Binswanger's Rehabilitation Institution Bellevue in Kreuzlingen until 1935.

During his stays abroad he remained member of the Munich Medical Faculty. When he returned to Germany in 1935 he went through the doctoral lecturer qualification process on a different subject. He joined the German army as sanitary officer and did research projects for the War Department. He died in Berlin around 1945.

Despite adverse conditions (repeated change in department management during the first years; disturbed work after outbreak of the First World War) the international reputation of the Chemical Laboratory grew. Unfortunately, the Chemical Laboratory was sorely neglected for several years after Wuth left. Later attempts were made to resurrect the laboratory to its former glory of Kraepelin's days (▶ Chapters 9–11); but continual biochemical psychiatric fundamental research never developed properly at the Munich clinic. It was not until the establishment of the Neurochemical Department in 1971 that things changed (▶ Chapter 13).

The Serological Laboratory, which had been built on Plaut's advice, went through a similar development. When Plaut – like Spielmeyer – resigned formally from the clinic to join the Research Institute at its opening, he did in fact keep rooms at the clinic until 1928, but with the move to the Research Institute's new building in Schwabing the serological immunological research at the clinic came to an end and was not reinstated until the fifties by K. Kolle (▶ Chapter 11).

The destinies of the Chemical and Serological Laboratories illustrate how the founding of the Research Institute caused a much more dramatic break for the clinic than it seemed from the outside.

In April 1918 the German Research Institute started work in the rooms of the clinic. At this time Spielmeyer, Plaut and Rüdin no longer belonged to the clinic, but were allowed to use rooms there for their work. In 1922 the Department for Experimental Psychology, the Genealogical Demographic Department and the archive moved out of the clinic and were located in a building on Bavariaring, which J. Loeb financed (▶ Chapter 8). An official residence for Kraepelin was also located in the building. Spielmeyer and Plaut moved out of the clinic with their work groups in 1928. Although it was advantageous for the clinic to have more room available in this way, the relocation of the German Research Institute's departments meant a reduction of scientific activity at the clinic (see above).

Literature

Grünthal, E. (1957): Eugen Kahn – zum 70. Geburtstag gewidmet. In: Claus, A., Grünthal, E., Heimann, H. et al (Ed): Beiträge zur Geschichte der Psychiatrie und Hirnanatomie. S. Karger-Verlag: Basle, New York, p. 5-9

Hoff, P. (1994): Emil Kraepelin und die Psychiatrie als klinische Wissenschaft. Springer-Verlag: Berlin, Heidelberg, New York

Jürgs, M. (1999): Alzheimer. List-Verlag, Munich

Kraepelin, E. (1988): Lebenserinnerungen, Ed.: Hippius, H., Peters, G., Ploog, D. Springer-Verlag: Berlin, Heidelberg, New York

Kraepelin, E.: Edition Emil Kraepelin. Ed.: Weber, M.M., Holsboer, F., Hoff, P., Ploog, D., Hippius, H.

Vol. 1 (2000): Persönliche Selbstzeugnisse, Ed.: Burgmair, W., Engstrom, E.J., Weber, M.M.

Vol. 2 (2001): Kriminologische und forensische Schriften, Ed.: Burgmair, W., Engstrom, E.J., Hoff, P., Weber, M.M.

Vol. 3 (2002): Briefe 1 (1868–1886), Ed.: Burgmair, W., Engstrom, E.J., Weber, M.M.

Vol. 4 (2003): Kraepelin in Dorpat (1886–1891), Ed.: Burgmair, W., Engstrom, Hirschmüller, A., Weber, M.M. Belleville Verlag Michael Farin: Munich

Leonhardt, M. (2004): Mehrdimensionale Psychaitrie: Robert Gaupp, Ernst Kretschmer und die Tübinger psychaitrische Schule. In: Hippius, H. (Ed.): Universtätskolloquien zur Schizophrenie. Vol II, Steinkopff-Verlag: Darmstadt (in print)

Maurer, K., Maurer, U. (1998): Alzheimer. Piper-Verlage: Munich, Zurich

Pokorny, A.D. (1973): Eugen Kahr, 1887–1973. Am J Psychiat 130: 7; p. 822

Weber, M.M. (1993): Ernst Rüdin. Springer-Verlag: Berlin, Heidelberg, New York

8

The Idea and Planning of the German Psychiatric Research Institute

In Emil Kraepelin's extensive life's work one aspect must be particularly emphasized: The founding of the »German Psychiatric Research Institute«. In the 20th century this psychiatric research institute became an example for many countries in the world, how psychiatric research could be planned, organized and put into practise in one independent institution: »Aims and methods of psychiatric research« will be defined via the inclusion, integration and coordination of different (scientific) »auxiliary sciences« into clinical research.

Kraepelin received his first impulses for scientific work in early years; firstly from his (by 9 years) older brother, then as a student in Wurzburg of F. von Rinecker and H. Emminghaus, and in Munich from B. von Gudden and his Munich circle. The biggest influence on Kraepelin's later development and his trend-setting preoccupation with the construction of an institution, attached to a clinic, but with independent psychiatric research facilities, relates to Wilhelm Wundt (▶ Chapter 7).

Kraepelin read Wundt's »Lectures on the human and animal soul« in his student days; they aroused his interest in psychological problems and were crucial for his decision to become a »doctor for the insane«, as it seemed to be the only way for him to »combine psychological work with a career that pays the bills«. His interest in psychological matters continued whilst Kraepelin was working for B. Gudden, although the emphasis of Gudden's circle was mainly on neuromorphological problems. When Kraepelin left Munich in 1882 to work with P. Flechsig in Leipzig as an assistant at the newly opened psychiatric university clinic there, he did so, because he saw a chance to work in Wundt's laboratory as well as in the clinic. Soon after arriving in Leipzig, Kraepelin realized that he would not be able to combine the two: clinical duties with Flechsig and research work with Wundt. Kraepelin even considered giving up his career as clinical psychiatrist, in order to work solely in Wundt's laboratory for experimental psychology, but abandoned this plan as well and returned to Gudden in Munich. Once back in Munich, he realized that he would have to turn in a totally new direction if he were to achieve his plans for psychiatric research. He considered the restriction of scientific, clinical-psychiatric research to neuromorphological methods to be less promising and was convinced that greater progress could be made with Wundt's concept of experimental psychological research. Consequently, he left Gudden's work group to carry out scientific, clinical studies with psychiatric patients. The facilities at his new jobs (Leubus; Dresden) were extremely limited; first and foremost he had to take care of his clinical duties. All the same, he tried to work scientifically but there were no staff available for research and in Leubus and Dresden there were no students who could be involved in the work. As a result his wife, who he had married shortly after leaving the Munich Mental Asylum, assisted him with the experimental psychological studies. It was during this phase that Kraepelin deliberated, how psychiatric research could be organized and how clinical research could be combined with experimental psychological research.

When Kraepelin took over the Psychiatric Clinic and the professorship for psychiatry at the university of Dorpat, thus returning to a university, he had considerably greater research possibilities at his disposal. His inaugural lecture was entitled »The directions of psychiatric research«. In Dorpat Kraepelin could unfold his organizational talent which was much admired in later years. In spite of the most difficult external conditions he managed to turn the clinic into a much reputed research institution. Students were involved in broadly based experimental psychological studies which had been restarted; a new mechanical test system was developed with an engineer; many of the doctoral candidates were trained to carry out individual scientific work.

Once Kraepelin had demonstrated in Dorpat how psychiatric research could be done with modest means, he continued his efforts to improve and further develop psychiatric research in Heidelberg and especially later in Munich.

During his time in Heidelberg, Kraepelin preferred to employ co-workers who »had not only worked scientifically on clinical-psychiatric subjects, but also in other areas, or at least had the intention to do so«. All such co-workers were entrusted not only with scientific activity, but also with extensive clinical duties. In Munich Kraepelin went one step further: He »created the class of scientific assistants, which included researchers who could use the means available in the clinic for their research, but would not be paid«, and they would not be encumbered with routine clinical work.

A. Alzheimer was the first »Scientific Assistant, who could dispose of his time freely«. After Alzheimer, Rüdin, Plaut and Isserlin had a similar agreement with the clinic (▶ Chapter 7). By connecting the »scientific assistant« to the clinic, they could also, as was the case for Alzheimer and Rüdin, later become senior consultants at the clinic. Hence, at the beginning of the 20th century, a model was developed at the Munich University Clinic for future psychiatric research institutions where fundamental researchers and clinicians could work together closely within one organizational unit; the clinic director himself and the senior consultants were responsible for the coordination of the various sectors.

During the same period suggestions for improvements in psychiatric research facilities were being made in other places: In the kingdom of Prussia the provincial associations – the supporting organization of psychiatric care, of the »provincial asylums« – proposed to create an independent, psychiatric research institution. This recommendation was supported by a large number of »asylum psychiatrists«; their spokesman was F. Siemens (1849–1935). Siemens, who had been director of the newly built provincial asylum Lauenburg in Pomerania, managed to convince the board of the German Psychiatric Association in 1913 that an exposé on a »Psychiatric Research Institute« should be prepared on their behalf. Due to his excellent national and international reputation, Emil Kraepelin was entrusted with the exposé. The association's board hoped the recently founded »Kaiser-Wilhelm-Gesellschaft zur Förderung der Wissenschaften« (Kaiser Wilhlem's Society for the Promotion of the Sciences) would support the plan; the plan's aim was to build a psychiatric research institute in Berlin-Dahlem. When Kraepelin presented his paper on the subject in 1915 the First World War had broken out and the Kaiser-Wilhelm-Gesellschaft was no longer interested.

Despite the Kaiser-Wilhelm-Gesellschaft's refusal and the adverse war situation, Kraepelin pursued his plans.

Via the discussions in the bodies of the Kaiser-Wilhelm-Gesellschaft Gustav Krupp von Bohlen und Halbach had been informed of Kraepelin's ideas on the building of a psychiatric research institute (◻ Fig. 8.1), was interested and visited him in late autumn 1915 in Munich. Together they looked at the possibilities to realize the plans without the support of the Kaiser-Wilhelm-Gesellschaft. In the meantime Kraepelin had prepared his trend-setting plans for publication. This publication about »A Psychiatric Research Institute« was released shortly after G. Krupp von Bohlen und Halbach and Kraepelin's meeting, in November 1915 in the »Journal for Psychiatry and Neurology«.

Kraepelin proposed to annexe the planned research institute to the Munich Psychiatric Clinic. Together with G. Krupp he came to the correct conclusion that by doing so the project would cost considerably less, no new building would need to be constructed and the expenses for the building

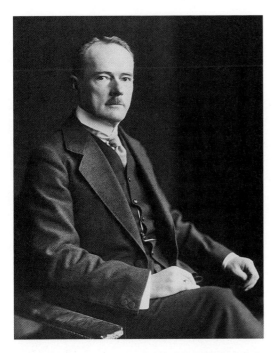

and running of the research institute would be considerably reduced.

G. Krupp assured his full support for the project, but suggested to wait until the end of the war before taking any further steps. Kraepelin and G. Krupp wrote to each other on the project continuously from December 1915 (■ Fig. 8.2) until 1925 (62 of these letters are in the psychiatric history collection of the Munich Clinic).

Shortly after the first meeting with Krupp, Kraepelin informed one of his patients about his plans and that they could only be realized after the war. The patient was James Loeb.

James Loeb (1867–1933, ■ Fig. 8.3) was born in New York as the son of Jewish parents. His family originated from the Palatinate; his father emigrated to America as a young man and became a very successful business man and banker. It was the explicit wish of his father that James Loeb studied economy and commercial law at Harvard from 1884 until 1888; he also used his 4 years at Harvard to study archaeology, which had particularly interested him since

his youth. In 1888 he joined the family company as banker and was apparently – like his father – very successful. In 1893 and then again in 1895 and 1897 he became mentally ill. As was later ascertained, he suffered from an affective disorder. In 1901 he resigned from the bank, in his own words due to a repeated »breakdown«. His considerable fortune enabled him to dedicate himself to archaeology and other interests in the arts. He acquired a collection of the ancient world, supported museums, founded – in remembrance of his mother – the American Institute of Musical Art which later became the Juilliard School of Music. In Athens he organized grants for young American archaeologists.

When Loeb became ill again in autumn 1903 and spring of 1905, he travelled to Europe, visited Sigmund Freud during a short stay in Vienna and finally became a patient of Emil Kraepelin in Munich.

Loeb lived in Germany as of 1905, mainly in Munich and in Murnau on Lake Staffel. Neither did he leave Germany on the outbreak of the First World War, but even stayed there when the United States joined the war in 1917. During this period Loeb suffered from a particularly strong and longer lasting nervous breakdown. (Medical notes on the course of illness are kept with the psychiatric history collection at the Munich Clinic.) At the end of the war Loeb's condition stabilized. He married the widow of a friend who had passed away, and continued to live in Munich and Murnau. He was a generous patron, who created the still famous »Loeb Classical Library« at Harvard University (translations of classical texts into English). For his scientific contributions to archaeology he received an honorary doctorate from Cambridge University. In Munich he was made honorary citizen of the university and given an honorary doctorate by the philosophical faculty.

All visitors to the collection of ancient art (Antikensammlung) in Munich will know »Loeb's Poseidon« and the other important objects from his excellent collection, exhibited in 14 glass cases, which he left to the State Museums of Bavaria.

Loeb died in Murnau on May 29, 1933, a couple of weeks after the death of his wife. Loeb had experienced the first months of national socialism. His death saved him from experiencing the disastrous developments which had started during his last months.

Post: Hügel Rheinprovinz.
Telegramme: Auf dem Hügel.

Auf dem Hügel
den 6. Dezember 1915.

Sehr verehrter Herr Professor,

Mit verbindlichstem Dank bestätige ich den
Empfang Ihres sehr gefälligen Schreibens vom 30. v.Mts.
nebst seiner Anlage, dem Nachtrage zu dem Plane eines
Forschungsinstitutes für Psychiatrie. Mit grossem In-
teresse habe ich von dem Inhalte beider Schriftstücke
Kenntnis genommen und durch denselben mich in meiner
Annahme bestärkt gesehen, dass durch die Verbindung
eines Forschungsinstitutes mit einer bestehenden Klinik
einem selbständigen, alle einschlägigen Gebiete umfas-
senden Forschungsinstitut in praktischer Weise vorge-
baut werden könnte. Ich werde die Angelegenheit im
Auge behalten und sehen, wie ich meinerseits zu einer
Ausführung Ihres wohldurchdachten Planes in ruhigeren
Zeiten beitragen kann.

Heute möchte ich die Gelegenheit be-
nutzen, Ihnen für die liebenswürdige und weitgehende
Auskunft, die Sie mir in unserer neulichen mündlichen
Unterhaltung zu erteilen die Güte hatten, erneut
meinen aufrichtigen Dank zum Ausdruck zu bringen.

In vorzüglichster Hochachtung verbleibe
ich, sehr verehrter Herr Professor,

Ihr ganz ergebener

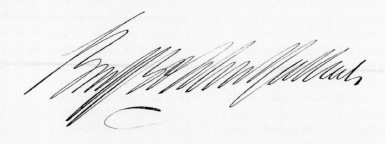

◨ **Fig. 8.2** Letter from G. Krupp to E. Kraepelin on December 6, 1915

Dear Professor

I herewith confirm receipt of your most agreeable letter of 30th of the month, together with enclosure, the appendix to the plan of a psychiatric research institute. I acknowledge my great interest in the content of both and see my assumption confirmed that by combining a research institute with an existing clinic, an independent research institute, covering all the necessary areas could be set up in a most practical manner. I will bear this matter in mind and see what I can do for my part to assist you and your well thought out plan in a calmer period.

Today, I would like to take the opportunity to once again thank you for the detailed information, which you kindly gave me in person on the occasion of our recent meeting.

I remain most respectfully yours, your most loyal

◻ **Fig. 8.2** *Continued*

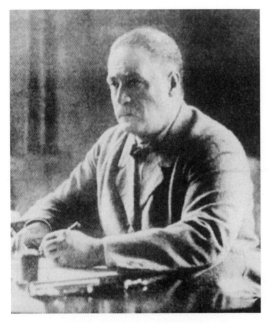

◻ **Fig. 8.3.** James Loeb (1867–1933)

After a couple of meetings Loeb informed Kraepelin on January 6, 1916, that he would be prepared to donate 500,000.- Goldmarks for the institute »if the same amount be donated by another party and the institute be built in Munich«. Kraepelin informed G. Krupp von Bohlen und Halbach immediately and convinced him that it would be detrimental to the plan to wait until the war was over. G. Krupp von Bohlen und Halbach assured his support for the plan to be put into being as quickly as possible and made sure that a further half a million Marks be given. At the suggestion of Emil Fischer (chemist and winner of the Nobel Prize 1902), the German Chemical Industry agreed to give 200,000.- Marks (later increased to 300,000,- Marks); and the Kaiser-Wilhelm-Gesellschaft also agreed to give an annual subsidy of 5,000.- Marks for the duration of 5 years.

The money was now available but the foundation's sponsor had not been determined. Neither was it clear how the Research Institute would be accommodated in the University Clinic. Nor had the problem been solved of embedding the research institute in the Munich clinic or its scope within the clinic (◻ Fig. 8.4).

Supported by the Bavarian Ministry for Science and Art, the following solution was found: The entire donation would be handed to King Ludwig the Third (◻ Fig. 8.5) with the request to mandate the establishing of the Psychiatric Research Institute, affiliated to the university. The foundation was set up on February 13, 1917, (◻ Fig. 8.6) by King Ludwig the Third, according to Bavarian law. At the beginning of 1917, the entire foundation capital had grown to 1,700,000.- Marks. On June 10, 1917, the first public meeting of the Research Institute took place in the presence of Ludwig the Third. Kraepelin gave a lecture on »A Hundred Years of Psychiatry«.

For the Research Institute to be able to start work as soon as possible, the use of the clinic rooms and the laboratories was set down in a precise contract. As Kraepelin was director of both the Psychi-

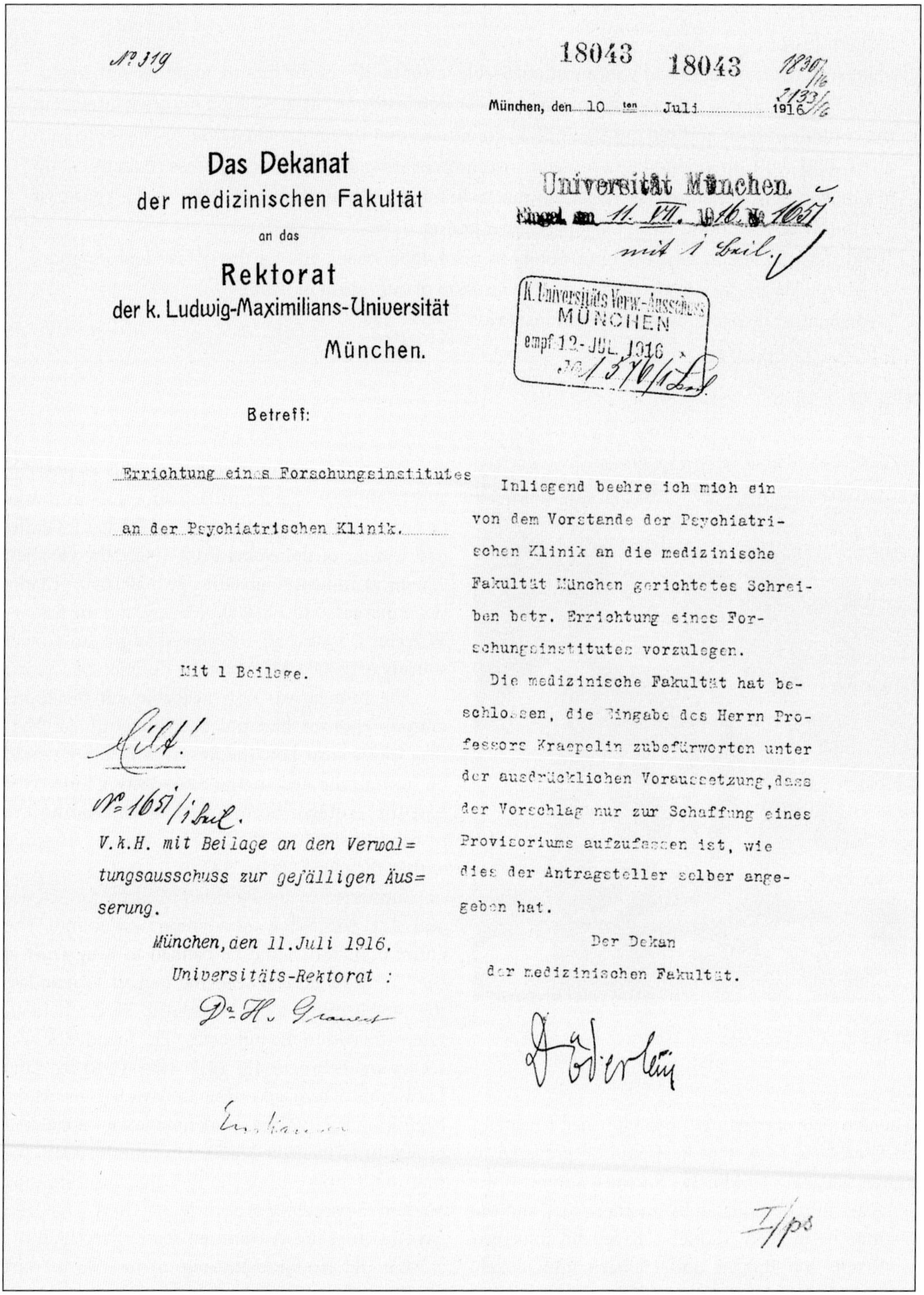

№ 319

18043 18043 1830/16 2133/16

München, den 10 ten Juli 1916

Das Dekanat
der medizinischen Fakultät
an das
Rektorat
der k. Ludwig-Maximilians-Universität
München.

Universität München.
Eingel. am 11. VII. 1916. № 1651
mit 1 Beil.

K. Universitäts Verw.-Ausschuss
MÜNCHEN
empf. 12. JUL. 1916
№ 1576/1 Beil.

Betreff:

Errichtung eines Forschungsinstitutes an der Psychiatrischen Klinik.

Inliegend beehre ich mich ein von dem Vorstande der Psychiatrischen Klinik an die medizinische Fakultät München gerichtetes Schreiben betr. Errichtung eines Forschungsinstitutes vorzulegen.

Die medizinische Fakultät hat beschlossen, die Eingabe des Herrn Professors Kraepelin zubefürworten unter der ausdrücklichen Voraussetzung, dass der Vorschlag nur zur Schaffung eines Provisoriums aufzufassen ist, wie dies der Antragsteller selber angegeben hat.

Der Dekan
der medizinischen Fakultät.
Döderlein

Mit 1 Beilage.

Eilt!

№ 1651/1 Beil.

V.k.H. mit Beilage an den Verwaltungsausschuss zur gefälligen Äusserung.

München, den 11. Juli 1916.
Universitäts-Rektorat:
Dr. H. Grauert

I/ps

Fig. 8.4. Permission from the University to set-up a research institute at the Psychiatric Klinik Munich, dated July 10, 1916 (from the university archives, signed: Sen 30711)

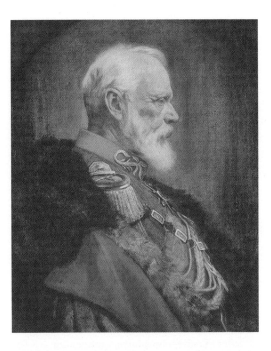

Fig. 8.5. Portrait of King Ludwig the Third

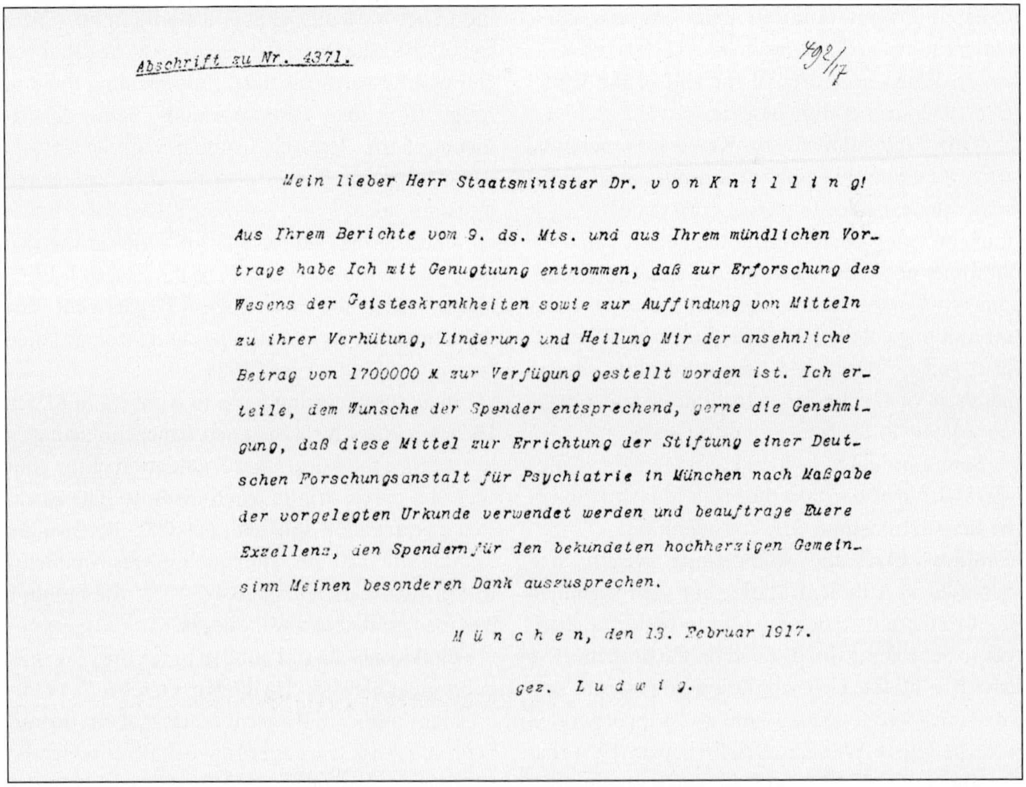

Abschrift zu Nr. 4371.

Mein lieber Herr Staatsminister Dr. v o n K n i l l i n g!

Aus Ihrem Berichte vom 9. ds. Mts. und aus Ihrem mündlichen Vor-
trage habe Ich mit Genugtuung entnommen, daß zur Erforschung des
Wesens der Geisteskrankheiten sowie zur Auffindung von Mitteln
zu ihrer Verhütung, Linderung und Heilung Mir der ansehnliche
Betrag von 1700000 X zur Verfügung gestellt worden ist. Ich er-
teile, dem Wunsche der Spender entsprechend, gerne die Genehmigung, daß diese Mittel zur Errichtung der Stiftung einer Deutschen Forschungsanstalt für Psychiatrie in München nach Maßgabe
der vorgelegten Urkunde verwendet werden und beauftrage Euere
Exzellenz, den Spendern für den bekundeten hochherzigen Gemein-
sinn Meinen besonderen Dank auszusprechen.

M ü n c h e n, den 13. Februar 1917.

gez. L u d w i g.

Fig. 8.6. Permission from King Ludwig the Third to set-up a German Psychiatric Research Institute in Munich, dated February 13, 1917 (from the university archives, signed Sen 307/1)

atric Clinic and the new Research Institute, it was possible to come to terms. It was assumed that the set-up was only for the time being, as Kraepelin had concluded a contract with the City of Munich in May 1917, which assured that the German Research Institute would be able to build its own institute on a piece of land with a building lease. It was hoped to fulfil these plans within a couple of years.

On April 1, 1918, the Research Institute began work in the clinic rooms. However, it took 10 years until June 1928 before the German Research Institute, which in the meantime had been incorporated into the Kaiser-Wilhelm-Gesellschaft, could move into its own building financially supported by the Rockefeller Foundation.

As long as Kraepelin was clinic director, the provisional arrangements for the German Research Institute to be located in rooms of the clinic caused relatively few problems. But problems did exist during this period because Kraepelin dedicated himself energetically to the development of the German Research Institute and left many pressing clinic matters to his senior consultants (G. Stertz and E. Kahn). When he retired at the end of the winter term 1922, further difficulties arose.

The negotiations with Kraepelin's potential successors were not only drawn out, because the candidates expected to receive exact details of their future working conditions at the clinic. The open questions not only related to the space problems; some co-workers of the Germany Research Institute (amongst others W. Spielmeyer, E. Rüdin, F. Plaut and O. Wuth) had jobs at the clinic, but as members of the Research Institute would not be subordinate to the future clinic director.

Solutions had to be found to protect the clinic's interests, but also to take the precarious situation of the Research Institute into consideration.

Since 1917 the foundation's wealth had increased to 3 million Marks, but then dwindled due to inflation; hence the idea to build the institute in Schwabing disappeared on the horizon. The existence of the German Research Institute was threatened and it was not until it was incorporated into the Kaiser-Wilhelm-Gesellschaft in 1924 that the situation seemed secure. As long as it remained unclear which plans the new clinic director would have, the situation at the clinic remained difficult.

Under the deanship of F. Sauerbruch, the medical faculty decided on a successor for Kraepelin in 1922. Bonhoeffer was offered the job at the beginning of the summer term in 1922. He negotiated and replied fast and in detail, but quickly turned the offer down and the medical faculty applied to the ministry in July 1922 to be able to offer the position to O. Bumke. On receiving the offer, Bumke presented his detailed plans in September 1922 and made it clear, to which conditions he would be prepared to accept the offer. Initially the problems seemed unsolvable. As both sides were conciliatory and the situation favourable, Bumke finally accepted the offer and took over the clinic on April 1, 1924.

In October 1922 the City of Munich gave the German Research Institute the right to set up a small psychiatric admission department at the Schwabing Hospital (managed by J. Lange, 1891–1938) which should later serve as clinical department of the Research Institute.

James Loeb set up a further foundation (»Solomon Loeb – Memorial Foundation«) in New York to pay the salaries of the department heads at the German Research Institute, thus enabling them to resign from their clinic positions. Some departments of the Research Institute were accommodated in private houses near the clinic sponsored by James Loeb. James Loeb organized for a house on »Bavariaring« (◻ Fig. 8.7) to be put at the disposal of the Clinical Archive of the Research Institute as well as the Psychological Department. The departments of neuropathology and serology could remain at the clinic until 1928.

In addition, during a trip to America in March 1925, organized by James Loeb, Kraepelin managed to convince the Rockefeller Foundation of the concept of a psychiatric research institute: The Rockefeller Foundation donated 1,000,000.- Reichsmark to build the institute. The building was completed within two years: On June 13, 1928, the building was inaugurated and work began.

Emil Kraepelin did not live to see the crowning of his great lifework. He died on October 7, 1926.

Many stories and anecdotes exist about the difficult and tense years after Kraepelin's retirement in 1922 and before Bumke took up office in 1924.

Bumke wrote rather acrimoniously, but also full of admiration, that »nothing happened with-

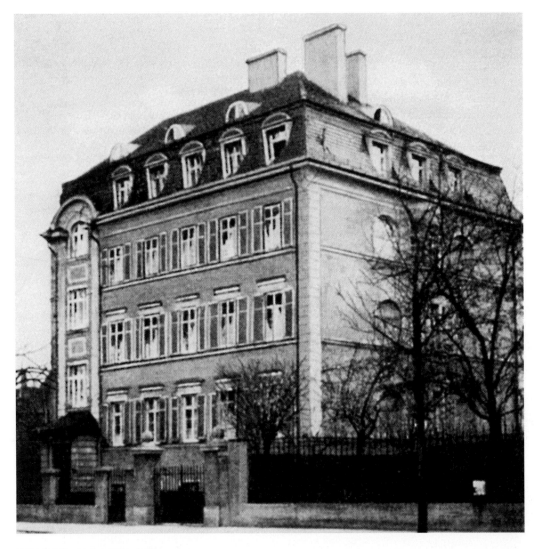

■ **Fig. 8.7.** Bavariaring 46 (ca. 1930)

out a fight«. »The weapons used varied; Kraepelin was used to a cudgel and I was used to the floret. Finally we came to an agreement and when I took over the clinic on April 1, 1924, it worked out quite well. Kraepelin was a person worth grappling with and anyway we were all building our work on his lifework.«

Admittedly, the two great psychiatrists both did everything in their power to realize their plans and ideas and whilst doing so, it was obvious that fric-

tion would occur. Each one of them made concessions – especially Bumke, who realized that if he reacted in a totally unyielding manner, he would endanger the existence of the Research Institute. On the other hand, he did not wish to limit the possibilities of the clinic. In September 1925 a contract was drawn up laying down the conditions in details which were adhered to by both sides until the last departments moved out of the clinic rooms in the Nussbaumstrasse in 1928.

During his last years Kraepelin and Bumke met regularly with their co-workers at clinical and scientific conferences.

E. Kahn was provisional director of the clinic during the particularly difficult years for both the clinic and the German Research Institute. He deserves special thanks for ensuring that the clinic fulfilled its duties to take care of the patients and train the students during this transitional phase, with the Research Institute occupying numerous clinic rooms due to its increasing activities. Kahn made a vital contribution to ensuring the smooth running and developing of the Research Institute whilst its staff worked successfully in the clinic's rooms.

Literature

Hippius, H., Hoff, P. (1986): Murnau and the History of Psychiatry. In: Hippius, H., Klerman, G.L., Matussek, N. (Eds): New Results in Depression Research. Springer-Verlag: Berlin, Heidelberg, p. 1-7

Kraepelin, E. (1887): Die Richtungen der Psychiatrischen Forschung. Vogel-Verlag: Leipzig

Kraepelin, E. (1916): Ein Forschungsinstitut für Psychiatrie. Z. Neur. 32, p. 1-38

Kraepelin, E. (1918): Ziele und Wege der psychiatrischen Forschung. Z. Neur. 42, p. 169-205

Scholz, W. (1961): Geschichte der Deutschen Forschungsanstalt für Psychiatrie (Max-Planck-Institut) Jahrbuch der Max-Planck-Gesellschaft 1961 (Part III), p. 662-686

Steinberg, H. (2001): Kraepelin in Leipzig. Eine Begegnung von Psychiatrie und Psychologie. Edition »Das Narrenschiff«, Psychiatrie-Verlag: Bonn

Steinberg, H. (Ed.) (2002): Der Briefwechsel zwischen Wilhelm Wundt und Emil Kraepelin. Verlag Hans Huber: Bern, Gottingen, Toronto, Seattle

Vierneisel, K. (1983): 50 Jahre Vermächtnis James Loeb. Verein der Freunde und Förderer der Glyptothek und der Antikensammlungen München e.V.

Weber, M. (1992): Die Deutsche Forschungsanstalt für Psychiatrie 1917–1945. Berichte und Mitteilungen der Max-Planck-Gesellschaft. Heft 2/1992, p. 11-33

Oswald Bumke and his Munich Workgroup

Changing the Psychiatric Hospital into a »Hospital for Nervous Disorders«

The Hospital during National Socialism

Once the consultations over Kraepelin's successor started at the beginning of the twenties, it was assumed that one of his pupils would be offered the chair for psychiatry int Munich. Most people presumed Robert Gaupp, who had moved from Heidelberg to Munich together with Kraepelin, would be chosen. He was Kraepelin's first senior consultant in Munich until he took over the chair for psychiatry in Tubingen in 1906. Karl Bonhoeffer (1868–1948), holder of the chair of psychiatry in Berlin, was also a possible candidate. Compared to Kraepelin and Gaupp, Bonhoeffer was of the opinion that the psychiatric university clinics should be transformed into clinics for nervous disorders by integrating neurological clinics. In spite of the differing views on the subject, Kraepelin would have agreed to Bonhoeffer as his successor. The medical faculty put Bonhoeffer at the top of their list at »primo loco« and he was offered the position in 1922, but turned it down a couple of months later after »considering the matter thoroughly«. Hence, Oswald Bumke received the offer, which surprised many.

Oswald Bumke
Professor of Psychiatry and Neurology
of the University of Munich (1924–1945)

Oswald Bumke (◻ Fig. 9.1) was born on September 25, 1877, in Stolp (Pomerania) as third of four sons of a general practitioner. His father died young; Bumke was aged 15 when he died. Because his mother came from a wealthy family Bumke and his brothers received academic education in spite of his father's early death. Both elder brothers became lawyers. Oswald Bumke had a special relationship to his brother, Erwin, who later became president at the Reich's law courts in Leipzig.

O. Bumke went to secondary school in Stolp and took his final school exams in 1896. When he began his studies in Freiburg, he was at first undecided whether to become maths teacher at a secondary school or doctor. Finally he decided for medicine. After one term in Freiburg, he studied in

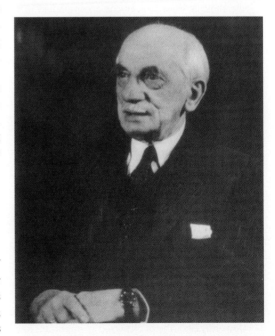

◻ **Fig. 9.1.** Oswald Bumke (1877–1950)

Leipzig for three terms. He completed his preliminary medical examinations and then spent a »lazy, fun summer term in Munich« before continuing his studies in Halle; he completed his final exams in Halle, but graduated in Kiel.

Bumke's first career stop was the Psychiatric Clinic in Freiburg. At that time, in the summer of 1901, Herrmann Emminghaus (▶ Chapter 7) was clinic director, but seriously ill. Bumke did not meet him personally. Following Emminghaus' death, the clinic was neglected for a couple of months; during this period Bumke noted that he found psychiatry »boring« and decided to look for another job. His attitude changed quickly once Alfred E. Hoche became head of the Freiburg clinic in 1902.

> A. E. Hoche (1865–1943) was the son of an evangelical vicar, who had died when Hoche was 13 years old. After studying medicine in Berlin and Heidelberg, Hoche graduated with Erb in Heidelberg, worked briefly as Erb's assistant at the outpatient clinic for internal medicine and then at the gynaecological and pediatric clinics in Heidelberg. In 1890 he joined C. Fürstner (1848–1906) at the psychiatric clinic in Heidelberg as co-worker. When Fürstner left Heidelberg in 1891 to take over the clinic in Strassburg, Hoche accompanied him, received his postdoctoral lecturer qualifications and remained in Strassburg as Fürstner's senior consultant until 1898. After working in a psychiatric practise in Strassburg for 4 years, Hoche was offered the chair of psychiatry in Freiburg in 1902 and remained there until his retirement in 1934. During the years prior to the First World War, Hoche was as scientist a prominent opponent of Kraepelin. Hoche considered Kraepelin's concept on the dichotomy of endogenous psychoses to be useless. He challenged Kraepelin's (in Hoche's opinion) dogmatically stiff nosological system with a »syndrome doctrine«. Hoche considered the postulated »disease units« to be speculation and for the description of psychiatric symptoms he acted on the assumption of psychopathological syndromes, a concept holding still ground today.
> Together with the lawyer K. Binding, Hoche wrote the article on »The Liberalization of Annihilation of Unworthy Life«. The book played an important role in the disastrous developments in psychiatry during national socialism: The national socialists used the book to legitimize their criminal handling of the mentally ill.
> Hoche was married to a lady of Jewish origin. In 1933 he requested retirement because he wanted to avoid reprisals for being married to a Jewish person. He retired in 1934, his wife died in 1937 and Hoche committed suicide on May 16, 1943.

A close personal relationship grew between Bumke and his teacher Hoche, which continued up to Hoche's death. In 1904 Bumke received his postdoctoral lecturer qualification whilst working with Hoche, became senior consultant at the Freiburg clinic in 1906 and was nominated extraordinary professor in 1910.

In 1914 Bumke received his first offer as ordinary professor and director of the Psychiatric Clinic and Clinic for Nervous Disorders in Rostock; the former »asylum Gehlsheim« had been turned into a university clinic. Bumke was very disappointed in Rostock. Later Bumke, who tended to be ironic and even sometimes sarcastic, referred to the clinic as the »prison of Gehlsheim«. He termed the conditions there as run down and corrupt; hence he was relieved when he received an offer from Breslau to become Alois Alzheimer's successor. Bumke found that the clinic in Breslau, which had been constructed according to Karl Boehoeffer's plans, had been built and equipped ideally; Bonhoeffer himself had managed the clinic from 1904–1912 excellently, as had Alois Alzheimer from 1912–1915. In Breslau Bumke made the acquaintance of Otfrid Foerster; they formed a lifelong friendship.

> Otfrid Foerster (1873–1941) came from Breslau; his father was professor for classical philology and archaeology at the local university. After studying medicine in Freiburg, Kiel and Breslau O. Foerster graduated in Breslau. Foerster's development was influenced decisively by C. Wernicke (1848–1905), who occupied the chair for psychiatry at Breslau and was responsible for the Breslau university clinic, located in wards at the Municipal Asylum for Mental Disorders. On Wernicke's advice, following his final medical exams and graduation, Foerster worked in France for two years (with Déjérine in Paris), in Switzerland (with H.S. Frenkel in Horn on

Lake Constance), returned to Breslau and became assistant to C. Wernicke in 1899, where he habilitated in 1903. Foerster's scientific interests were completely concentrated on neurology; therefore, whenever possible, he worked at the department of neurology at a Breslau hospital alongside his work with Wernicke. When the Breslau Psychiatric Clinic had its own building constructed and inaugurated in 1906, Foerster kept his senior functions at the neurological department of the Breslau hospital. When the Department of Neurology at the Wenzel-Hancke-Hospital finally became University Clinic for Neurology, Foerster received the chair for neurology in 1921.

During his time in Breslau Bumke was determined that the psychiatric clinics should be turned into »Clinics for Nervous Disorders«. Foerster pleaded emphatically that neurology should be separated from psychiatry. It was expected that the two differing opinions would lead to conflicts, but this was not the case. Bumke saw Foerster as the »greatest neurologist ever in Germany«. The collegial collaboration between Bumke and Foerster continued without friction and later (as of 1924) they published together the supplementary volumes to M. Lewandowsky's (1876–1918) (■ Fig. 9.2) »Handbook of Neurology«. From 1935 to 1939 they also published the 17 volumes of their own, famous »Handbook of Neurology«.

Bumke considered the personal relationship to Foerster and their collegial collaboration to be »one of the most precious gifts« of his life; in this connection he also emphasized that the »broad overlapping of the two work areas do not necessarily have to lead to strain between those involved«.

After being in Breslau for two years, Bumke received an offer for the chair of psychiatry in Heidelberg. He turned the offer down because he feared that there he would not be able to combine psychiatry with neurology according to his expectations. Apart from that, Bumke also enjoyed being in Breslau from a personal and professional perspective. All the same, he did accept the offer to Leipzig in 1921. In Leipzig he took over the clinic from Paul Flechsig (1847–1929), who justified his 42 years at Leipzig through his work on neuroanatomy and pathology of the brain.

During his time at Leipzig Bumke travelled to Moscow to the bedside of W. I. Lenin. The journey took place in 1923 together with G. Henschen, M. Nonne, O. Minkowski, O. Foerster and A. Strümpell and lasted a couple of weeks (■ Fig. 9.3). The stay entailed meetings and often daily contact with Lenin, Trotzki, Bucharin and Stalin. As a result, Bumke was one of the first West Europeans to get intimate insight into the leading circle of the Soviet Union. The trip was particularly important for Bumke, because he met up with Foerster again and their personal friendship grew deeper.

Like Bonhoeffer, Bumke was a determined advocate of the concept of **psychiatry** and **neurology** being combined into one subject at university and to have it accommodated in one »**clinic for nervous disorders**«, headed by **one** professor. Bumke presumed that psychiatric and neurological diseases affected the same organ system. Affliction of the nervous system could lead to psychiatric and/or neurological disorders. Bumke thought lesser neurological diseases to be psychic disorders with neurological symptoms (e.g. conversion syndromes). He considered it possible for these diseases to have a relatively favourable course. On the other hand at Bumke's time, psychiatric diseases which needed in-patient treatment, were generally considered to have an unfavourable course of illness.

By combining psychiatry and neurology into »medicine for nervous diseases«, Bumke hoped to achieve several aims: For psychiatric patients it should be easier to get treatment. By admitting psychiatric and neurological patients to the same clinic, the stigmatization of psychiatric patients should be overcome. Doctors for both psychiatry and neurology should have easier access to the lesser neurological diseases. In particular, Bumke saw the combination of psychiatry and neurology as an important basis for the training of doctors responsible for such patients. Without the connection to neurology the danger existed that »pure« psychiatry would fall too strongly into a field of speculation. Only the in-depth examination of patients, taking special neurological knowledge into consideration, would allow for over-hasty and »purely« psychiatric diagnoses to be avoided.

HANDBUCH
DER NEUROLOGIE

BEARBEITET VON

G. ABELSDORFF-BERLIN, R. BÁRÁNY-WIEN, M. BIELSCHOWSKY-BERLIN, R. DU BOIS-REYMOND-BERLIN, K. BONHOEFFER-BRESLAU, H. BORUTTAU-BERLIN, W. BRAUN-BERLIN, K. BRODMANN-BERLIN, O. BUMKE-FREIBURG I. B., R. CASSIRER-BERLIN, T. COHN-BERLIN, A. CRAMER-GÖTTINGEN, R. FINKELNBURG-BONN, E. FLATAU-WARSCHAU, G. FLATAU-BERLIN, E. FORSTER-BERLIN, H. GUTZMANN-BERLIN, H. HAENEL-DRESDEN, FR. HARTMANN-GRAZ, K. HEILBRONNER-UTRECHT, R. HENNEBERG-BERLIN, S. E. HENSCHEN-STOCKHOLM, E. JENDRASSIK-BUDAPEST, O. KALISCHER-BERLIN, S. KALISCHER-BERLIN, M. KAUFFMANN-HALLE A. S., FR. KRAMER-BRESLAU, LÉRI-PARIS, M. LEWANDOWSKY-BERLIN, O. MARBURG-WIEN, P. MARIE-PARIS, FR. MOHR-COBLENZ, E. NEISSER-STETTIN, E. PHLEPS-GRAZ, F. H. QUIX-UTRECHT, E. REDLICH-WIEN, K. SCHAFFER-BUDAPEST, A. SCHÜLLER-WIEN, P. SCHUSTER-BERLIN, W. SPIELMEYER-FREIBURG I. B., H. VOGT-FRANKFURT A. M., W. VORKASTNER-GREIFSWALD, O. VULPIUS-HEIDELBERG, E. WEBER-BERLIN, J. WERTHEIM SALOMONSON-AMSTERDAM, J. WICKMAN-STOCKHOLM, K. WILMANNS-HEIDELBERG

HERAUSGEGEBEN VON

M. LEWANDOWSKY

ERSTER BAND
ALLGEMEINE NEUROLOGIE

MIT 322 TEXTABBILDUNGEN UND 12 TAFELN

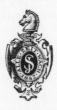 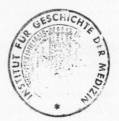

BERLIN
VERLAG VON JULIUS SPRINGER
1910

▢ Fig. 9.2. First volume of the »Handbook of Neurology« from 1910, edited by M. Lewandowski

When it seemed possible to Bumke that he would be offered the chair in Munich in 1922, it was clear to him that he would only accept if the clinic would be changed according to his plans. The extension of the clinic was also a pre-condi- tion for him going to Munich. During negotiations the extension was agreed to and the problems in connection with the merger of the university clinic with the German Research Institute, which had existed since 1917 (▶ Chapter 8), were solved.

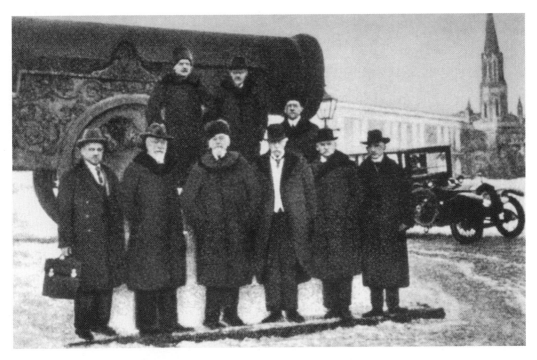

Fig. 9.3. Doctors, who were called to Lenin: (front row from left to right) Semashko, Soviet Minister for Public Health, Minkowski from Breslau, Struepell from Leipzig, Henschen from Stockholm, Nonne from Hamburg, Bumke from Leipzig. (back row from left to right) Kramer from Moscow, Foerster from Breslau and Koshevairoff

Bumke finally accepted and took up office in Munich on April 1, 1924.

Bumke's plans for the re-organization and change of the clinic into a »clinic for nervous diseases« were supported emphatically by the medical faculty. Important and influential faculty members, such as the internal specialist, Friedrich von Müller, and the surgeon, Ferdinand Sauerbruch, gave him advice and helped him settle in.

Bumke soon began to enjoy life in Munich. He lived in the »director's villa« with his wife who originated from Munich and was pleased to return there, and their two children. It did not take long before his reputation grew in the entire university. In 1928 he was voted rector to the university and in the same year became president of the German University Association; he remained in this office, which was important for his entire academic life, until 1933 (see below).

The »Medical Reading Hall« which is situated close to the clinic on Beethovenplatz, still reminds us

today of Bumke's great influence during the first decade of being in office in Munich (Fig. 9.4). The building had been designed by the architects, Gabriel von Seidel, in a late art noveau style for the operetta tenor Franz Joseph Brakl, who was well known at the time. Brakl lived in the house and kept his large art collection there; the spacious building was also used for art exhibitions (e.g. for the painters of the »Blaue Reiter« (»blue riders«) and auctions.

As Brakl lost the greater part of his wealth due to inflation after the First World War, his tax debts forced him to sell his house. He asked the director of the neighbouring clinic for his advice and, as university rector, Bumke was able to arrange that the house was purchased for the university via a foundation, set up by a wealthy German-American doctor, Sophie A. Nordhoff-Jung. The house was put at the disposal of the university as »Reading Hall«. Brakl and his wife received a life annuity and right of abode in an adjacent building (now, the Institute for the History of Medicine).

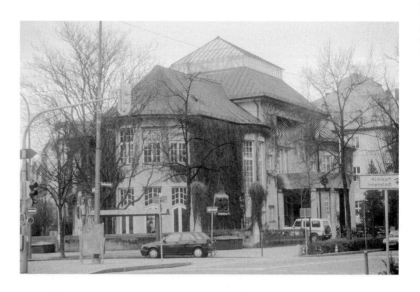

◘ Fig. 9.4. Medical reading hall (recent photo)

Bumke succeeded in combining the two fields of psychiatry and neurology not only at the Munich medical faculty, but also in the entire German speaking realm, proving it further by publishing the 11-volume »Handbook of Mental Diseases« (Handbuch der Geisteskrankheiten) (1928–1939 (◘ Fig. 9.5) and the 17-volume »Handbook of Neurology« (Handbuch der Neurologie) (1935–1937; together with O. Forerster). These handbooks were famous at home and abroad and further secured Bumke's reputation, which had already been achieved by him being offered the chair at three universities in quick succession before coming to Munich. Bumke's lectures were very popular with the students; his lectures for members of all faculties were always overcrowded. Bumke's »Handbook of Mental Diseases« (seven volumes 1922–1948) (◘ Fig. 9.6) was a standard textbook at all the German universities.

Although Bumke admired and valued Kraepelin as founder of scientific psychiatry, he was often strongly critical of Kraepelin's understanding of psychiatry. He considered Kraepelin's postulations on disease units to be »phantoms«; in the clinical reality he did not see clear boundaries between »healthy and ill«, but smooth transitions. In Bumke's opinion, for psychiatric science to develop in a prolific manner it would be necessary to overcome the »pompous idling in experimental psychology far from reality«. His goal was to achieve an »understanding psychiatry« by avoiding »unreal laboratory psychology« as well as the speculative efforts of psychoanalysis. He looked for his »own way« between Kraepelin and Freud, as outlined in critical statements on psychoanalysis (1930–1938) in his book »Thoughts on the Soul« (Gedanken über die Seele) (1941–1948).

Bumke headed the Munich clinic for almost 22 years. The first few years were a most successful and happy time for him. The early death of his wife in 1937 left a deep scar, and not only in his personal but also in his professional life a difficult time lay ahead: Bumke was responsible for the Munich clinic during national socialism, the Second World War and during the months following the war (► see below and Chapter 10). In December 1945 he was suspended from the clinic management (► Chapter 10). He was put through a denazification process and in 1947 was reinstated as university professor and clinical director. In the meantime he had turned 70 years old and retired.

Oswald Bumke died in Munich on January 5, 1950.

Extension of the Clinic Building under O. Bumke

As soon as Bumke had taken up office in April 1924, construction work began. The east wing which was originally planned to be two storeys

HANDBUCH DER
GEISTESKRANKHEITEN

BEARBEITET VON

K. BERINGER · K. BIRNBAUM · A. BOSTROEM · E. BRAUN · A. v. BRAUNMÜHL
O. BUMKE · H. BÜRGER-PRINZ · J. L. ENTRES · G. EWALD · E. GAMPER
F. GEORGI · HANS W. GRUHLE · E. GRÜNTHAL · J. HALLERVORDEN
A. HAUPTMANN · A. HOMBURGER † · F. JAHNEL · W. JAHRREISS · A. JAKOB
H. JOSEPHY · V. KAFKA · E. KAHN · F. KEHRER · B. KIHN · H. KORBSCH
E. KRETSCHMER · E. KÜPPERS · J. LANGE · W. MAYER-GROSS · F. MEGGEN-
DORFER · K. NEUBÜRGER · P. NITSCHE · B. PFEIFER · F. PLAUT · M. ROSEN-
FELD · W. RUNGE · H. SCHARFETTER · K. SCHNEIDER · F. SCHOB · W. SCHOLZ
J. H. SCHULTZ · H. SPATZ · W. SPIELMEYER · J. STEIN · G. STEINER · F. STERN
G. STERTZ · A. STRAUSS · W. STROHMAYER · R. THIELE · W. VORKASTNER †
W. WEIMANN · A. WETZEL · K. WILMANNS · O. WUTH

HERAUSGEGEBEN VON

OSWALD BUMKE
MÜNCHEN

NEUNTER BAND
SPEZIELLER TEIL V

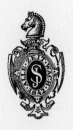

BERLIN
VERLAG VON JULIUS SPRINGER
1932

Fig. 9.5. First page of the »Handbook of Mental Diseases« by O. Bumke (1932)

9

LEHRBUCH DER
GEISTESKRANKHEITEN

VON

PROF. OSWALD BUMKE

DIREKTOR DER PSYCHIATRISCHEN UND NERVENKLINIK
IN MÜNCHEN

★

MIT EINEM ANHANG:

DIE ANATOMIE DER PSYCHOSEN

VON DR. B. KLARFELD

260 ABBILDUNGEN IM TEXT

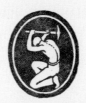 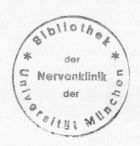

ZWEITE, UMGEARBEITETE AUFLAGE
DER DIAGNOSE DER GEISTESKRANKHEITEN

MÜNCHEN / VERLAG VON J. F. BERGMANN / 1924

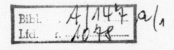
◨ Fig. 9.6. First page »Textbook of Mental Diseases« by O. Bumke (1924)

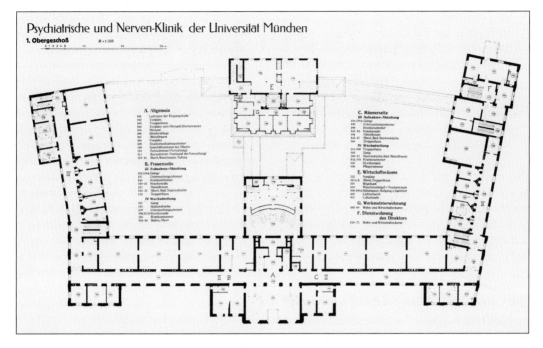

Psychiatrische und Nerven-Klinik der Universität München
1. Obergeschoß

☐ Fig. 9.7. Floor-plan with tract for the auditorium (1st floor) during Bumke's time in office

high (ground and first floors), was extended and increased by a further floor. In the new part of the building a conclave and refectory for the sisters was located and a chapel for the clinic. As a result, the rooms originally used by the sisters (in the part of the east wing built in 1904) were freed up for a ward for the »nervously ill«.

In 1926 Bumke also managed to move the »Clinical Department« of the German Research Institute for Psychiatry«, which occupied the ground floor of the building on the Nussbaum-strasse, into a house on Bavariaring. Consequently, at the end of 1926 the clinic had a further 53 beds.

The extension was authorized in 1924 and inaugurated on February 7, 1927. At the inauguration Bumke explained his motives for restructuring the clinic into a »psychiatric hospital and clinic for nervous diseases«. By setting up »wards for nervous diseases« and enlarging the out-patient clinic, it was Bumke's intention to overcome the »mistrust in the population with respect to a pure mental asylum«. In his opinion, he had come close to his target by renaming the clinic. The number of annual in-patient admittances increase from 1,750 to 2,500

and the number of patients treated at the out-patient clinic increased from 626 to almost 1800.

In 1928 the space situation in the clinic improved futher: Once the new building for the Research Institute in Schwabing was finished, it was no longer a guest at the clinic. Spielmeyer and Plaut (▸ Chapter 8) moved with all their departments and Bumke now had use of all floors at the clinic (☐ Fig. 9.7).

The Research Institute's department of histopathology, headed by W. Spielmeyer, remained in the clinic until 1928. Together with the laboratory for neuropathology, this part of the Research Institute was located on the 3rd floor of the clinic, in the rooms with the large microscopy laboratory which Alois Alzheimer had put at the disposal of the department for neuropathology since the opening of the clinic. It was here that W. Spielmeyer – assistant at the clinic since 1912 – worked together with Alzheimer, later with K. Brodmann and F. Nissl. When Brodmann and Nissl died shortly one after the other (August 1918 resp August 1919), Krae-pelin gave Spielmeyer communal use of staff and the management of the clinic's laboratory for neuropathology and the Research Institute's department of histopathology. Until moving into the new building in Schwabing, which was financed by the Rockefeller Foundation, Spielmeyer was able to use the clinic rooms for his department of histopathology until 1928, although the German Research Institute had been integrated into the Kaiser-Wilhelm-Association (before Kraepelin's death).

Despite the fact that the clinic's rooms were forced to accommodate more and more patients during the thirties and in particular after the outbreak of the Second World War, and due to the ensuing damage, after 1928 the clinic would not be extended further for the next 60 years (▶ Chapter 13).

The Co-Workers of Oswald Bumke in Munich

In April 1924 Bumke was accompanied to Munich by his senior consultant from Leipzig, **August Bostroem**. Bumke gave Bostroem the position of first senior consultant which he was until 1932. Apart from Bostroem **Eugen Kahn** was senior consultant at the clinic. Following Kraepelin's retirement, Kahn had managed the clinic provisionally; Bumke kept him on. In spite of what must have been a difficult situation for Kahn, he and Bostroem worked together well as Bumke's senior consultants. In 1930 Kahn was offered a position at Yale University (▶ Chapter 7). His successor in Munich was **Kurt Blum** (1895–1932), who had received his postdoctoral lecturer qualifications in Cologne in 1928 with G. Aschaffenburg (1866–1944). Blum worked in Munich for three years and then died at the age of 37 years. Bostroem left the Munich clinic the same year (1932) and went to Koenigsberg.

August Bostroem (1886–1944) (◻ Fig. 9.8), son of a pathologist, studied medicine in Freiburg and Giessen, worked at a pathological institute, then worked for Max Nonne (1861–1959) in Hamburg and afterwards for Karl Kleist (1879–1960) in Rostock. Bumke called Bostroem to the Leipzig clinic as senior consultant in 1921. Bumke and Bostroem agreed on professional matters and had a good personal relationship, which continued whilst working together for 11 years in Leipzig and Munich.

In 1932 Bostroem became E. Meyer's (1871–1931) successor on the chair for psychiatry and nervous diseases at the University of Koenigsberg.

The correspondence between Bostroem and Bumke during the years prior to Bostroem's death in 1944 illustrates the considerable mutual trust between the two. Bostroem asked Bumke for his advice; he regularly reported to Bumke about his personal situation and his family. Bumke was reserved with regard to personal matters, but did contact Bostroem confidentially about the difficult professional problems connected with the seizure of power by the Nazis (e.g. regarding the law of 1933 on the »prevention of offspring with hereditary diseases«).

During his time in Munich Bostroem was mainly interested in problems at the border between neurology and psychiatry (diseases of the extrapyramidal motoric system; neurological and psychiatric syndromes in cases of neurolues and encephalitis). In 1929, together with Johannes Lange (1891–1938) Bostroem founded the journal »Progress in neurology, psychiatry and their border areas« (Zeitschrift der Neurologie, Psychiatrie und ihre Grenzgebiete).

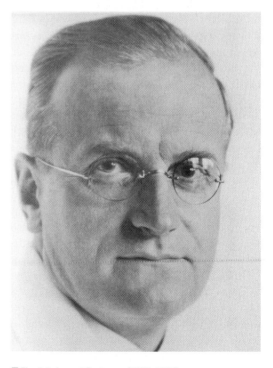

◻ **Fig. 9.8.** August Bostroem (1886–1944)

Bostroem headed the clinic in Koenigsberg from 1932 until 1939, accepted an offer to Leipzig and in 1942 he joined the University of Strassburg, where he died of a heart attack in 1944.

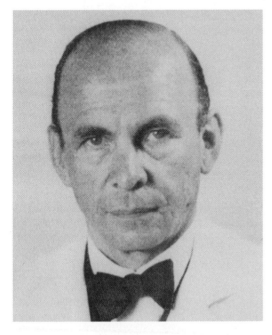

◘ **Fig. 9.9.** Kurt Beringer (1893–1949)

When Bostroem left the clinic in 1932 and Blum had died, **Kurt Beringer** became senior consultant at the Munich clinic.

After his medical studies and participation in the First World War from 1920 until 1933 K. Beringer (1893–1949) (◘ Fig. 9.9) became assistant and later senior consultant to K. Wilmanns (1873–1945) at the Heidelberg clinic. In Wilmans' Heidelberg workgroup Beringer emerged – as is tradition in Heidelberg – with studies on the problems of schizophrenia and the »schizoid« and in particular with his work on »model psychoses« (harmine, mescaline, haschisch). Together with K. Hansen, W. Mayer-Gross and E. Straus, Beringer founded the journal »Der Nervenarzt« (The Doctor of Psychiatry and Nervous Diseases) in 1928. Beringer only worked in Munich briefly; in 1934 he was appointed Alfred Hoche's successor in Freiburg, where he stayed until his death, although he received several offers from other universities.

Following Beringer's appointment to Freiburg, one after the other **F. Kant, K.H. Stauder, A. Bannwarth, M. Mikorey** and **V. Ziehen** were senior consultants at the Munich clinic (◘ Fig. 9.10).

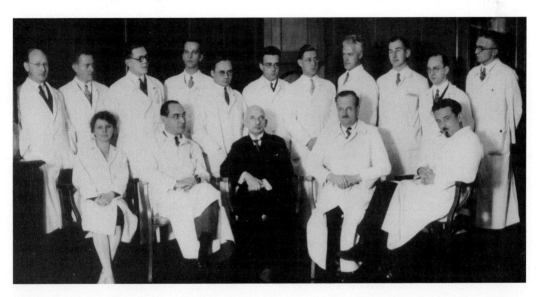

◘ **Fig. 9.10.** Oswald Bumke with his co-workers: back row, standing 1. Jahrreis, 2. Zech, 3. Krapf, 4. Kant, 5. Kothe, 6. Mikorey, 7. Mann, 8. v. Stähr, 9. Römer, 10. Müller, 11. Stauder, front row, sitting 12. Kuhl, 13. Kahn, 14. Bumke, 15. Bostroem, 16. Spatz

After graduating in Tubingen with a thesis on schizophrenic symptom complexes and a short job as internal specialist at the Medical Out-Patient Clinic in Berlin, Fritz Kant (born 1894) joined Bumke in 1925 at the Munich clinic. In Munich his main topics of interest were intoxication and symptomatic psychoses due to drug and alcohol consumption. In 1928 he published his own experiences with haschisch from a psychopathological point of view and in 1932 he became postdoctoral lecturer with a thesis on alcohol psychoses. In 1937 Kant had to emigrate to America, where he continued his clinical psychiatric and scientific work on psychopharmacological topics and alcoholism in Madison/Wisconsin.

K.-H. Stauder (1905–1969) was son of the First Chairman of the German Medical Fraternity and Harmann Association, Alfons Stauder. In addition to his medical studies and interests, Stauder soon discovered his talent as journalist and author. He joined the clinic in 1929 at the young age of 24 and had a wide spectrum of scientific interests with a main focus on research into epilepsy as well as neuro- and psychopharmacology. Despite his broad scientific oeuvres Stauder gave up his scientific career; he refused to join the NSDAP or one of their organisations. In 1937 he resigned from the clinic and opened a practice for psychiatry and neurology. He wrote numerous scientific publications and books and from 1951–1961 edited one of the important medical journals of the time, the »Medizinische Klinik« (Clinic for Internal Medicine). Under the pseudonym Thomas Regau he wrote stories as well as travel and other specialized books.

Alfred Bannwarth (1903–1970) (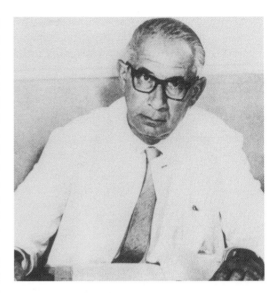 Fig. 9.11) first studied music after leaving school and then changed to medicine. After the state exams and graduation in Munich he became assistant to Max Nonne in Hamburg. In 1933 he joined the Munich clinic. As assistant to Bumke he worked on neurological research topics; his studies on the diagnostics of brain tumours marked the beginnings of x-ray diagnostics at the Munich clinic. Under A. Bannwarth's guidance the x-ray department made fast progress; in 1938 12,000 x-rays were taken. Because Bannwart was not a member of the NSDAP, he wrote a thesis as postdoctoral lecturer, but did not receive the qualifications from

◻ **Fig. 9.11.** Alfred Bannwarth (1903–1970)

the Bavarian Ministry of Education and Culture. In 1940 he joined the NSDAP. In 1941 he wrote a 92-page long paper in the »Archive für Psychiatrie und Nervenkrankheiten« (Archive for Psychiatry and Nervous Diseases) on »Chronically lymphocytous meningitis, inflammatory polyneuritis and rheumatism«, which contained a detailed description of the »Bannwarth syndrome«, later named after Bannwarth. As military doctor Bannwarth was stationed in the valley of Lake Tegern; he was captured by the Americans (held prisoner until June 1946). During the denazification process he was classified as exonerated and in 1949 he started worked again at the clinic. In 1950 he was nominated extraordinary professor. In 1955 he set up the neurosurgical department and also his own neurological department at the Municipal Hospital Rechts der Isar (on the right bank of the river Isar) becoming head of the latter.

Max Mikorey joined the clinic in 1929, became senior consultant in 1934 and remained in the same position, with intervals, until 1968 (▸ Chapter 10).

Vult Ziehen (1899–1975) was son of the psychiatrist and neurologist, Georg Theodor Ziehen (1862–1950), who was ordinary professor for psychiatry at the Charité in Berlin from 1904 to 1912, and one of the founders of child psychiatry in Germany. Georg Ziehen later changed to philosophy, worked in Wiesbaden for some years as a private teacher, and until his retirement in 1930 was full professor for philosophy in Halle. As his father had done, Kurt Viehen worked on developmental psychology and psychopathology of infants. He joined the clinic in 1933 and became deputy head of Haar in 1946. Later Viehen became publicly known due to some options he furnished some of which had caused a sensation.

Hugo Spatz had a special position in the clinic as senior consultant.

On completion of his medical studies in Munich and Heidelberg and after graduation with a thesis on »Contributions to the normal histology of the spinal cord of newly born rabbits«, Hugo Spatz (1888–1969) (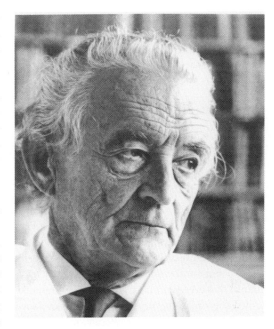 Fig. 9.12) worked at the Heidelberg clinic as assistant to F. Nissl. When Nissl left the Heidelberg clinic in 1918 to take over the department for histopathology at the German Research Institute for Psychiatry, Spatz followed him one year later. Nissl died shortly afterwards and Spatz kept his job at the Research Institute. He became assistant to Spielmeyer and received his postdoctoral lecturer qualifications under Spielmeyer's guidance. When Spielmeyer moved to Schwabing with his department for histopathology in 1928, Spatz remained in the clinic. Bumke made him senior consultant and gave him the responsibility for the neuro-anatomical laboratory of the clinic.

Spatz worked at the clinic from 1928 until 1937; in 1937 he became successor to O. Vogt (1870–1959) and director of the Kaiser-Wilhelm-Institute for Brain Research in Berlin-Buch. The extensive scientific studies of H. Spatz impressively reflect how productive the combination of clinical and neuropathological research can be. The topics Spatz worked on ranged from the detection of special neurochemical findings in neurolues to the description of a peculiar form of extrapyramidal motoric disorders (the Hallervorden-Spatz disease) from studies on system degeneration to descriptions and classifications of encephalitis and encephalomyelitis according to their spreading patterns. Spatz also dealt with fundamental questions on the evolution of brain development.

Fig. 9.12. Hugo Spatz (1888–1969)

Once Spatz left the clinic, Bumke brought **Eduard Beck** (1892–1876) to Munich as head of the laboratory for neuropathology; Beck had worked in Berlin for O. Vogt as neuropathologist and trained clinically with K. Kleist. Beck left the clinic in 1945 and opened a practise for psychiatry and neurology.

The tradition of neuropathology at the Munich clinic – during the time of Kraepelin and Bumke and linked to the great names of Alzheimer, Nissl, Brodmann, Spielmeyer and Spatz – drew to a close at the end of the Second World War.

Under K. Kolle another attempt was made at setting up a laboratory for neuropathology with J.E. Meyer (1917–1998) (▶ Chapter 11). When J.E. Meyer left the Munich clinic in 1968 to take over the chair for psychiatry in Gottingen, no further attempts were made to open a neuropathological laboratory. During the war and after Spielmeyer's early death (1935), the German Research Institute established neuropathological research with Spielmeyer's successor W. Scholz (1889–1960). In 1961 Scholz's successor, the neuropathologist G. Peters (1906–1987), became director of the Germany Research Institute for Psychiatry, which had been integrated into the

Max-Planck-Association as an institute. At the medical faculty of the university an independent chair of neuropathology was set up in 1965 (O. Stochdorph, 1914-1999; P. Mehrain, born 1931).

The Hospital During National Socialism

The appointment to Munich was a challenge for Bumke, especially since great things were expected from Kraepelin's successor. In particular, Bumke had to take into consideration that the development of the clinic after the founding of the German Research Institute (1917) and in the years following the First World War had been neglected to a certain extent. During his last years in office (until 1922) Kraepelin was occupied with building up the Research Institute. In the seven years (1917–1924) up until Bumke joined the clinic, the Research Institute developed into a scientific institution of international standing. As it had been decided that two departments of the Research Institute should remain in the rooms of the clinic for quite some time, Bumke was faced with a difficult task. He hoped soon to be able to solve all difficulties with diplomatic and organizational talent. On the whole he succeeded (see above), but Bumke did not forsee that he would be confronted with disproportionately greater problems: Bumke was responsible for the clinic during the Nazi regime.

In Munich – the movement's main city – political developments were in the making, which finally led to Hitler »seizing power« and in the following period to the more and more disastrous involvement of psychiatry in the Nazi ideology. As early as July 14, 1933 the »Law on the Prevention of Offspring with Hereditary Diseases« (law on sterilization) was passed and came into force in 1934. E. Rüdin was the co-author of the commentary on the law which was the basis for probably 360,000 people (predominantly forced sterilizations) to be sterilized from 1934 to 1945. With the »sterilization law« the doctors (as well as some other professionals, such as midwives) were forced to register any »hereditary diseases«. According to the definition this included among other things »inherited mental deficiencies, schizophrenia, circular madness, inherited epilepsy« and »serious alcoholism«. In the summer of 1939

the Reich's Ministry of the Interior issued a secret decree for the registration of offspring with »serious abnormalities« and »mongolism«. Five thousand such children were killed. Due to a decree from the »Fuehrer«, backdated to the same day the Second World War broke out, from 1939–1941 more than 80,000 mentally ill persons (»ballast existences«) were killed (by »euthanasia«) with the assistance of psychiatrists. During the following years up until the end of the war, several thousands of patients died in psychiatric hospitals due to »hunger«.

Bumke and his doctors at the Munich clinic were contemporary witnesses of the events. It is unclear whether and to what extent they were informed of the developments and whether the situation was influenced by their deeds. There was no open and fundamental resistance.

It is desirable that all available sources (case histories, reports on transferrals, correspondence etc) be accessed and processed. Only then will it be possible to judge the role of the Munich clinic during national-socialism, like in the report, issued in 1999 (M. v. Cranach and H. Siemen), on the Bavarian healing and caring institutions.

In 1946 Bumke began to write his »Memoirs and Observations«, in which he gave a retrospective on »Medicine in the Third Reich« from his point of view. The memoirs were published in 1952 – after his death. Whilst writing his memoirs Bumke was embittered that – following the publication of a newspaper article in Switzerland, condemning him for his close collaboration with the Nazis – he was relieved of his duties and had to wait until the end of a long denazification process which finally proved his innocence; in 1947 he was put back into office. Bumke's personal situation at the time he wrote his »memoirs« explains why the »Memoirs« do not have the significance of a true record of the Munich clinic in the years 1933–1945.

Contradictory assumptions have been made retrospectively regarding Bumke's attitude towards national-socialism. By no means is it justified to count him as one of the psychiatrists who were precursors and committed advocates of national-socialism. Allusions to the fact that after all he was a pupil of A. Hoche and the brother of the Reich's president of the courts of justice, Erwin Bumke (who committed suicide in Leipzig in April 1945) give little accurate insight into Bumke's role during the Nazi regime.

At an early stage as a scientist and in other aspects, Bumke already stood in opposition to those concepts in psychiatry, which the Nazis later used to justifiy the racial ideology and ensuing criminal acts.

In his study on »Nervous Degeneration« in 1912 Bumke gave his opinion critically and effectively against the much discussed (amongst others by Kraepelin) and generally heeded »degeneration doctrines«. Although he approved of research into genetics, Bumke disapproved of Rüdin's – at that time Kraepelin's co-worker at the Munich clinic – hereditary-biological theories of »eugenics« and »racial hygiene«. In the twenties he expressed himself critically and in a warning tone towards those in favour of sterilization and abortions in psychiatric patients. Whilst Rüdin was already seriously considering the idea of forced sterilization, Bumke rejected the idea entirely. In 1930 Bumke forbid the transfer of patients to the German Research Institute for genealogical-anthropological studies, which Rüdin was performing on a large scale following his return from Basle in 1928.

In the second half of the twenties and at the beginning of the thirties, Bumke experienced how the political life in Munich changed radically. As rector he faced demonstrations by NS students against him because he had forbidden the wearing of uniforms in the university rooms. He observed the developments at the German Research Institute under Rüdin carefully. In January 1933 he was of the opinion that the worst was over and said to his secretary: »Don't worry, it will all be over in three months.«

But it turned out differently and Bumke himself was affected. In 1933 the German University Association, of which he was president, was dissolved. When O Foerster was forced by the new powers that be to give up the chairmanship of the »Association of German Psychiatrists and Neurologist« (Gesellschaft Deutscher Nervenärzte), Bumke became his successor. He was not able to stop this scientific association – as ordered by the Reich's Ministry of the Interior – from being »united«

with the »German Association for Psychiatry« to become the »Association of German Neurologists and Psychiatrists« in 1935 under the presidency of E. Rüdin. This »unification« was one of the Nazis measures intended to »consolidate«. Bumke also had to accept that on orders of the Reich's governor for Bavaria, Rüdin was bestowed with a personal professor's chair at the Munich medical faculty.

Once the »Law on the Prevention of Offspring with Hereditary Diseases« came into force (January 1, 1934), the Munich clinic was obliged to report patients with »hereditary diseases«. It was commonly known that Bumke – as opposed to Rüdin – was against broadening the range of indications for sterilization and was against forced sterilization. He confined himself to pointing out to the Bavarian State Ministry for Education and Culture (in a letter written in May 1934) that »some parts of the population seem to avoid the clinic in order to avoid sterilization, and that it would therefore be advisable to rid the clinic of its character as a closed institution. Thereby the clinic would no longer file applications for sterilization, but it would report any hereditary diseases. The patients and their relations would only be informed that the respective public health officer had filed for sterilization«. As Bumke was worried that the »old mistrust against this clinic« (i.e. against the Psychiatric and Neurological Clinic) would start to »flare up« in the population, he also requested that the clinic would only be called »Clinic for Nervous Diseases« in the future (◘ Fig. 9.13).

In June 1934 Bumke requested to resign as professor and clinic director; his request was not granted. It is presumed that under Bumke's responsibility (as of 1934) the patient diagnoses were in such a manner that the compulsory registration could be by-passed. However, it is known that in 1934/1935 female patients were transferred to the gynaecological clinic for sterilization.

Due to a change in the »Law for Hereditary Health« as of 1935 not only sterilization, but also abortions became »legal«. Bumke commented openly and as a warning in 1935 and 1936 on the law. In the »Guidelines for Abortion and Sterilization for Health Reasons« (◘ Fig. 9.14), published by the Reich's Medical Association, he wrote that in his opinion there was no indication to abort a pregnancy in cases of mental illness.

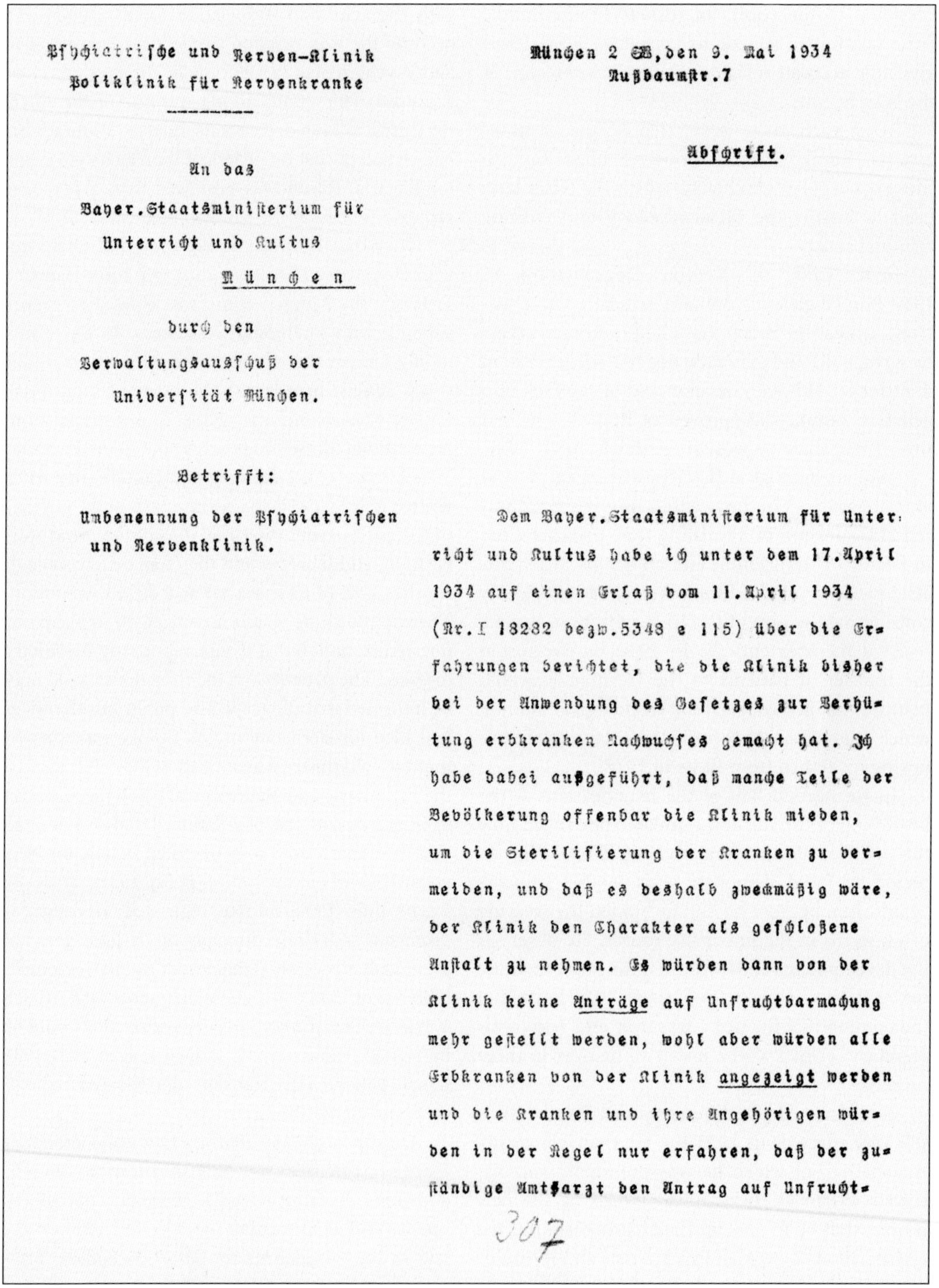

Psychiatrische und Nerven-Klinik   München 2 NW, den 9. Mai 1934
Poliklinik für Nervenkranke   Nußbaumstr. 7

Abschrift.

An das

Bayer. Staatsministerium für

Unterricht und Kultus

M ü n c h e n

durch den

Verwaltungsausschuß der

Universität München.

Betrifft:

Umbenennung der Psychiatrischen
und Nervenklinik.

Dem Bayer. Staatsministerium für Unterricht und Kultus habe ich unter dem 17. April
1934 auf einen Erlaß vom 11. April 1934
(Nr. I 18282 bezw. 5348 e 115) über die Erfahrungen berichtet, die die Klinik bisher
bei der Anwendung des Gesetzes zur Verhütung erbkranken Nachwuchses gemacht hat. Ich
habe dabei ausgeführt, daß manche Teile der
Bevölkerung offenbar die Klinik mieden,
um die Sterilisierung der Kranken zu vermeiden, und daß es deshalb zweckmäßig wäre,
der Klinik den Charakter als geschloßene
Anstalt zu nehmen. Es würden dann von der
Klinik keine Anträge auf Unfruchtbarmachung
mehr gestellt werden, wohl aber würden alle
Erbkranken von der Klinik angezeigt werden
und die Kranken und ihre Angehörigen würden in der Regel nur erfahren, daß der zu-
ständige Amtsarzt den Antrag auf Unfrucht-

307

Fig. 9.13. Letter of May 9, 1934, from O. Bumke to the Bavarian State Ministry. The »Psychiatric and Clinic for Nervous Diseases« should be renamed »Clinic for Nervous Diseases«. Also, in his letter Bumke makes reference to the sterilizations taking place at the time (from: University Archive Munich, signed: 307/1)

- 2 -

darmachung geſtellt hat.

Inzwiſchen iſt durch die Verfügung des Staatsminiſteriums des Innern vom 25. April 1934 (Nr.5348 e 115) beſtimmt worden, daß die Univerſitäts= kliniken für Pſychiatrie nicht als "geſchloſſene" Anſtalten zu gelten haben.

In meinem Bericht vom 17. April 1934 habe ich es dann weiter für wünſchenswert erklärt, die Pſychiatriſche und Nervenklinik in Zukunft nur noch Nervenklinik zu nennen. Zur Begründung habe ich geſchrieben: "Eine mehr als dreißigjährige Erfahrung hat mir gezeigt, daß Kranke und An= gehörige ſich immer wieder an dem Wort 'Pſychiatriſch' ſtoßen. Gerade jetzt, wo ein altes Mißtrauen gegen dieſe Kliniken zu ſehr ungelegener Zeit wieder aufzuflackern beginnt, wäre es vielleicht gut, dem auch durch eine ſolche Änderung des Namens entgegenzutreten." Hinzufügen möchte ich noch, daß das Wort 'pſychiatriſch' von der Bevölkerung beinahe niemals richtig gebraucht wird und daß es ſchon deshalb zweckmäßig wäre, eine für jeden verſtändliche Bezeichnung zu wählen.

Heute habe ich in einer Unterredung mit den Herren Profeſſor Schittenhelm und Profeſſor Stepp deren Zuſtimmung zu einem formulierten Antrag dieſer Art erhalten. Beide Herren erheben keine Einwendungen dagegen, daß die Pſychiatriſche und Nervenklinik in Zukunft nur noch Nervenklinik heißt.

                                        B u m k e .

»To the decree from April 11, 1934 (No. I 18282 resp 5348 e 115), I informed the Bavarian State Ministry for Education and Culture on April 17, 1934, about the experiences I have had with the law on the prevention of genetically ill offspring. I reported that certain parts of the population seem to avoid the clinic in order to avoid the sterilization of patients and that it would therefore be advisable to release the clinic from its status as a closed institution. No further requests for sterilization would be made by the clinic, however, the genetically ill would be notified and the patients and their relations would only know that the responsible public health officer had made the proposal for sterilization.

In the meantime it has been decided in a motion by the State Ministry for the Interior on April 25, 1934 (No. 5348 e 115), that the University Clinic for Psychiatry is no longer a »closed« institution.

Furthermore, in my report of April 17, 1934, I declared it desirable that the Psychiatric and Clinic for Nervous Diseases be only referred to in future as the Clinic for Nervous Diseases. I quote my reasons: »More than 30 years of experience have shown me that patients and their relations continually object to the word »psychiatry«. Particularly now, when the old mistrust of this clinic is beginning to flare up again at a most inconvenient time, it would perhaps be advisable to counter this tendency with such a name change.« I would also like to add that the word »psychiatry« is almost never applied correctly by the population and for this reason it would be appropriate to use a more generally understandable term.

In a discussion today with Professor Schittenhelm and Professor Stepp, I received their agreement to this request. Both gentlemen have no objections against the Psychiatric and Clinic for Nervous Diseases being known in future as the Clinic for Nervous Diseases.

Bumke«

◼ **Fig. 9.13.** *Continued*

In 1940 when it leaked out that psychiatric patients had been killed in certain psychiatric institutions, Bumke discussed these atrocities with his very close former colleague, A. Bostroem, who had become head of the hospital in Leipzig in the meantime.

Both men had been informed in writing by K. Jaspersen, who worked as assistant to Bumke from 1924–1927. As head of the department of neurology at the deaconess asylum in Bethel, Jaspersen had been asked to fill out »forms«, but rejected this request and tried to get prominent psychiatrists to give statements against »euthanasia«. Bostroem informed Jaspersen that he agreed and that Bumke »would definitely give his opinion if asked«. Nothing is known about this. Bumke did, however, not allow his patients to be transferred to the asylum Haar-Eglfing, as it had become known that patients from Haar were transferred to »death asylums« (Grafeneck, Brandenburg, Hartheim, Sonnenstein). Without being able to transfer patients, the clinic very quickly became overcrowded and finally patients had to be transferred to Haar-Eglfing.

It seems that Bumke became more and more of the opinion that it was useless to say what he thought in public and to resist, as »it would not have been helpful to anyone«. It is also most likely that in case of Bumke's resignation, Ernst Rüdin, who already belonged to the Munich medical faculty as ordinary professor of psychiatry and who had great political clout due to his ideas on racial hygiene, would have become Bumke's successor (▶ Chapter 7).

Bumke was later criticized for his conduct. The time between his dismissal as clinic director and his reinstatement as ordinary professor – which actually did not happen due to his age – was dominated by a very controversial discussion on the matter, typical for the post-war period. Bumke was not reproached for being directly involved in the activities of the Nazis, or in the various campaigns against the mentally ill, but was criticized for not having taken a determined, public stand against the activities of the Nazi regime. In the opinion of his critics, his position as occupant of the »first and foremost psychiatric chair in Germany« and his reputation meant that his public support for the rights of the mentally ill would not only have strengthened the cause, but the Nazis would not have dared to do anything against him. This controversial debate was held in public and partly in the press. Most of Bumke's earlier assistants, but also former patients and their families took his side.

It is also well-known that the hospital doctors ignored rules from the authorities in favour of the patients. For example, the use of insulin for the treatment of the mentally ill – the insulin »cure« was mainly used in cases of schizophrenia – was stopped with a resolution of the Reich's Minister for Science and National Education of 04.02.1942 and could only be used for diabetics. All the same, the insulin treatments – although in a reduced form – were still given at the clinic until the summer of 1944 and beyond – as long as insulin was available.

The End of the War

During the war the various university clinics had been considerably damaged by air raids: certain clinics (e.g. the Dental Clinic) was almost completely destroyed. The building of the »clinic for nervous disorders« survived the bombardments better than most of the other neighbouring clinics (the Medical, Surgical Clinics and Ophthalmic Clinics); but the psychiatric clinic was affected and had to offer space to the other clinics more damaged than itself.

One explosive bomb did considerable damage to the east wing of the clinic (constructed in 1926), with the clinic chapel and the floor below including the living and sleeping rooms for the nuns. Fire bombs also hit the clinic on several occasions and caused a fire in various attic areas. The living quarters of the clinic director were also badly damaged by a large air mine which struck Goethestrasse 55 (south of the west wing). The worst damage was caused by a liquid fire bomb which luckily did not explode, but hit the roof, attic and the underlying floors in the west part of the main building, right behind the doors to the wards for male patients, and created a hole, 9-meters in diameter, through all the floors.

In 1943 parts of the clinic were moved to the cure and care asylum Haar. Bumke made sure that the wards and function areas of the clinic remained separate from those of the asylum. In 1944 the removals

Sonderabdruck aus:

Richtlinien für Schwangerschaftsunterbrechung und Unfruchtbarmachung
aus gesundheitlichen Gründen

Herausgegeben von der

Reichsärztekammer

Bearbeitet von
Dr. Hans Stadler

Mit 94 Abbildungen

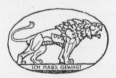

J. F. Lehmanns Verlag / München 1936

◨ **Fig. 9.14.** O. Bumke writes in »Guidelines on abortion and sterilization for health reasons«, 1936, that he sees no indication for abortion in the mentally ill

7.

Unterbrechung der Schwangerschaft aus medizinischen Gründen bei Geistes- und Nervenkranken.

Von Oswald Bumke, München.

Es soll hier nur über die medizinischen Indikationen gesprochen werden, die Geistes- und Nervenkrankheiten für die Unterbrechung einer Schwangerschaft abgeben können. Dies ist ausdrücklich zu betonen, denn es gibt kein Gebiet der klinischen Medizin, in dem sich medizinische, soziale und eugenische Gründe für die Schwangerschaftsunterbrechung so vielfach durchflechten wie hier, und zugleich keines, in dem medizinische Gründe so häufig zu Unrecht vorgeschützt werden, wenn man eugenische oder soziale nicht nennen kann oder will.

Daß medizinische Indikationen für die Schwangerschaftsunterbrechung jetzt gesetzlich anerkannt sind, ist auf das wärmste zu begrüßen; denn es ist sinnlos, eines Paragraphen wegen eine Frau sterben und ihr Kind mit ihr zugrundegehen zu lassen, und es ist nicht viel besser, wenn eine Mutter siech werden muß, nur damit vorher noch ein gewöhnlich auch nicht widerstandsfähiges Kind zur Welt kommen kann. Aber wir wollen nicht vergessen, einmal: auch das Kind im Mutterleib ist ein lebendiger Mensch, und weiter: auch durch Aborte sind unendlich viele Mütter siech gemacht, d. h. körperlich und seelisch schwer geschädigt worden. Namentlich wenn eine Frau mehrere Aborte hintereinander über sich ergehen lassen muß, wird sie körperlich und seelisch auf das äußerste geschwächt. Ihr Gefühlsleben wird verändert; jede normale geschlechtliche Einstellung und jedes natürliche Verhältnis zur Frage der Mutterschaft werden erstickt, und so werden Ehe und Familienglück auch da untergraben, wo die Mutter nicht zugleich früh gealtert, verbraucht und für spätere Geburten ebenso unfähig gemacht worden ist wie für die Arbeit und für die Erziehung schon vorhandener Kinder.

Aber wir werden das Problem der Abtreibung noch in einem viel weiteren Rahmen sehen, es viel allgemeineren Gesichtspunkten unterordnen müssen. Vor bald fünfundzwanzig Jahren habe ich in einem Referat auf der Naturforscherversammlung in Karlsruhe[1]) gefragt: Woran gehen denn Völker zugrunde? „Wenn wir die Kette der Erscheinungen" (beim Untergang der Griechen und Römer), hieß die Antwort, „rückläufig verfolgen, so bildet ihr letztes Glied unzweifelhaft das Aussterben, die quantitative Abnahme der Bevölkerung. Die Nation verliert die physische Kraft, ihre Stellung äußeren Feinden gegenüber zu behaupten. . . . Entscheidend war für Rom und Hellas der gleiche Vorgang, der das heutige Europa wieder

---

[1]) Über nervöse Entartung. Berlin, Springer. 1912. S. 76.

▫ **Fig. 9.14.** *Continued*

»7. Abortion during pregnancy for medical reasons in the mentally ill.

By Oswald Bumke, Munich

Only the medical indications for aborting a pregnancy in cases of mental disease will be discussed here. This must be emphasized in particular, as there is no other area in clinical medicine, where the medical, social and eugenic grounds as so complicated as here, and at the same time no other area, where medical reasons are quoted so incorrectly, in order to avoid mentioning social or eugenic reasons.

It must be welcomed that medical indications for an abortion are now anchored in the law; as it is senseless to let a woman and her child die just because of a paragraph, and it is not much better that a woman must suffer in order to deliver a healthy child. But we do not want to forget, that firstly the child in the mother's womb is a living being, and furthermore, that with abortion countless women become seriously ill, e.g. physically and mentally. Especially when a woman has had to have several abortions, one after the other, she will become physically and mentally very weak. Her emotional life changes: every normal sexual attitude and every natural relationship to motherhood is suppressed and thus, the marital and family life erodes, whereby the mother ages prematurely and becomes incapable of work and bringing her up existing children.

But we must see abortion in a much broader context and not just according to general aspects. About 25 years ago in a talk given at a scientists' meeting in Karlsruhe* I asked: What was the cause of the downfall of various races? The answer was: »If we follow the chain of events (on the downfall of the Greeks and Romans), the last occurrence was most definitely extinction, the reduction of numbers of a race. The nation loses its physical power, its ability to compete with the external enemy….. The same process, which is affecting Europe today, was decisive for Rome and Hellas«….

* About nervous degeneration. Berlin, Springer. 1912, p. 76«

◨ **Fig. 9.14.** *Continued*

continued and finally 150 patients were placed in Haar. But these measures remained insufficient and the situation for the patients and staff in the building on the Nussbaumstrasse became more and more difficult. In the autumn of 1944 and the beginning of the winter 1944/1945 the clinic staff was often more occupied with taking care of or provisionally repairing damage to the building (broken pipes due to the cold, damage to the heating, cracks in the building, damage to windows and doors) than taking care of the patients. The back up capacity in Haar was already over the limit and other buildings for clinic use had to be found. Finally in the last winter of the war, the clinic's neurological wards and the army's neurological hospital, which had been located in the clinc, were relocated. The necessary space was found in the valley of Lake Tegern. The clinic patients were accommodated in the »Bahnhotel« (station hotel) in Tegernsee, later also in Hotel Bachmair in Rottach-Egern. The clinic's x-ray equipment was relocated to Tegernsee and in January 1945 Bumke himself moved to Tegernsee. Dr. H. Bitterauf (Mrs) stayed behind in the damaged clinic as senior consultant. She was in charge of a small admissions department and an out-patient department. In Tegernsee Drs W. and H. Grohmann, a married couple, were in charge

of the neurological department of the clinic, which had been moved there. The neurological military hospital was managed by K.F. Scheid.

Karl Friedrich Scheid (◨ Fig. 9.15) was born in 1906 and became assistant at the German Research Institute for Psychiatry in 1931. In the same year

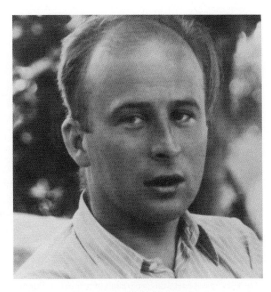

◨ **Fig. 9.15.** Karl Friedrich Scheid (1906–1945)

Studien
zur pathologischen Physiologie des Liquor cerebrospinalis.

I. Mitteilung.

Elektrische (kataphoretische) Trennung der Eiweißkörper im Liquor cerebrospinalis von entzündlichen Erkrankungen des Nervensystems, ein Beitrag zur pathologischen Physiologie der meningealen und cerebralen Blutgefäße.

Von

K. F. und L. Scheid.

Mit 23 Textabbildungen.

(Eingegangen am 11. November 1943.)

A. Einleitung.

Die Liquordiagnostik verdankt ihren großen Aufschwung der Einführung der heute gebräuchlichen *Laboratoriumstechnik*, die seit fast drei Jahrzehnten nur wenig modifiziert, unentbehrliches Hilfsmittel der Klinik geworden ist. Wenn sich auch die Beschreibung der Liquorbefunde bei den einzelnen Nervenkrankheiten im Laufe der Zeit erheblich vervollkommnet hat, so fehlte uns aber bisher jede Sicherheit, wenn es sich darum handelte, diese Befunde pathologisch-physiologisch zu erklären und damit mittelbar zu einem tieferen Verständnis der pathologischen Vorgänge bei jenen Erkrankungen zu kommen.

Eine solche Vertiefung unserer Erkenntnis ist wesentlich an die Einführung und den Ausbau *neuartiger Untersuchungsmethoden und experimenteller Möglichkeiten* [1] gebunden, da die bisher vorliegende Technik wichtige Fragen nicht sicher zu entscheiden vermag. Es sei nur auf das Problem der Herkunft der Eiweißkörper im Liquor und die sich daraus ergebenden Folgerungen für die pathologische Physiologie der cerebralen und meningealen Blutgefäße hingewiesen. Eine Klärung dieser Frage würde gerade der Klinik neue Anregungen geben.

Es hat in den letzten beiden Jahrzehnten nicht an Versuchen gefehlt, neue experimentelle Wege für die Liquorforschung zu suchen. Die Ausbeute an neuen Erkenntnissen blieb aber im allgemeinen gering [2]. *Das methodische Rüstzeug der normalen und pathologischen Liquorphysiologie ist bemerkenswert rückständig und starr geblieben*, wenn man die moderne

---

[1] Herrn Geheimrat *Bumke* sind wir für die großzügige Unterstützung unserer Arbeiten zu ganz besonderem Dank verpflichtet. Außerdem wurde die Arbeit durch Mittel der Münchener Universitätsgesellschaft unterstützt.

[2] Siehe z. B. *F. Roeder:* Die physikalischen Methoden der Liquordiagnostik, Berlin 1937.

◻ **Fig. 9.16.** Publication by K. F. Scheid and his wife, L. Scheid, on »Studies on the pathological physiology in liquor cerebrospinalis« (Arch. Psychiat. Nervenkr. 117, p. 219–250 (1944)
»Electrical (cataphoretical) separation of proteins in liquor cerebrospinalis in inflammatory diseases of the nervous system; a contribution on the pathological physiology of meningeal and cerebral blood vessels«

Kurt Schneider (1887–1967) had taken over the clinical departments of the Research Institute from J. Lange (see above) which was the psychiatric department of the municipal hospital Schwabing at the same time. K.F. Scheid became senior consultant to K. Schneider. On the outbreak of war Scheid was drafted as health officer. He was put to work in various military hospitals and finally transferred in 1940 to the »military hospital for nervous disorders«, which was accommodated in rooms of the Munich clinic. A. Bannwarth was the head of this »military hospital for nervous disorders« as well as Bumke's clinical senior consultant and head of the x-ray department at the Munic clinic. When K. F. Scheid was transferred to the »military hospital for nervous disorders«, the Munich clinic was almost laid bare of medical staff and consequently K.F. Scheid took over the additional function of clinical senior consultant, and in addition Bumke gave him the job of head of the chemical and serological laboratories. By combining his various functions, K.F. Scheid worked at the Munich clinic from 1940 until 1945.

Scheid managed to reanimate research activities at the clinic, which had become more difficult from year to year: Together with his wife, Lotte Scheid-Seidl, he did »studies on the pathological physiology of liquor cerebrospinalis« (amongst others by using the first »electrophoretic (cataphoretic) separation of protein in liquor cerebrospinalis«), which were even published during the war in 1944 (◘ Fig. 9.16). These ground-breaking, first electrophoretic studies of proteins in liquor, done by K.F. Scheid, were never really appreciated in the light of their historical importance.

K.F. Scheid's destiny was linked to the war in a most tragic way. At the beginning of May 1945, when the American army reached the valley of Lake Tegern from the north, which was overcrowded with military hospitals, hospital wards and refugees, K.F. Scheid, accompanied by a doctor and translator with a white flag, walked towards the approaching Americans. His aim was to negotiate the capitulation of the valley with the Americans. During his courageous attempt to save the valley of Lake Tegern from any type of military action, K.F. Scheid was shot in the back on May 4, 1945, probably by SS-troops, and died from his wounds shortly afterwards. The valley was spared any further aggression.

In memory of K.F. Scheid, the saviour of the valley of Lake Tegern, a square in Schwabing/Munich has been named after him: »Scheid-Platz«.

Literature

Bumke, O. (1927): Die Psychiatrische und Nervenklinik in München. MMW 47, p. 332-333

Bumke, O. (1952): Erinnerungen und Betrachtungen. Der Weg eines deutschen Psychiaters. Richard Pflaum-Verlag: Munich

V. Cranach, M., Siemen, H.-L. (Eds.) (1999): Die Bayerischen Heil- und Pflegeanstalten in der Zeit des Nationalsozialismus. R. Oldenbourg Verlag: Munich

Klee, E. (1983): Euthanasie im NS-Staat. Die »Vernichtung lebensunwerten Lebens«. S. Fischer Verlag: Frankfurt/Main

Schimmelpenning, G.W. (1993): Oswald Bumke (1877–1950). His life and work. History of Psychiatry 4, p. 483-497

10

The Post-War Period and Beginning of the Hospital's Reconstruction under Georg Stertz

When the Americans occupied Munich on April 30, 1945, only a provisional, emergency set-up was running in the building on the Nussbaumstrasse.

In 1943/44 several of the clinic's wards had been transferred to the asylum in Haar. In January 1945 the rest of the clinic had been moved to the valley of Lake Tegern. Oswald Bumke had also moved to Lake Tegern and managed the clinic, parts of which were located in different places.

The situation in the Nussbaumstrasse only normalized slowly after the war. The most necessary repairs were carried out with simple means and only on parts of the building essential for the running of the clinic. Beds were put up and slowly, but surely the clinic received new patients. During the last months of war Dr. H. Bitterauf (Mrs) was senior consultant and responsible for the admission ward and the out-patient clinic in the Nussbaumstrasse. O. Bumke returned from the valley of Lake Tegern at the beginning of June 1945 and managed the clinic in Munich.

Shortly after the war had ended, former doctors returned to Munich to start work again. They were only allowed to start work once they had been checked with regard to their political attitude; there was a general hiring-stop and only a few exceptions were made. It was not until a denazification process proved without doubt that a candidate was politically »innocent«, that a person could be considered for a re-employment or new employment as assistant doctor.

Like in other German universities, students in Munich, returning from the war, urged to be accepted for study in the winter term 1945/1946.

Since O. Bumke (▶ Chapter 8) was considered to be politically »innocent«, was been asked – in agreement with the occupying forces – to assist with the reconstruction of the university.

In the autumn of 1945 a newspaper article was published in Switzerland, seriously accusing Bumke of allegedly having close contacts to the Nazis. Consequently at the beginning of December 1945, the occupying forces suspended Bumke as director of the clinic and all other university offices. A denazification process began. Because it was clear from the beginning that the denazification process would be a lengthy matter, the university and medical faculty had to look for a replacement immediately: a professionally suitable, politically correct university lecturer who would be capable of taking over the clinic provisionally and be competent with regard to the rebuilding as well as giving lectures on psychiatry and neurology of students.

A solution was found quickly. In February 1946 Georg Stertz became provisional head of the clinic.

O. Bumke's denazification process lasted until 1947. When the accusations proved to be without grounds, he was rehabilitated and reinstated in office as of April 16, 1947 as ordinary professor and director of the clinic for nervous diseases. Since he was 70 years old now he turned down the reinstatement and went into retirement, keeping the official residence at the clinic until his death on January 5, 1950.

With O. Bumke's retirement, G. Stertz's two-year provisional management of the clinic came to an end, he became ordinary professor for psychiatry and nervous diseases and director of the Munich clinic for psychiatry and neurology. He headed the clinic for a further 5 years, in total 7 years, until 1952.

Georg Stertz
Professor of Psychiatry and Nervous Diseases of the University of Munich (1946–1952)

Georg Stertz (◘ Fig. 10), oldest son of a business man, was born in Breslau on December 19, 1878. After school and studies in Freiburg, Munich and Breslau he graduated in 1903 in Breslau. He began his clinical training at the institutes for pathology at the universities of Hamburg and Freiburg. He became assistant doctor to Max Nonne for two years (1904–1906) at the Eppendorf hospital in Hamburg.

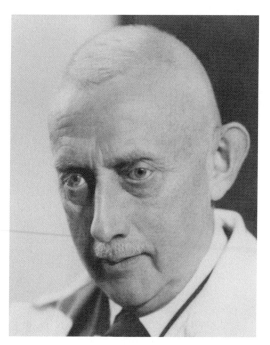

◘ **Fig. 10.1.** Georg Stertz (1878–1959)

At this time, Max Nonne's clinic was one of the most important research institutions in the field of neurology; after the founding of the University of Hamburg in 1919, it became one of the first separate university clinics for neurology in Germany.

> Max Nonne (1861–1959), the best of his year (1879) at the humanistic secondary school, Johanneum, in Hamburg, studied in Heidelberg, Freiburg and Berlin. He set up a practice as psychiatrist and neurologist and was also an external assistant at the clinic for dermatology in Hamburg where he acquired in-depth knowledge of all forms of syphilis and neurolues. Prior to this he was the youngest student of Wilhelm Heinrich Erb (1840–1921) in Heidelberg; in Hamburg he was the founder of neurology: as of 1896 he he was the head of the 2nd department for internal medicine at the Eppendorf hospital, which later became the »Department of Neurology«. When the Hamburg university was founded, Nonne became personal professor in ordinary in 1919, regular professor in ordinary in 1925 as well as director of the clinic for neurology. Nonne retired in 1934; he died at the age of 99 years.

M. Nonne considered G. Stertz to be one of his best students; as Nonne emphasizes in his memoirs, he noticed Stertz's »serious will to research and absolute reliability«. As Nonne had no possibility of giving his assistants postdoctoral lecturer qualifications prior to the founding of the university, and as the regulations of »General Hospital Eppendorf« only allowed for assistants to work there for up to two years, Stertz could only stay for two years with Nonne. Following Eppendorf and his time with Nonne, Stertz had »learnt the basics of neurology and psychiatry« and had »discovered his appreciation of this special subject«, Stertz went to the Charité in Berlin temporarily and then finally to Breslau in 1907. In his home-town Breslau Stertz became assistant to K. Bonhoeffer (1868–1948), who had taken over the Breslau clinic in 1904 as successor to C. Wernicke. Under Bonhoeffer's influence in Breslau, Stertz worked mainly on psychiatric problems. In 1910 he joined Alexander Westphal (1863–1941) in Bonn, received his postdoctoral qualifications there and returned to the Breslau clinic in 1912, where Alois Alzheimer had become director in the meantime. G. Stertz became

Alzheimer's senior consultant and managed the clinic provisionally after Alzheimer's early death in 1915 until O. Bumke took over the chair of psychiatry at Breslau in 1917. G. Stertz remained a further two years in Breslau as Bumke's senior consultant, before receiving an offer from E. Kraepelin in 1919 to go to Munich.

Following the founding of the German Research Institute (▶ Chapter 9), E. Rüdin remained clinical senior consultant in addition to his duties at the Research Institute and consequently Kraepelin looked for a clinically, particularly experienced co-worker to replace E. Rüdin. By filling this job, Kraepelin also wanted to fulfill a further plan: He wanted to employ a senior consultant with experience in neurology. He considered Stertz to be very suitable, based on his clinical and scientific development with M. Nonne, K. Bonhoeffer, A. Westphal and A. Alzheimer. Stertz accepted Kraepelin's offer, although he only stayed in Munich for two years; in 1921 he was offered a job in Marburg and became director of the clinic for nervous diseases there.

When Stertz left Munich in 1921, he did not realize that his later professional life and personal destiny would be tied to Munich and finally take him back there.

During his time in Brelau Stertz made the acquaintance of Alzheimer's eldest daughter and shortly afterwards (1915) they married. Therefore, Stertz's ties to the Alzheimer family were very strong and remained so even after Alzheimer's death. When Stertz worked for two years in Munich after the First World War, he and his family had the use of a beautiful, large house on the Lake of Wessling, where they could relax and enjoy themselves. A. Alzheimer had purchased the house and it remained family property after his death. Stertz did not realize that this house would become a refuge in bad times for his family and himself.

After leaving the Munich clinic in 1921, Stertz followed the further developments with particular interest, sympathy and sometimes most likely with apprehension.

In Breslau a very good collegial and personal relationship lasting for years, had developed between A. Alzheimer's successor, O. Bumke, and G. Stertz. Bumke and Stertz were about the same age and on the whole had complementary opinions from a professional point of view. Both of them were of the opinion that psychiatric clinics should develop into »clinics for nervous diseases« through the inclusion of neurology. However, in this matter they did not agree with Kraepelin. All the same, Kraepelin was Stertz's admired »master«, in particular after two years of working together. From his position in Marburg Stertz watched on as it came to tensions between Kraepelin and Bumke concerning the matter of succession. In the letters to Bumke during this time it is evident how Stertz tried to make Bumke understand Kraepelin's comments and reactions and it is obvious how these must have irritated Bumke (15 such letters are in the Psychiatry-Historical Collection of the Munich Clinic).

In this situation Stertz proved to be a person, who – with great loyalty, as Nonne had already noticed – tried to find a solution and mutual understanding in a reliable and altruistic manner.

G. Stertz managed the clinic in Marburg from 1921 until 1926 when he took over the chair for psychiatry in Kiel; in 1931 he turned down an offer to go to Bonn as successor to his tutor, Alexander Westphal, and remained in Kiel.

Georg Stertz worked on many topics in the border regions between psychiatry and neurology (amongst others clinical problems of symptomatic psychoses and aphasias). He gained an ever increasing reputation with his studies on »Periodical fluctuation of the brain function«, in particular with studies on the »Extrapyramidal symptom complexes« and the »Functional organization of the extrapyramidal system«. With a study »On the lowering of the personality level as a functional disorder and as a defect symptom« and finally with the publication of the »Interbrain syndrome« he worked on problems, still of topical interest nowadays, although the name of Georg Stertz is often left unmentioned.

Since the beginning of the Nazi regime Stertz had been confronted with increasing difficulties, which finally culminated in his being forced to leave office. He would have had to inform the Reich's Ministry for Education that his wife, Gertrud, and daughter of Alzheimer, had a Jewish mother. In a letter to Bumke in Munich at the beginning of September 1937 (◘ Fig. 10.2) Stertz wrote that he had »prematurely reached the end of his professional career«: »Around mid May I

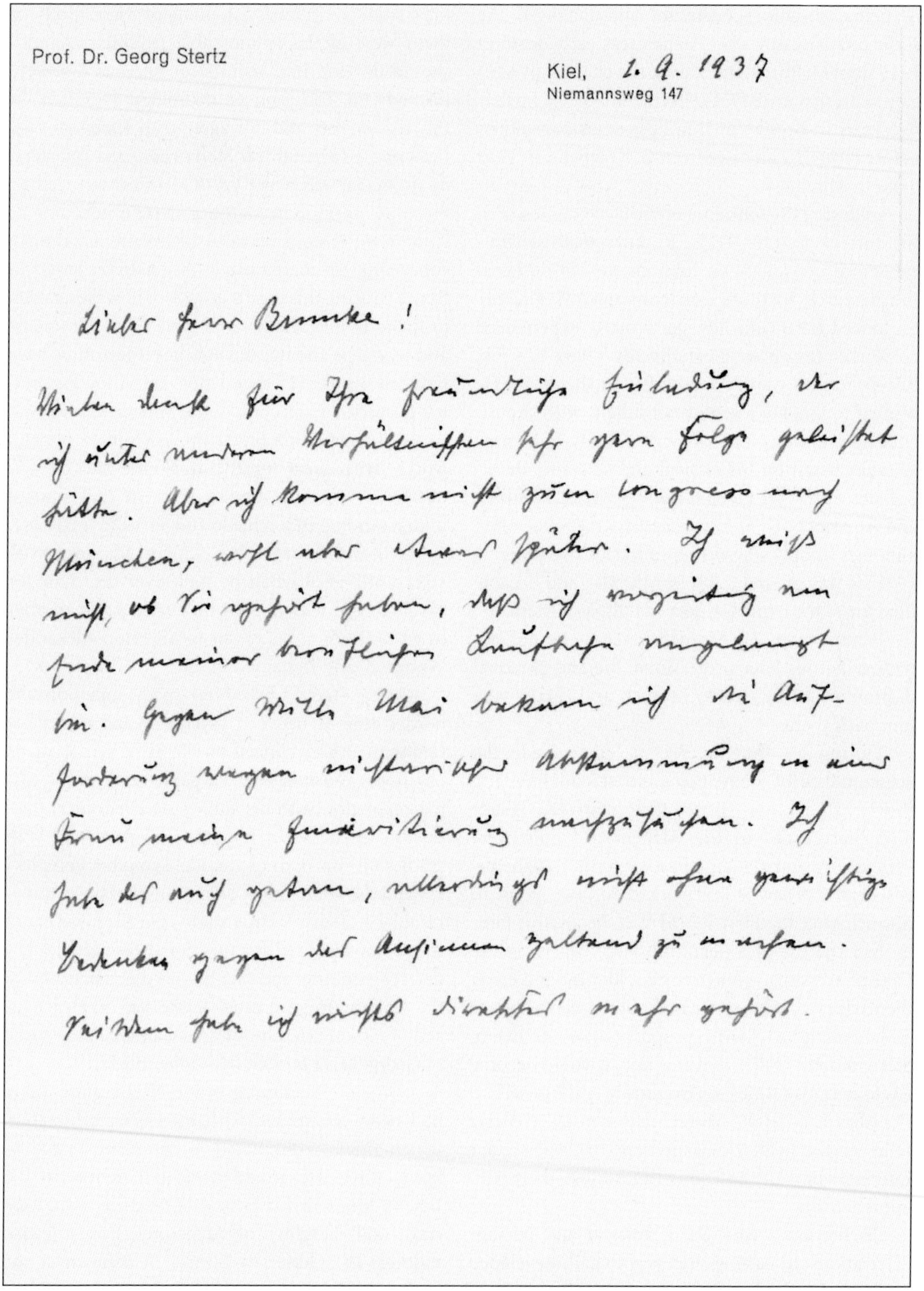
Prof. Dr. Georg Stertz

Kiel, 1. 9. 1937
Niemannsweg 147

Lieber Herr Bumke!

Vielen Dank für Ihre freundliche Einladung, der ich unter anderen Verhältnissen sehr gern Folge geleistet hätte. Aber ich komme nicht zum Kongress nach München, wohl aber etwas später. Ich weiss nicht, ob Sie gehört haben, dass ich vorzeitig am Ende meiner beruflichen Laufbahn angelangt bin. Gegen Mitte Mai bekam ich die Aufforderung wegen nichtarischer Abstammung meiner Frau meine Pensionierung nachzusuchen. Ich habe das auch getan, allerdings nicht ohne gewichtige Bedenken gegen das Ansinnen geltend zu machen. Seitdem habe ich nichts darüber mehr gehört.

Fig. 10.2. Letter of September 1, 1937 from G. Stertz to O. Bumke, informing him that he had been forced to retire due to his non-Aryan wife

Indirekt ist mir das delphische Orakel bekannt geworden, daß die „Marktstützung u. Hesses Lungenzustand sei, daß aber ein „Fernmeldeärztliche" schwieriger Fall vorliege. Dieser Meinung bin ich für meinen Teil zwar nicht, wohl aber wirkt sich die Verzögerung der Entscheidung – als Termin war der 1. Oktober gedacht – natürlich für uns sehr unangenehm aus. So befinden wir uns augenblicklich in einem Freiballon-artigen Zustand und wissen nur, daß wir in Wessling landen werden, wo unser Haus als dauernder Wohnsitz hergerichtet wird. Auch lernt meine Frau das Auteln, damit wir – soweit erforderlich – mit der größeren Welt in Verbindung bleiben. Da alle Dinge 2 Seiten haben, sind wir mit unserem Schicksal schon ganz ausgesöhnt.

Das ist also in Kürze der Grund, weshalb ich im September nicht nach München komme und weshalb ich auch nicht an den [illegible] Ehrungen teilnehmen kann, durch welche der [illegible] einer 70 jährigen Jubiläums bei Ihnen gefeiert werden wird.

Lassen Sie uns Ihnen schon heute unsere herzlichsten Glückwünsche dazu aussprechen. Sobald wir unsere Residenz in W. bezogen haben, werde ich mich bei Ihnen melden und werde Sie in Erinnerung alter schöner Zeiten um gute Nachbarschaft mit uns bitten. Mit vielen guten Wünschen und Grüßen an Sie beiden

Stets Ihr getreuer

G. Hertz

Fig. 10.2. *Continued*

»Kiel, 1.9.1937

Dear Mr. Bumke!

Many thanks for your kind invitation, which I would have gladly accepted under different circumstances. However, I will not be coming to Munich for the congress, although I may come a bit later. I am not sure if you have heard that I have prematurely arrived at the end of my professional career. Around mid May I was ordered to apply for retirement due to my wife's non-Aryan origin. So, that is what I did, although not without considerable doubts about the whole matter. Since then I have received no further or direct information.

Indirectly, I have made the acquaintance of the oracle of Delphi, who let me know that the »esteem« of my person is untouchable, but that it is »technically and legally« a difficult matter. Of course I am not of the same opinion, but the delay with respect to the decision – the deadline was October 1 – is very inconvenient for us. We find ourselves in a kind of floating-balloon-situation and only know that we will land in Wessling, where our house is equipped as a long-term domicile. My wife has also learned how to type, so that we – as far as possible – can remain in touch with the outside world. There being two aspects to all these things, we have reconciled ourselves with our destiny. That is also the reason why I am not coming to Munich and why I cannot participate in the probable distinctions to celebrate another annulus. We would like to express our best wishes. As soon as we have taken up residence in Wessling, I will be in touch and in remembrance of the good old times will remain your good neighbour.

Yours sincerely

G. Stertz«

◻ **Fig. 10.2.** *Continued*

was requested to retire due to my wife's non-Arian origins. I have done this, although not without mentioning my serious doubts about this request«. On October 1, 1937, Georg Stertz – not even 60 years of age – went into forced retirement. He left Kiel and led a secluded life with his family in the Alzheimer's house at Lake Wessling.

During the last months of the war he no longer received salary payments and for economic reasons Stertz had to consider starting work again as a doctor. A job as a psychiatrist at one of the Munich hospitals seemed to be most promising; in June 1945 he asked O. Bumke for his advice and assistance (letter of June 24, 1945), but without success.

Bumke's dismissal in December 1945 led to a surprising turn in fortune for Stertz; in February 1946 he was given the provisional management of the Munich clinic. At the end of 1947 he – who had retired from Kiel in 1937 under humiliating circumstances – was given a full professorship by the Munich faculty. He retired when he was almost 74 years of age. He died in Munich on March 19, 1959.

Together with his co-workers Georg Stertz initiated the re-building of the clinic during the most difficult post-war period (◻ Fig. 10.3).

Beginning of the Clinic's Rebuilding

In August 1947 the psychiatric wards, which had been relocated to Haar in 1943, were brought back to the Munich clinic. In 1947 the backup clinic at the station hotel in Tegernsee was dissolved. Room had to be made for neurological patients to be once again admitted to the clinic in the Nussbaumstrasse. The X-ray department, which had also been moved to Tegernsee, also had to be brought back to Munich; in order to make room, what had formerly been Alzheimer's microscopy laboratory was turned into a large ward.

Work began on the rebuilding of the east wing in 1947. Half of the entire ground floor was used by the dental clinic (until 1950), as it would be a while before the new building for the dental clinic in the Goethestrasse would be complete. The con-

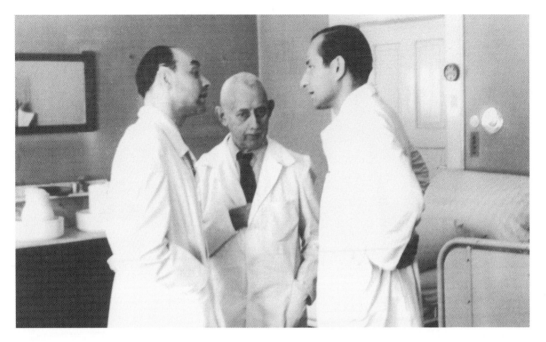

◻ **Fig. 10.3.** G. Stertz with co-workers (on the right: P. Matussek)

crete safety screens, which had been erected in the ground floor rooms of the clinic, were not taken away until the dental clinic moved out.

In spite of the constantly increasing shortage of rooms, more and more patients had to be admitted. During 1950 almost 5,700 patients were treated as in-patients.

From 1948 until 1950 all crates containing all kinds of equipment, such as books from the library and a large part of the case histories and files were finally returned to the clinic. Unfortunately, by storing the crates in different places, a large amount of clinic belongings disappeared (e.g. case histories from the years prior to 1926).

During the post-war years lectures were in great demand. Following the currency reform 400 to 500 students attended lectures and as the lecture theatre did not have capacity to hold such numbers, the lectures during the terms of 1948 to 1950 had to be given twice.

G. Stertz did all he could to lessen any plight and in this manner did all he could to enable those, who returned from the war or even internship, to begin or continue their training in psychiatry and neurology. All former co-workers of the clinic, who returned to Munich, were reinstated at the clinic. Stertz employed more than 70 assistants, which was a problem, because many of the assistants could not be paid appropriately for their work. Stertz used the additional income from the constant inflow of patients to pay the staff and the construction work on the clinic.

Co-Workers of Georg Stertz in Munich

Max Mikorey (1899–1977) (◻ Fig. 10.4) came from a well-known Munich artist family. After studying medicine, he became assistant in 1929 and later (1935) senior consultant to O. Bumke at the clinic for nervous diseases. He qualified as professor in 1942. During the Second World War he was consultant psychiatrist on the East Front where he was taken prisoner. After a daring escape it took him a while to return to Munich from Russia. Stertz immediately gave him back his old job as senior consultant, which he kept until 1968. Mikorey had a particularly good reputation in post-war Munich due to his work as an expert to the courts and his

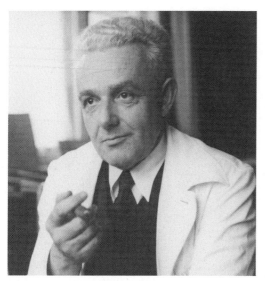

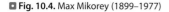
Fig. 10.4. Max Mikorey (1899–1977)

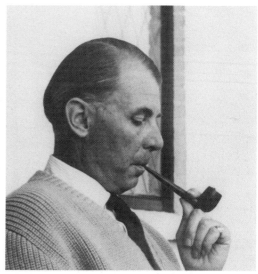
Fig. 10.5. Werner Wagner (1904–1956)

very popular lectures on medical psychology and forensic psychiatry. It has since been forgotten that at about the same time as I.L. von Meduna (1896–1964) and U. Cerletti (1877–1963) Mikorey also pointed out the therapeutic possibilities of shock therapy for schizophrenics.

From 1948–1949 Werner Wagner (1904–1956) (**Fig. 10.5) worked at the Munich clinic as a senior consultant to Stertz. Wagner, who had qualified as professor in 1930 in Breslau with J. Lange, became provisional director of the Breslau clinic for two years after Lange's death. In 1940 he went to A. Bostroem in Leipzig as senior consultant and, following Bostroem's departure for Strassburg in 1942, he was provisional head for the second time. After the war, Wagner left Leipzig for Munich and become senior consultant to Stertz. Wagner had manifold interests, in particular the fundaments of psychiatry with regard to the humanities, with psychopathological phenomena and with existential analysis. He tried to characterize his clinical home position with his concept of »brain psychopathology«. In 1949 he became successor to Kurt Schneider as director of the Clinical Institute of the German Research Institute for Psychiatry in Munich.

Shortly after the war Bumke employed Max Kaess (1907–1994) (**Fig. 10.7) as assistant; he became a close co-worker of Stertz and promoted to university lecturer in 1950. Kaess worked at the clinic for 25 years. Later he became the first ordinary professor of psychiatry and held the chair of psychiatry at the medical faculty of the Technical University of Munich (▶ Chapter 11 and 12).

In 1951 Ludwig Baumer (1908–1977) qualified as professor with Stertz. With an interval for military service Baumer had worked for K. Schneider in the clinical department of the German Research Institute at Schwabing Hospital from 1936–1947, before he became senior consultant with Stertz in 1947. In 1951 Baumer became Head of the Municipal Clinic for Nervous Diseases in Bamberg, where he stayed for 25 years.

Hubert Tellenbach (1914–1994) worked at the Munich clinic from 1945 until 1950 and then joined K. Schneider in Heidelberg. Tellenbach had already worked for Bumke as a voluntary doctor and was reinstated by him immediately after the war.

Helmut Stolze (born 1917) was also employed by Bumke as voluntary doctor immediately after the war, but left the clinic again a few months later. Stolze graduated at the clinic during the war. In 1948 he returned to the hospital only and worked as scientific assistant to Stertz for four years (1948–1952). He then opened a practice as psychiatrist and neurologist and made a considerable contribution to the development of psychotherapy in Munich; he was responsible for the organization of the »Psychotherapy Weeks in Lindau« for many years.

In the Munich clinic's staff records numerous names appear from Stertz's term of office of doctors who made a considerable contribution to the re-establishment of psychiatry in Munich and Upper Bavaria during the decades after the war – some were practising psychiatrists (L. Broichhausen, H.F. Eiden, F. Eisheuer, E. Goebel, I. Lehle, K.-Th. Ruckdeschel and many others), others took over managerial positions in district hospitals (L. Achner, E. Schinner), the Heckscher Clinic (F. Meinnertz), in a clinic for persons with brain injuries (O. Mistler), at the health authorities (H. Keller) and other public authorities. One is also confronted with names having nothing to do with the Munich clinic during Stertz's term of office, like for example the psychoanalyst Paul Matussek, and the neurochemist Horst Jatzkewitz, who became known as prominent scientists and members of the Max-Planck Institute.

Stertz's term of office was really the starting point for two working directions, which would define the profile of the Munich Clinic for Nervous Diseases for a long time:

Robert Weber set up an EEG laboratory in 1951. Weber remained at the clinic until Stertz's retirement in 1955 and then left to take over a job with the technical monitoring instance for Upper Bavaria in Munich; he later opened a practice in Innsbruck. The EEG laboratory set up by Weber was later taken over by Johannes Kugler (born 1922) during Kolle's term of office, he developed it into a training instance for clinical neurophysiology of national and international renown (▶ Chapter 11 and 13).

Kurt Decker also played a considerable role in the development of the Munich clinic after the war.

Kurt Decker (1921–1985) (◘ Fig. 10.6) became assistant to G. Stertz in 1946. When the »X-ray department« (originally founded by Bannwarth), which had been relocated to Tegernsee during the war, returned to the clinic in the Nussbaumstrasse and had to be reinstalled there under difficult circumstances, G. Stertz handed over the task to young assistant, K. Decker. Under Decker's guidance the »X-ray department« quickly became

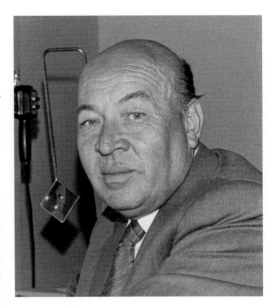

◘ **Fig. 10.6.** Kurt Decker (1921–1985)

a »department for neuroradiology«, which soon became well-known outside Germany's borders. Decker qualified as professor with Stertz and under Kolle further expanded the »department for neuroradiology«. With his workgroup for neuroradiology Decker sporadically performed brain-surgical and radiotherapeutical treatments.

Not only doctors, but also the nursing staff contributed decisively to the reconstruction of the clinic and these include not only the nuns, but also voluntary sisters as well as the male nurses, who returned from the war or internship.

It was particularly important for the clinic that Stertz dealt with both staff and patients in a kind and friendly manner. All who witnessed this period and are still alive enjoy remembering these good old times. In this context Alma Kreuter (born 1906) played a special part; she began work in 1922, during Kraepelin's term of office, became secretary to director Bumke, experienced national-socialism, the war years and remained in her position as Stertz's secretary during the reconstruction phase. She continued working for Kolle and for Kaess during the transition period (▶ see Introduction and Chapter 11).

The clinic staff especially appreciated Stertz's understanding and kind manners towards patients

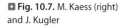 **Fig. 10.7.** M. Kaess (right) and J. Kugler

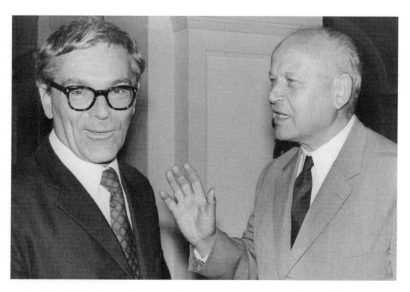

and that he demonstrated considerable tolerance and a liberal and co-operative attitude.

Thanks to Stertz, scientists with completely differing interests were able to come together and work scientifically at the Munich clinic. Stertz and his staff managed the reconstruction work and set down the foundations for further developments at the Munich clinic.

Literature

Nonne, M. (1971): Anfang und Ziel meines Lebens. Hamburg: Hans Christians Verlag

Christiani, K. (2006): Georg Stertz. In: Hippius, H., Holdorff, B., Schliack, H. (Ed.): Nervenärzte. Vol. 2. Georg Thieme Verlag – Stuttgart, p. 179–185

11

Kurt Kolle and Plans for a New Hospital Building in Grosshadern

Once the main damage to the clinic and institutes had been repaired five years after the war, thoughts were given to the future of the medical faculty, whether the building activity should be of a repair and interim nature or whether long-term solutions should be sought. Unclear was also whether the entire medical faculty should be located on the site of the old hospital on the left bank of the River Isar or in its vicinity. Neither had a plan from the thirties been forgotten, to move the university clinics out of the inner city to the outskirts.

Originally, the opinion was that it would be useful to keep the clinics and institutes in the inner city, taking possible and necessary expansions into account. For this reason, the Free State of Bavaria purchased parts of the hospital »Links der Isar« from the owner, the city of Munich. It was assumed that this could satisfy the needs of the medical faculty for quite some time. However, it soon became clear that the clinical and clinical-theoretical teaching and research institutions would grow much larger and faster than originally expected. It was also feared that in spite of the best possible use of all available space capacity in the inner city, the development of the medical faculty would soon be impeded by lack of space. Consequently, the plans to place the clinics (and possibly some institutes) on the western border of the city were resumed. To clarify the location, a tender was organized in 1954. The result supported the decision to move the clinics to the city's border and the Bavarian Council of Ministers decided in August 1955 to build new clinics in Grosshadern.

During the planning stages in 1952, K. Kolle accepted the offer to become successor to the 74-year old, retired G. Stertz in Munich.

Kurt Kolle
Professor of Psychiatry in Munich (1952–1966)

Kurt Kolle (◘ Fig. 11.1) was born on February 7, 1898, in Kimberley, South Africa. His father, the

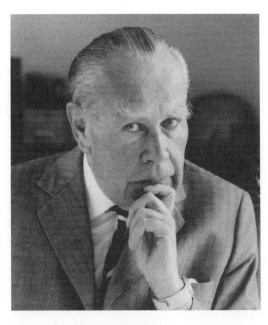

◘ **Fig. 11.1.** Kurt Kolle (1898–1975)

bacteriologist Wilhelm Kolle (1868–1935), was a co-worker of Robert Koch at the Imperial Public Health Department of the Reich at the end of the previus century in Berlin. As head of a department W. Kolle researched into means to combat cattle plague (»Rinderpest«) and this task took him South Africa for a longer period of time; Kurt Kolle and his younger brother Helmut were born there.

On return of the Kolle family to Berlin (1904), K. Kolle went to school for two years. His father was offered a job as professor for hygiene and bacteriology at the university of Berne. Kurt Kolle spent the rest of his school time in Berne.

From 1916 until 1918 Kolle participated in the war. Immediately after the war he intended to start studying law in Bonn or Jena, but soon abandoned this plan. At the beginning of 1919 he went to Frankfurt/Main to study medicine. In 1917 his father became successor to Paul Ehrlich in Frankfurt as director of the Paul-Ehrlich-Institute.

Following his studies in Frankfurt, Kolle also studied in Jena and Munich; he graduated in 1923 in Jena and wrote a thesis on »The concept of natural healing forces in changing times«. His development as a student during the period following the First World War is reflected in his choice of title for his memoirs: »Student and Revolutionary«. He later referred to himself as a non-conforming liberal.

Kolle began his psychiatric training as assistant at the Mecklenburg institution Sachsenberg, with a pupil of Ideler, F. Matusch (1856–1942), whose daughter he married in 1926. During his first years as assistant Kolle gave his critical opinion on E. Kretschmer's ideas of the connection between »character and physique«. At that time Kretschmer had already gained a reputation as senior consultant to R. Gaupp at the clinic for nervous diseases in Tubingen. The disputes with Kretschmer continued for quite a while, until K. Jaspers advised him to spend his time in a more »fruitful occupation«.

In 1925 Kolle became assistant to Hans Berger (1873–1941), the founder of electroencephalography, at the clinic for nervous diseases in Jena. Kolle remained at the clinic only for a short time and then joined G. Stertz in Kiel where he spent seven years as assistant doctor, qualifying as university lecturer in 1928. Whilst with Stertz, Kolle began

studies on paranoid psychoses and continued this work during a study visit to the German Research Institute for Psychiatry in Munich in 1932.

When Kolle returned to work in March 1933 in Kiel, polemic articles were published in March 1933 in what had become the national-socialistic Kiel press; the article was about the »Conditions at the German University Clinic for Nervous Diseases in Kiel« and Kolle was referred to by name. Consequently, Kolle took leave, left Kiel and opened a practice as psychiatrist and neurologist in Frankfurt. He had a hard time coming to terms with Frankfurt: The panel practice took a while to pick up and contact with the medical faculty in Frankfurt did not develop, as Kolle had left Kiel without taking care that his status as university lecturer would be recognized in Frankfurt. Kolle's father who had a good reputation in Frankfurt as the director of the Paul-Ehrlich-Institute, was able to help him transfer the qualifications from Kiel to Frankfurt and made sure that he would receive the title of professor. This was particularly important for Kolle, as he had been very involved in student training in Kiel and highly enjoyed giving lectures. His work as panel doctor only gave him little time during the day, so he organized »Psychiatric, Neurological Colloquiums« held at 8 p.m. in his apartment. To be more effective as an academic teacher in Frankfurt, in the years prior to the outbreak of the Second World, Kolle wrote the textbook »Psychiatry – for Students and Doctors«. This book was published for the first time in 1939, later six further editions were published and translated into several languages. (A further book by Kolle which was published after the war, entitled »Introduction to Psychiatry«, came out in six editions and was translated into English and Japanese.) (◻ Fig. 11.2).

Kolle was not particularly successful with the panel practice in Frankfurt; he only had a few patients. Without support from his father he and his family would not have survived. When his father died in 1935, Kolle was forced to look for a better way to earn money. He applied as sanitary officer with the army, but his application was turned down. He moved his practice from the west of Frankfurt into the inner city and soon profiled from the change in location.

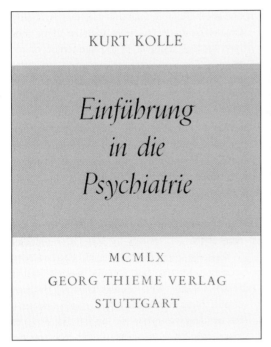

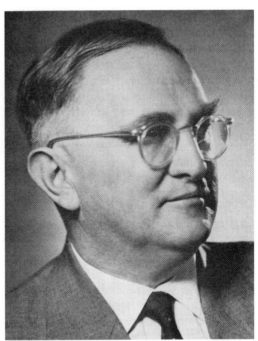

◻ **Fig. 11.2.** K. Kolle's »Introduction to Psychiatry« (1960)

◻ **Fig. 11.3.** Gustav Bodechtel (1899–1983)

At the beginning of the Second World War Kolle was drafted into the army. He became military doctor, head doctor of a military hospital and finally consultant psychiatrist to a sector of the army; he continued to work now and then at the military hospital. Once the war was over, he returned to his practice.

Kolle resigned himself to the fact that he would never manage to continue his university career which he had begun in the thirties, when – together with K. Schneider, E. Kretschmer and E. Straus – he was short-listed as candidate to succeed G. Stertz. It also made a good impression that K. Jaspers from Basle warmly recommended him. Kolle was offered the job in Munich and took up office in September 1952, at the age of 54 years.

Right from the start, Kolle took part in the consultations on the future development of the medical faculty and the respective plans to move the clinics to Grosshadern. He supported the concept to move the clinics there in an integrated form. The most important prerequisite for him to support the plan was the assurance that psychiatry

and neurology would be bound together structurally. As dean of the medical faculty (1958/1959), Kolle could use his influence and agreed that the »clinic for nervous diseases« at Grosshadern would be a closed unit in the first building phase, but in a later (third) phase would have a greater amount of space available. In the summer of 1959 Kolle gave his precise demands to his successor as dean (H. Schwiegk) in writing. During the following ten years Kolle's proposals and demands had to be re-thought and could not be put into practice (▶ Chapter 12).

Although Kolle had always implicitly emphasized the need for a close connection between psychiatry and neurology and was not prepared to make concessions, he and the Munich neurologist **Gustav Bodechtel** (1899–1983) (◻ Fig. 11.3), never let their opinions impair their good personal and working relationship.

Bodechtel and Kolle had known each other since working at the German Institute for Psychiatry during the thirties.

After taking up office in Munich, Kolle recommended that Bodechtel be offered the position of professor for internal medicine (as successor to the professorships of F. von Müller and A. Schittenhelm) and that he left Dusseldorf for Munich.

Bodechtel's opinion of Kolle's intention to keep psychiatry and neurology together was well known: According to Bodechtel neurology belonged to internal medicine and should remain so even a certain independence if given.

Kolle insisted on his point of view for many years and did not change his mind when he retired; he considered the resolutions of the faculty, the university and the Bavarian Ministry of Science to divide psychiatry and neurology into two separate clinics to be wrong. However, Bodechtel changed his mind and became convinced that the scientific development of neurology would be restricted if it remained a sub-area of internal medicine. Influenced by the negotiations at an international congress for neurology in Rome in 1963, Bodechtel worked towards the separation of neurology from both internal medicine and psychiatry. Bodechtel's opinion not only had a decisive effect on the Munich faculty, but on the whole of Germany.

In spite of differing opinions on such an important subject, neither Kolle nor Bodechtel resented one another during their time together in Munich. On the contrary: For more than 20 terms they held lectures together in the auditorium of the Munich clinic and there are numerous anecdotes from these legendary meetings, still remembered today!

When Kolle joined the clinic, most war damage had been repaired, but there was still a serious shortage of space. Kolle realized that it was his most urgent task to make sure that the situation for both staff and patients improved without delay.

The clinic had been planned and built at the beginning of the 20th century for 100–120 in-patients. In Kraepelin's time the number of beds had been increased to 180, but without making further space available. When Bumke changed the psychiatric clinic into a »clinic for nervous diseases«, the building was expanded (on the east wing) to make room for neurological patients. However, the actual capacity did not improve much due to these changes, as the number of beds was increased at the same time to 250. During the war and the first post-war years the clinic was overflowing. All the patients' dayrooms and the large microscopy laboratory were turned into wards.

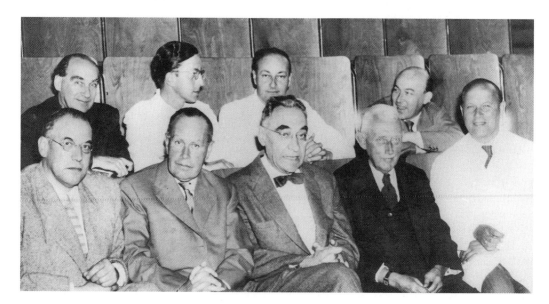

◻ **Fig. 11.4.** K. Kolle with colleagues and co-workers in the auditorium (from left to right, back row): H. Koebcke, J.E. Meyer, H. Tellenbach, K. Decker; front row: A. v. Braunmuehl, K. Kolle, E. Kahn, G. Stertz, M. Kaess

In 1952 an average of 370 patients were admitted to the clinic. In 1954 Kolle reduced the number of beds to 300 and in 1955 to 250. Due to the reduction in patients to one third, a reduction in the number of doctors also took place. Consequently, more work space was made available for the many doctors (mainly badly paid or completely unpaid).

During his 14 years in office and through his choice of co-workers, Kolle strove to show (■ Fig. 11.4) that both psychiatry and neurology were of equal importance at the clinic for nervous diseases.

When Kolle joined the clinic, **M. Mikorey** and **M. Kaess** were the senior consultants in charge of the psychiatric and neurological wards; their main scientific work concentrated on psychiatric topics.

During Stertz's time in office, K. Decker had developed this X-ray department – originally set up by the neurologist A. Bannwarth who in the meantime worked at the Hospital »Rechts der Isar« – into the leading neuroradiology department in Germany. Kolle promoted the expansion of the X-ray department and had rooms made available for neurosurgical operations and radio therapeutical treatments.

To follow-up on the considerable neuro-anatomical research begun by B. von Gudden, a laboratory for neuro-pathology was set up. J.E. Meyer, who came to Munich in 1954 from Freiburg, took over the laboratory and was also senior psychiatric consultant at the clinic.

J.E. Meyer (1917–1998) (■ Fig. 11.5) was born in Koenigsberg. His father was professor of psychiatry; his grandfather was the first professor on the chair of psychiatry in Gottingen.

Following his medical studies, J. E. Meyer worked as assistant to W. Scholz at the department for neuro-pathology at the German Research Institute for Psychiatry in Munich (1945–1949). Similar to his brother, H.H. Meyer (1910–2000; full professor for psychiatry at the Saarland University from 1959 until 1978), J.E. Meyer also wanted a clinical career. He began training with Kurt Beringer in Freiburg. After Beringer's early death (August 1949) J.E. Meyer remained in Freiburg, but became a co-worker in R. Jung's Department for Clinical Neurophysiology. In 1952 in Freiburg J.E. Meyer qualified as university lecturer for psychiatry and neurology. In 1954 Kolle offered him a job in Munich.

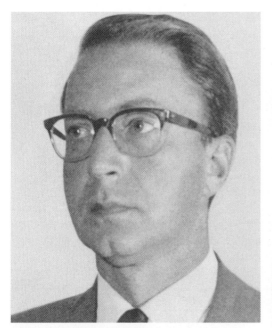

■ **Fig. 11.5.** Joachim-Ernst Meyer (1917–1998)

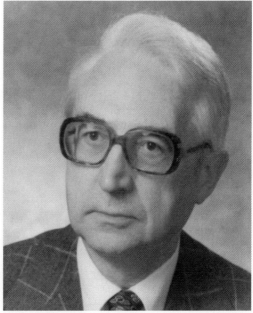

■ **Fig. 11.6.** Ewald Frick (born 1919)

Kolle hoped that apart from his job as senior psychiatric consultant J.E. Meyer would revive the clinic's tradition for neuro-morphology going back to B. von Gudden's times. Since the departure of H. Spatz in 1932, nothing had been done in this area.

Apart from his studies on neuro-pathology, J.E. Meyer also dedicated his time in Munich to clinical-psychiatric issues (amongst others: studies on depersonalization experiences; adolescent psychopathology; anorexia nervosa) and tried to integrate psychotherapeutic concepts into psychiatry. In 1963 J.E. Meyer was offered the chair for psychiatry in Gottingen. When J.E. Meyer left Munich, Kolle was upset that he would take H. Lauter with him as senior consultant soon after (see below). J.E. Meyer headed the Psychiatric Clinic of the University of Gottingen until his retirement in 1985. He died in Gottingen on June 5, 1998.

Kolle employed E. Frick who had worked with H. Pette in Hamburg, in the serological laboratory.

> Ewald Frick (■ Fig. 11.6), born in 1919, was Kolle's senior neurological consultant. After studying and graduating in Hamburg in 1944, Frick had been taken prisoner. On his release from war captivity Frick joined H. Pette in Hamburg and worked as assistant for 8 years at the Neurological University Clinic in Hamburg-Eppendorf, before accepting Kolle's offer in Munich.

Frick took over the well-equipped and well-staffed chemical and serological laboratories and used the opportunity to broaden his training in psychiatry, as he had been restricted to neurology until this time. In 1959 he qualified as university lecturer in psychiatry and neurology.

Frick continued the work he had started with Pette and followed-up on the studies K.F. Scheid had carried out at the clinic during the war: through Frick's work, studies on the immunology and chemistry of CSF proteins became a focal point of the clinic's research. On separation of the clinics in 1971, Frick opted for the Neurological Clinic where he worked for A. Schrader as senior consultant until his retirement.

▬ At the same time as Frick, H. Häfner (■ Fig. 11.7) joined Kolle as assistant. He had worked previ-

ously for E. Kretschmer in Tubingen and left Munich in 1958.

▬ In 1955 H. Koebcke, long-time secretary of the German Medical Weekly, was given a lectureship at the clinic.

▬ From 1955 until 1960 H. Oepen was assistant at the clinic. Following his clinical training he went to Marburg's Institute for Genetics, qualified as university lecturer there and later became full professor for human genetics.

▬ In 1956 J. Kugler and H. Lauter became assistant doctors at the clinic.

H. Lauter (born 1928) (■ Fig. 11.8) was born as son of a doctor in Dusseldorf; he grew up in Berlin. After his medical studies in Zurich and Munich he was assistant doctor to Kolle for eight years. Lauter's scientific interests covered gerontology and dementia. After leaving Munich, he qualified as university lecturer in Gottingen in 1964 with a thesis on the clinical symptoms of Alzheimer's and Pick's disease. From 1972 until 1978 Lauter was Medical Director of the General Hospital Ochsenzoll and head of the psychiatric department there. In 1978 he was offered the position of full professor

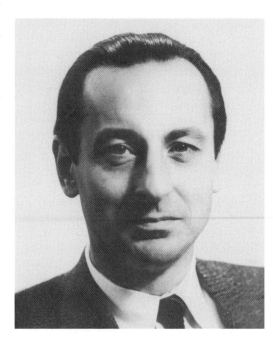

■ **Fig. 11.7.** Heinz Häfner (born 1926)

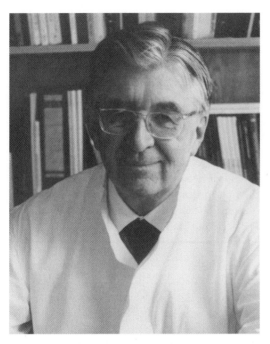

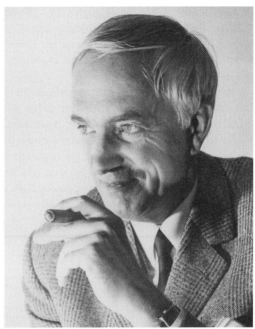

Fig. 11.8. Hans Lauter (born 1928)

Fig. 11.9. Heinz Dietrich (born 1918)

at the University of Homburg, but went to Munich instead where he was professor of psychiatry and director of the Psychiatric Clinic of the Technical University Munich.

▬ In 1958 **H. Dietrich** joined Kolle from the Charité Hospital in Berlin.

H. Dietrich (◘ Fig. 11.9) was born in Berlin in 1918, spent his school days there and following school exams, wanted to study medicine in his hometown. As Dietrich's grandmother on his mother's side was Jewish, he was not allowed to matriculate at a German university. Consequently, he began his medical studies in Innsbruck, but had to go to Switzerland in 1938 to continue studying. On outbreak of the Second World War he was allowed to continue his studies in Berlin. In the summer of 1945 Dietrich became assistant to R. Thiele (1888–1960) at the clinic for nervous diseases at the Charité Hospital in Berlin. He qualified as university lecturer for psychiatry and neurology in 1951.

Initially Dietrich worked scientifically on neurological topics (in particular neuroradiological ones). He was especially interested in psychiat-

ric-psychopathological and forensic-psychiatric subjects. When K. Leonhard took over the psychiatric/neurological clinic at the Charité in 1957, Dietrich became one of his close co-workers. A year later Dietrich had to give up the very fulfilling work with Leonhard and leave the Charité, after being accused in the German Democratic Republic of having a »middle-class, reactionary attitude«. When »cleansing« activities against »opponents of democratic socialism« began at the universities in the spring of 1958, Dietrich was publicly attacked. He went to Munich in October 1958 and became scientific assistant and later senior consultant to Kolle. On separation of psychiatry and neurology, Dietrich opted for the psychiatric clinic; he became the first and the most senior consultant. He retired in 1983, but remained a forensic-psychiatric expert and opened a practice as psychiatrist and neurologist in Bad Aibling.

During Kolle's 14 years in office two of his co-workers qualified as professor: E. Frick (1959) and J. Kugler. It was also planned that H. Lauter would habilitate, but before negotiations with the

Munich faculty could be finalized, J.E. Meyer, who had been offered the chair of psychiatric in Gottingen, asked Lauter to join him there. Lauter accepted and received his professorial qualifications in Gottingen.

With Kugler's qualification as professor, the EEG Laboratory achieved a special standing within the clinic, similar to that of Decker's X-ray department. Kugler turned the EEG laboratory into a center of clinical neurophysiology soon gaining importance in Germany, but also abroad. The training courses for EEG assistants, which were set up during Kolle's term in office, soon achieved a good reputation not only in Munich.

To improve the care of the clinic's patients, Kolle supported the **department of physiotherapy** and also **occupational therapy**.

Kolle's primary scientific interest was in psychiatric problems. He continued where he had been forced to leave off in 1933 when he left the hospital in Kiel. He revisited the topic of his first monograph (»The Primary Madness«, 1931) in 1957 with a book entitled »The Person Suffering from Delusions in the Light of Old and New Psychopathology«. After the war Kolle was one of the first to deal with the problem of »Victims of National-Socialist Persecution from a Psychiatric Perspective« (1958).

GROSSE NERVENÄRZTE

21 LEBENSBILDER

IN GEMEINSCHAFT MIT H. J. de BARAHONA FERNANDES
J. F. FULTON · E. GRÜNTHAL · G. R. HEYER · G. HOLMES
M. JANTSCH · R. JUNG · J. KLAESI · M. MINKOWSKI
G. de MORSIER · M. NONNE · R. de SAUSSURE
L. SCHÖNBAUER · J. H. SCHULTZ · TH. SPOERRI
G. STERTZ · R. THIELE · K. J. ZÜLCH

HERAUSGEGEBEN VON

KURT KOLLE
MÜNCHEN

MIT 21 ABBILDUNGEN

19 56

GEORG THIEME VERLAG · STUTTGART

☐ **Fig. 11.10.** Three-volume work by K. Kolle: »Famous Psychiatrists and Neurologists«

Kolle's inaugural lecture was about »The Endogenous Psychoses – The Oracle of Delphi in Psychiatry«. As far as he was concerned, phenomenology according to Karl Jaspers, and psychopathology according to the Heidelberg School were the foundations of clinical psychiatry. He was also interested in the philosophical and historical aspects of psychiatry and was of the opinion that, without reviewing history, living science could not flourish. Accompanied by this conviction, from 1956 until 1963, he published three volumes of biographies »Famous Psychiatrists« (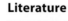 Fig. 11.10).

Thanks to Kolle's interest in history, the »Golden Kraepelin Medal« has been awarded (Fig. 11.11) for exceptional achievements in Munich psychiatry since 1956.

> In 1928 the Kraepelin Medal was awarded to O. Vogt (1870–1959) on the occasion of the opening of the German Research Institute for Psychiatry's new building. In 1956 Kolle organized a ceremonial act in the auditorium of the clinic on Kraepelin's 100th anniversary. Together with the managing director of the German Research Institute W. Scholz, Kolle set up an international panel to revive the medal's tradition. It was decided that the Golden Kraepelin Medal would be awarded jointly by the directors of the Psychiatric University Clinic

and the German Research Institute for Psychiatry and that on the advice of well-known psychiatrists from various countries the award would be only given to outstanding achievements in psychiatry. In 1956 the Kraepelin Medal was given to Ernst Kretschmer and Ludwig Binswanger. Later, during Kolle's term of office it was given to M. Reichart (1964), also K.T. Neubuerger, K. Schneider and W. Scholz (1966) received this honour.

Kolle retired at the end of the winter term 1965/1966. He left the official residence on the same day and moved to Starnberg with his wife. As an »outsider«, he remained keenly interested in developments in psychiatry and neurology even though he found some of the decisions made were wrong. He also took time for things he had neglected during his time at the clinic and spent time tracking down the expressionist pictures by his brother who had committed suicide in 1924. Some of these pictures were hunging in his house in Starnberg long before Helmuth Kolle was re-discovered as an important expressionist painter (exhibition in Lenbachhaus in Munich, 1991).

After his wife's death (1969) Kolle led an increasingly solitary life in Starnberg. He became ill and invalid at 75 years of age and had himself admitted to the clinic in the Nussbaumstrasse where he was treated and cared for by »his« nuns. He died in the clinic on November 21, 1975.

Literature

Kolle, K. (1972): Wanderer zwischen Natur und Geist. Das Leben eines Nervenarztes. Lehmanns Verlag, Munich

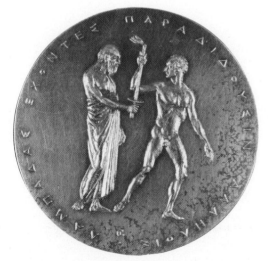

 Fig. 11.11. Kraepelin medal

Division of the »Hospital for Nervous Diseases« into a Psychiatric Hospital in the Inner City and a Neurological Hospital in Grosshadern

After Kolle's retirement in 1966, Max Kaess (1907–1995) was entrusted with the provisional management of the Munich Clinic for Nervous Diseases.

Kaess was born in Augsburg (■ Fig. 12.1) and began his psychiatric training with K. Schneider at the Schwabing Hospital. Immediately after the war he became assistant doctor with O. Bumke. He worked at the Munich clinic for 25 years without interruption, first with Bumke, then with Stertz,

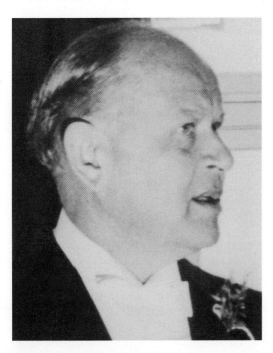

■ **Fig. 12.1.** Max Kaess (1907–1995)

under whom he qualified as university professor for psychiatry and neurology in 1950. After Stertz's retirement Kaess remained co-worker of Kolle and managed the clinic provisionally, following Kolle's retirement, from 1996 until 1970. In 1971 Kaess took over the professorial chair for psychiatry at the Technical University of Munich. He retired in 1975 and died in 1995.

When Kolle retired, the medical faculty seriously debated the alternatives of either looking for a successor to the chair of psychiatry and neurology, or of dividing the professorship into two, one for psychiatry and the other for neurology. Much to Kolle's discontent, the faculty decided to divide the professional chair and by doing so, followed the trend already in motion at many German universities.

Following a resolution of the Bavarian council of ministers in 1955, the decision on the future academic organization of psychiatry and neurology coincided with the first building activities to move some of the inner city clinics to the site at Grosshadern on the outskirts of Munich. It was inevitable that negotiations with Kolle's successor would be with a psychiatrist and a neurologist and that space for both would have to be taken into consideration as part of negotiations. It was assumed that the old clinic on the Nussbaumstrasse needed a thorough renovation and that additional need for space would arise. It remained open whether it would possible from a long-term perspective to accommodate two clinics in the old building, even if extensions were made.

During Kolle's time as dean (1958/1959) plans had been drawn up for a third building phase in Grosshadern, where one entity for a clinic containing both psychiatry and neurology would be accommodated (by means of extending the basic substance of the clinic building above the auditorium segment to the west). Since the sixties it had been obvious that the plans could not be financed. The first part of the building, which had begun in 1967/1968, was already so expensive that any plans for further building projects in Grosshadern had to be abandoned. In reducing the plans for Grosshadern, the university and the Bavarian state government agreed in the mid seventies to divide the medical faculty's clinics into two locations (city centre and Grosshadern):

- In the city centre, the inner city clinics (the hospital »Links der Isar«) and
- on the edge of the city, the newly built clinic Grosshadern.

All the clinics in the inner city with two clinics per specialist area (e.g. internal medicine, surgery and gynaecology) would have to move one of their clinics to Grosshadern. Also, any hospital in the inner city occupying rented buildings (e.g. neurosurgery) were to move to Grosshadern as well. It was clear right from the start that some speciality areas (e.g. neurosurgery) would only be located in Grosshadern, whilst others (e.g. dermatology, paediatry, ophthalmology) would be solely in the inner city. For some clinical subjects (e.g. anesthesiology, radiology, ENT) it was obvious that they would have to work in both locations. These plans also foresaw that the psychiatric clinic would remain in the inner city, whilst neurology was intended to be housed in Grosshadern – although sufficient rooms in Grosshadern would only be available from the mid seventies.

On December 4, 1968 the medical faculty asked to the Senate of the University of Munich to propose to the Bavaria State Ministry for Education and Culture that Hanns Hippius be appointed as chair of psychiatry in Munich. (▶ Chapter 13).

H. Hippius was born in 1925 in Muhlhausen/Thuringia and had been full professor and held the chair of psychiatry of the Free University of Berlin since February 1968 and was director of the »Psychiatric Clinic« there.

Hippius studied medicine and chemistry in Freiburg/Breisgau, Marburg and Berlin (FU). After graduating in medicine in 1950, he wrote a thesis on post-icteric encephalopathy in neonates (nuclear icterus) due to Rh-incompatibility and became scientific assistant to the immunologist, H. Schmidt (1882-1974) at the »Institute for Experimental Therapy Emil von Behring« in Marburg. In 1952 he built up a research laboratory at the Clinic for Psychiatry and Neurology of the Free University Berlin which was headed by H. Selbach (1909–1987). Following his clinical training as doctor of psychiatry and neurology, he qualified as university lecturer with a thesis on »Immunological findings from neurolues« and became Chief Senior Consultant at the Berlin Clinic.

At the beginning of 1967 he was offered the professorial chair for psychiatry at the medical faculty of the Technical University of Aachen, but at the same time received an offer to join the newly founded chair for psychiatry in Berlin. When he received the assurance by the Berlin senate that a new building was planned for the »Psychiatric Clinic II«, he remained in Berlin. In July 1968 he was offered the ordinary chair of psychiatry at the University of Hamburg as successor to H. Bürger-Prinz (1897–1976), which he turned down, on being offered the chair of psychiatry in Munich.

Because the situation in Munich was becoming problematic, Hippius began negotiations with the medical faculty and its deans (F. Marguth and E. Kraft) in summer 1969. Following Kolle's retirement at the end of the winter term 1965/66, there had been a long vacancy in Munich. Term by term, every decision dealing with problems and faculty tasks with respect to psychiatry and neurology had been postponed. In particular regarding student teaching, it had become urgently important to man the posts as soon as possible. If the negotiations with the psychiatrist last for a long time of fail, it was likely to be difficult to find a neurologist who would be prepared to start work, prior to the completion of the neurological clinic in Grosshadern.

On the other hand, it was a difficult situation for Hippius: During retention negotiations the senate in Berlin assured him that a completely new building would be constructed with 100 beds and a rather generous amount of staff. They also offered him two departmental heads (for geronto-psychiatry and psychiatric epidemiology/social psychiatry), as well as research laboratories combined with the neighbouring university clinic for neuropharmacology.

Although the potential for future clinical and scientific research work in Berlin seemed promising, the general situation at the universities had to be taken into consideration. In the late sixties there was unrest at the German universities, some were less affected than others.

At the Free University of Berlin it soon came to a rather radical upheaval in 1967/68 also affecting the medical faculty and its clinics (change from the traditional rectorate constitution to a politicized presidential assembly: Separation of the medical faculty into seven areas; establishment of many time-consuming, often insufficient and incompetent advisory bodies; student demonstrations: Boycott of lectures, etc).

In the clinics, representatives from all staff groups formed »co-management bodies« (with a biased right to vote). The situation was particularly unfortunate at the Free University of Berlin, where the resolutions of these bodies, demands by the »assistants' councils« and student representations far outweighed the objective and functional proposals for development of the medical faculty and the clinics and institute managements they represented.

When Hippius began negotiations with the scientific senate and the medical faculty in Hamburg at the end of 1968, the situation in Hamburg was far more factual than that in Berlin. Only some assistant and student delegations made demands for future psychiatrists to agree to a »comtemporary and progressive social psychiatry«.

Bavaria remained untouched by the developments, which had set in at the end of 1968. In Munich the medical faculty had remained a unit and the splitting of individual clinics into a multitude of autonomous departments did not occur. In the Munich Psychiatric Clinic the preoccupation with daily clinical work and care of the patients

was of utmost importance in spite of the (in some respects not particularly good) working conditions (▶ Chapter 13).

With regard to the university situation and the working atmosphere, Munich was given preference, although both sides claimed insurmountable difficulties in the details. Finally, a satisfactory solution could be found for everyone involved: The professorial chair for neurology would be occupied by the internal specialist and neurologist **Adolf Schrader** (1912–2002) (◻ Fig. 12.2), a pupil of Bodechtel and head of a municipal hospital.

Schrader came to Munich from Dusseldorf in 1953 and was co-worker of G. Bodechtel, when Bodechtel took over the chair for medicine as director of the 2nd Medical Clinic of the medical faculty. Schrader qualified as lecturer for internal medicine in 1954. In 1962 he became head of the 2nd Medical Department of the Municipal Hospital Harlaching: According to a tradition started by Bodechtel in Dusseldorf and continued in Munich, Schrader's department in Harlaching treated both internal and neurological patients.

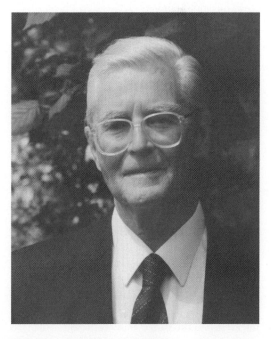

◻ **Fig. 12.2.** Adolf Schrader (1915–2002)

Hippius and Schrader quickly got in contact with each other, discussed all the difficulties, were soon assured of their mutual and complete loyalty and together were able to find solutions for many problems.

Hippius wrote an exposé to illustrate the various complexities and matters to be addressed in Munich:

- Extension work to be done on existing buildings, as well as completion of considerable renovation and reconstruction work, in particular with respect to the wards.
- Organizational restructuring of the clinic with the establishment of several independent,special departments and working areas, connected to the wards and under a central clinic management.
- Improvement of the staffing, both in nursing and medical areas, with specific attention to the heads of departments (H3, respectively C3 professorships).
- Improvement in the equipping of the clinic with respect to the co-workers' research activities.
- Planning of a large out-patient clinic (with consiliary services) and
- planning of partial out-patient clinics (day-clinic, night-clinic).

The plans in Hippius' exposé were accepted by the faculty without reservations, in particular by G. Bodechtel, and also by the deans F. Marguth (1969/1990), E. Kraft (1970) and W. Spann (as of winter term 1970/1971 until summer term 1989), and continued to be supported for many years to come.

The Ministry of Culture supported the proposals and used them a basis for further negotiations with the Ministry of Finance.

In the Ministry of Culture the senior legal secretary Dr. F. Hunger, was in charge of the negotiations and was an especially strong lobby for the successful conclusion of Hippius' negotiations. Whenever important questions remained open. In particular, with respect to the extent and financing of the necessary building activity, the head of the university department, Dr. J. von Elmenau, intervened and ensured that »sufficient« financial means would be available for the necessary con-

struction work during a period of six to (maximum) ten years: This would also be the case before the detailed conditions had been drawn up. During a meeting at the Ministry of Culture in July 1970 J. von Elmenau told H. Hippius: »In Bavaria you can rely on this promise. After all we are talking about the professorial chair of E. Kraepelin!«

The general agreement on the rebuilding and extension work was finalized. Firm consent for 48 staff positions was given (including four positions for departmental heads) as well as for financing to improve research equipment. The departments for psychiatric epidemiology and geronto-psychiatry could not be financed, neither could the night- and day-clinics.

Hippius accepted the offer to go to Munich and started work on January 1, 1971; Schrader joined the university on July 1, 1971. Schrader was responsible for the nucleus of the future Clinic of Neurology in Grosshadern which, to begin with, was located in the ground-floor rooms of the clinic's west wing on the Goethestrasse (rooms for the management and a ward with 20 beds; rooms for the neurological out-patient clinic and the EEG department).

The space available for the Neurological Clinic was so modest at the beginning because Schrader had agreed with the Free State of Bavaria and the City of Munich that he could keep his position as Head of the Department for Internal Medicine at the Municipal Hospital Harlaching (200 beds) until the Clinic Grosshadern opened in 1976.

When Schrader moved with the entire Neurological Clinic to Grosshadern in 1976, the rooms he had occupied in the Nussbaumstrasse became available and were taken over by the Psychiatric Clinic.

The allocation of staff within the separate clinics also worked smoothly. Hippius and Schrader each negotiated separately with the Ministry on the subject of clinic staffing.

With the exception of a few jobs for doctors, the entire staff (nursing staff, psychologists, staff from the occupational therapy, physiotherapists, laboratory staff and secretaries, administration, technical staff, etc) were allocated to the Psychiatric Clinic. Based on the existing »supply of staff«, negotiations were held to fortify the staff supply in several stages over a period of four years. Until the move to Grosshadern Schrader would be provided with all the clinical staff necessary.

Regarding the doctors' positions, Hippius and Schrader agreed (in particular for those professors and doctors who had been working at the clinic for quite some time) that they would leave it up to the employees themselves to decide in which clinic they would like to work. There was a certain risk in this process since the main objective was for a predominant number of academic co-workers to remain at the Psychiatric Clinic and for a smaller number to be allocated to the Neurological Clinic. Surprisingly enough, the process went smoothly. E. Frick became senior consultant of the Neurological Hospital; and J. Kugler with his EEG laboratory belonged to the Neurological Hospital (until 1976).

The following opted for the Psychiatric Clinic:

- K. Decker, who had been at the clinic since 1946 (under G. Stertz and later under K. Kolle) (▶ Chapter 10)
- H. Dietrich who had joined K. Kolle in 1958 from the Psychiatric and Neurological Clinic of the Berlin Charité (▶ Chapter 11)
- R. Meyendorf, who had been assistant during the provisional directorship by M. Kaess since 1966 and later became senior consultant at the clinic in 1968.

The EEG laboratory which actually belonged to the Neurological Clinic and was headed by J. Kugler, did not move to the Neurological Clinic at Grosshadern in 1976. It had been negotiated that J. Kugler would be a C3-professor at the Psychiatric Clinic and integrate his work group into the Psychiatric Clinic as of 1976. From this moment on, Kugler's work group was entitled »EEG Diagnostics and Psychiatric Neurophysiology«.

The Psychiatric Hospital 1971–1994

For the »Clinic on the Nussbaumstrasse«, which is well-known even outside Munich, the beginning of 1971 brought important changes: From 1904 until 1926 the clinic had been a psychiatric clinic, from 1926 until 1970 it had served as a hospital for nervous diseases, combining psychiatry and neurology and now it had been changed back into a pure »Psychiatric Clinic«.

The restructuring of the Munich clinic, with its long tradition, was a difficult task, not unusual when two clinics are separated from one another:

- Planning and implementation of extensive building measures.
- Organizational restructuring to modernize the clinic.
- Adaptation of education, training and further education for students, doctors and other staff (psychologists, nurses, social workers, physiotherapists, occupational therapists etc) to conform with contemporary standards, rules and guidelines.
- Revival of scientific work at the clinic – in particular to encourage and foster the interest of young academics in psychiatry. (Since 1950 not one clinic co-worker had written a thesis with a psychiatric theme in order to gain university lecturer status; only J. Kugler had done so, but with a thesis on »Clinical Neurophysiology.)

In spite of the diversity of the task, at all stages the main objective was to maintain the clinic's atmosphere of an ideal place of treatment for the mentally ill.

It was also advantageous in the situation that H. Hippius (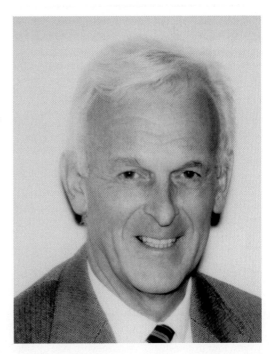 Fig. 13.1), who took on these tasks when he came into office on January 1, 1971, was also a member, and from 1972 onwards deputy chairman of the Commission which was to report on the situation of psychiatry and psychotherapy in the Federal Republic of Germany. The Commission

Fig. 13.1. Hanns Hippius (born 1925)

was also referred to as the »Psychiatry Evaluation« and had been constituted by the German Federal Government. The Commission was to review the situation and to make proposals on improvements.

> When the »Evaluation Commission« started work, it was obvious that 25 years after the end of the war the situation for psychiatric in-patients was deplorable and that the development of out-patient care of psychiatric patients was insufficient.
>
> The report was finished in 1974 and handed over to the Federal Government. It denounced that a large number of mentally ill and disabled patients had to live in inhumane conditions; it pointed out that »the buildings were partly dilapidated and the wards catastrophically over-filled, that the sanitary equipment was unacceptable, as were the general living conditions of the patients«. Worst affected were the large psychiatric institutions, but also some psychiatric university clinics were affected.
>
> The Evaluation Report attracted much interest amongst the responsible political bodies and authorities, as well as the general public and led to a considerable improvement in psychiatric patients' care in all parts of the Federal Republic of Germany. For this reason, the »Psychiatry Evaluation« can rightly be considered one of the milestones in the development of psychiatry in Germany during the last 30 years.

It was definitely an advantage for the Munich Psychiatric Clinic that the new structuring and restructuring coincided with the report. As far as the construction work was concerned, the building and its quality was clearly below the standard of some of the district institutions in Bavaria.

At the beginning of 1971 the clinic had eight wards with room for 208 patients. A large part of the beds were located in rooms for 10 to 18 patients; on the »closed wards« the toilets were in the middle of the bedrooms only separated by a type of screen. The nursing staff had either no or insufficient working rooms: either the writing-desk of the ward sister was in one of the bedrooms or on the corridor; on a few wards the nurses' offices were only separated by a glass screen from the corridor. In the few, usually hall-size large doctors' rooms four or five doctors had to work side by side. The doctors had to carry out the examination and

exploration of their patients or speak to patients' relatives under these conditions. All kinds of jobs had to be done in the ward corridors. The patients had no dining room at their disposal, no sitting or group room neither was there a room for visitors or any kind of cafeteria. Nor was there room for student training, apart from the large auditorium.

Staff was sparse: in 1971 there were 123 jobs for nursing staff, who were not only responsible for the 208 in-patients, but also for the provisional admittance of 20 neurological patients and all other out-patients.

In spite of all this and in comparison to the bad conditions at other university clinics, the Munich clinic's doctors and nursing staff were motivated and gave good clinical care!

Many factors contributed:

The good atmosphere at the clinic was upheld by the entire staff – even by the porters and the handicraftsmen – and their personal identification with the »Clinic on the Nussbaumstrasse«.

At the beginning of 1971 the clinic still had 32 nuns (Sisters of Mercy of the Order of St. Vincent of Paul). These nuns worked mainly on the wards and in cases of emergency were at disposal around the clock.

The other nursing staff had often been working at the clinic for many years and, although justified complaints of understaffing or of work with non-nursing character (e.g. cleaning) existed, they were highly motivated to take care of the patients.

The doctors were also very motivated in spite of a high workload; often they were still on the wards with patients until late at night, in order to be able to speak to them in peace and quiet and undisturbed when the other doctors had left the room. The doctors did not work by the book or check on each other with respect to working hours; the patients' well-being was their main concern: This meant much over-time, but without calculating the over-time, as had become practice in certain German psychiatric clinics as a result of the events in 1968.

The insufficient staffing of the clinic had improved since 1960, as two and sometimes three doctors and up to ten nursing staff had to do their military duty in the clinic. In exchange the clinic was obliged to have up to 20 beds available for mentally ill relatives of army staff.

The Rebuilding and Expansion of the Hospital

At the start of negotiations between Hippius and the Bavarian State Ministry for Education and Culture in 1969 it had been made clear that extensive building work would be necessary and that the university's building authorities would be involved in consultations at an early stage. The plans also had to take into consideration that the clinic's functioning« could not be restricted by building activities:

- Patient care including physiotherapy, occupational therapy etc (at the same time maintaining the 200 in-patients to be treated).
- Out-patient services
- Consiliary services for all clinics
- Documentation of case histories (secretarial services) and archives
- Administrative tasks (including the catering, kitchen, purchasing, washing, workshop and internal services
- Tuition for 250 to 300 students per term
- Diagnostic work for patient care in the laboratories and special departments (clinical chemistry, neuroradiological diagnostics, ECG and EEG diagnostics)

During the entire building period the research work on the wards and out-patient department – in cooperation with six special departments – needed to be activated and expanded.

Originally, it had been planned to complete all building work within 5–7 years; according to this plan, building would be finished at the end of the seventies. But already the planning stage starting in 1969, took much longer than intended. For various reasons the plans had to be changed over and over again. The actual building work could only begin, once the housekeeping building had been torn down in 1983, would be carried out in several steps (see below) and not be finished until 1983 (▶ Chapter 15).

- The original building concept proved to be unsuitable.
- The plans for the Psychiatric Clinic had to be adjusted to fit in with the phases and developments of the construction work in Grosshadern.

- The Neurological Clinic remained in the inner city until the opening of Grosshadern in 1976.
- Once Grosshadern had been opened, its management began to negotiate with the Ministry on whether the Psychiatric Clinic should be moved to Grosshadern after all. The construction work on the Psychiatric University Clinic was once again debated at the Bavarian parliament.

The »Grosshadern solution« was certainly worth considering since a completely new building would bring advantages for the clinic: Until the move to Grosshadern was possible, the old building on the Nussbaumstrasse would be able to continue functioning without any kind of disturbance or disruption. This solution would also have meant that all clinics would be close to one another; however, a new building in Grosshadern would only have been possible in a completely separate building, a smaller building near to the main building. From a psychiatric point of view this solution would have been disadvantageous, because the Psychiatric Clinic would not have been integrated into the new Grosshadern building and would have become an »outsider«, something to be avoided in the past as well as the future. Psychiatric institutions should not be isolated but easily accessible by in- and out-patients, and their relatives. Consequently, it was taken into consideration that in the long run the transport connections would remain unsuitable and the intended building site on the west side of the Grosshadern clinic would mean long distances for the patients to travel. This was only one of the reasons why – after consultations between the faculty and the responsible ministries – the Bavarian parliament decided to follow the recommendations made by the Psychiatric Clinic to remain at its location within the city. Finally, the decision was made that the clinic could stay on its historical site on the Nussbaumstrasse!

With a letter to the building authorities of the Ministry of the Interior, the State Ministry for Education and Culture gave its permission for the rebuilding and expansion plans (from 9,000 square meters to 11,500 square meters). At the time the building expenses were estimated at DM 55 million (without equipment/furnishing). The necessary ground space surrounding the clinic was found near Goethestrasse in the street leading to the »Ziemssen block« and close to the garden of the nuns' mother house.

In 1983 the Ministry decided that the university's building authorities should commission an independent group of architects (G.A. Roemmich, H.J. Ott, A. Zehentner and U.A. Brunner; followed by: H.J. Ott, G. Geiselbrecht, A. Peek and Partner) to draw up the final plans.

Step by step in the subsequent 15 years in collaboration with the architects, the university's building authorities and the clinic's management, the plans for the rebuilding and expansion work (including the necessary new furnishing) were developed and completed. At the beginning of the project all plans, which had been drawn up prior to 1983 were reviewed, but only certain details were transferred into the new plans.

Before the architects were called in, all previous plans had considered the necessary enlargement of general space and on the whole the expansion of the building had been for general rooms. The wards, however, were to remain in the thoroughly renovated old building.

Once the collaboration with the architects started, this concept was changed: The **new buildings** would be planned and built to serve the entire **in-patient needs**. The substance of the **old building** should be renovated and rebuilt to serve all needs not directly linked with in-patient care.

During the entire planning, building and equipping phase the university's building authorities (headed by H. Franz, W. Dilg, D. Naumann, G. Schmidt and P. Pfab, together with H. Rudolf, F. Vogt, Mrs U. König-Friedl, Mrs. A. Funk, Mrs. D. Holle, K. Stelzl, A. Brüggemann and many others, who were responsible for the Psychiatric Clinic) worked closely with the responsible members of the clinic (P. Buchheim, G. Laakmann, H.-P. Kapfhammer and N. Müller) (◘ Fig. 13.2).

All plans to enlarge the entire floor space were abandoned in 1983, in particular those which would have considerably changed and disfigured

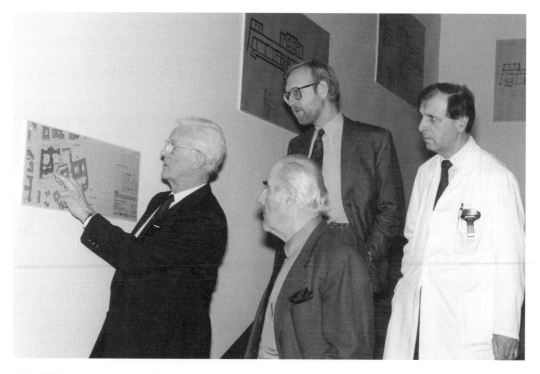

◘ **Fig. 13.2.** During the planning of the reconstruction and expansion of the clinic (from left to right) H. Hippius, G.A. Roemmich (architect), (behind) N. Müller, G. Kochinke (head of administration)

the architectural character of the original building. Fortunately, the following plans were discarded irrevocably:

▬ Destruction of the annex attached in 1904 (the director's villa) on the Goethestrasse and the construction of a modern, long, four to five storey high function building along the Goethestrasse.

▬ Destruction of housekeeping building in the middle wing of the clinic and construction of a five to six storey, tower-like extension (with underground parking in two cellars).

▬ Construction of two three-storey connecting buildings between the east, middle and west wings, whereby the two gardens for the patients would have been reconstructed as inner courtyards.

▬ Re-modeling of the façade along the Nussbaumstrasse by constructing a extension building in front of the old façade, whereby the »face« of the Psychiatric Clinic would match the ward buildings of the medical clinic, built in the fifties.

Although it was regrettable that the first planning phase had been so long before any architects were involved, it actually meant that any wrong planning had been avoided:

▬ In 1970 the generally predominant idea on the future structure of student tuition for medicine meant that the auditorium building would be torn down to make room for the extensions. A new auditorium would not be built, as the culture authorities of the time were of the opinion that »large lectures« had finally become obsolete; all tuition would be done in »small groups« and therefore only small seminar rooms would be needed.

▬ At the same time the authorities demanded more parking space and intended to use the patients' gardens for this purpose.

Both ideas were discarded. Kraepelin's auditorium was renovated and remained a place with historic character for lectures and other scientific meetings. The patients' gardens were retained and to a large part still contain the same trees planted during Kraepelin's time (◙ Fig. 13.3). For the patients and their

relatives the gardens are just as important a place for relaxation as the sitting areas on the new wards.

Based on the new concept, the building plans had to be re-thought and re-applied between 1983 and 1998. A prerequisite for fast realization of the plans was that the university administration and faculty find alternative solutions, respectively space, in the surrounding area for departments, which had to move out (rental of various floors in a building on Beethovenplatz from an insurance company; rental of apartments in the Goethestrasse; use of the »Cube« building within the inner city clinic complex, once the Second Gynaecological Clinic had been transferred to Grosshadern; use of rooms in the old dental clinic building, once the new dental clinic building had been completed). The inner city clinics' kitchen took over the catering and as a result it was possible to tear down the housekeeping building in the clinic's middle wing.

> The space allocation plan was quickly revised with the architects and two subsequent building phases were laid down:
>
> **First building phase** (complete new construction of three building sections B, C and D):
> The first building phase was carried out in two stages, one following the other.
> After demolition of the old housekeeping building (F):
> Building of the new construction B with three wards, gym and day clinic.
> Chronologically, one after the other and following demolition of the old west wing:
> Construction of the new building C with five wards; construction of new building D with two research wards.
> Basement construction of the new buildings B, C and D for the occupational therapy, logistics, housekeeping departments, maintenance department and archives.
> **Second building phase** (building A):
> Renovation of the old building (with entrance area and auditorium (G)) to accommodate all function departments, management, the private out-patient department, the senior consultants' offices and their secretaries, the out-patient clinic with special departments, the department of psychotherapy, management of the nursing staff, Kraepelin's library,

◻ Fig. 13.3. View of the interior garden (previously the men's garden)

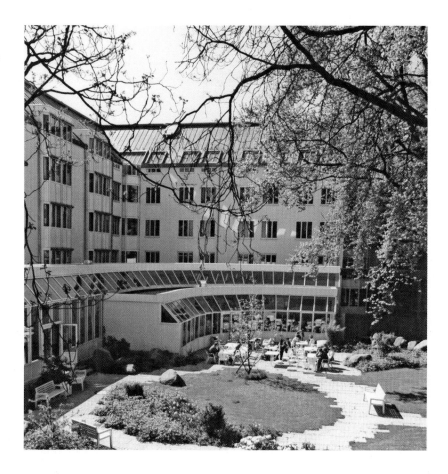

Alzheimer's microscopy laboratory as a lecture room and Museum for the History of Psychiatry.

Connection of the renovated old building (building A) with the new buildings B, C and D; on one side via the building D with the research wards and on the other side on the ground floor level with an arch-shaped glass corridor (◻ Fig. 13.3) and a cafeteria for patients with a view to the clinic gardens. The old east wing (E) was allotted for demolition.

The plan to transfer the heating system from the original building of 1904 (building A) into a newly constructed basement, in order to gain additional space, was abandoned due to costs (◻ Fig. 13.4, 13.5).

The eight wards in the new buildings B and C with 20 to 24 beds each, have angular floor plans (◻ Fig. 13.6). The »angular shape« of the wards avoids an optical impression of the usual, long cli-

nic corridors with bedrooms on both sides. At the external partings of the angle are the nursing staff bases (directly attached to the staff rooms). On the inside of the angle the »communication surfaces« are located (the eating and free-time areas, as well as the group rooms for patients); the patient and doctors' rooms are located on the arms of the angle. The bedrooms have two to four beds; the rooms for two beds can also be used as single rooms. The bathrooms are right next to the bedrooms and are generally arranged in such a manner that they can be accessed from the rooms and the toilets from the corridors.

The clinic's chapel is located on the fourth floor of building B, as is the staff canteen. There is also a large and well-equipped video studio (for training and scientific purposes).

The topping-out ceremony for the first part of the first building phase (building B) was held in

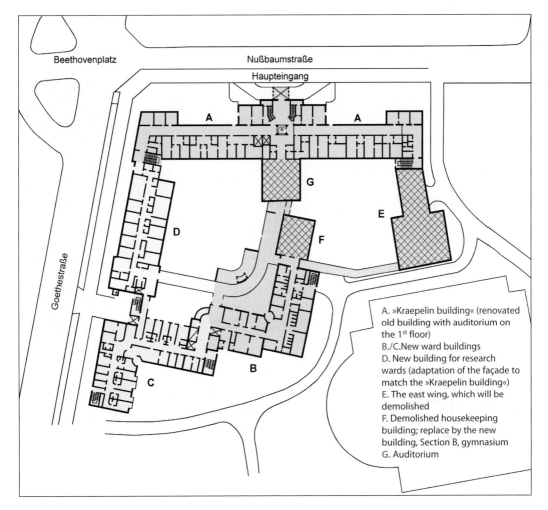

Beethovenplatz

Nußbaumstraße

Haupteingang

A   A

Goethestraße

D   F   G   E

B   C

A. »Kraepelin building« (renovated old building with auditorium on the 1st floor)
B./C.New ward buildings
D. New building for research wards (adaptation of the façade to match the »Kraepelin building«)
E. The east wing, which will be demolished
F. Demolished housekeeping building; replace by the new building, Section B, gymnasium
G. Auditorium

◼ **Fig. 13.4.** Site plan of the Psychiatric Clinic at the Nussbaumstrasse (Graphics: J. Christan)

July 1986. Once the interior had been equipped and furnished, the building was occupied during the last months of 1988 and the official opening ceremony took place on February 21, 1989.

The building and equipping measures for the second part of the first building phase (building C and D) were carried out and completed between 1988 and 1992. The architecture of building C (including the roof) matches building B. The old plans from 1902 until 1904 were put into use for the construction of the new building D (in place of the demolished west wing of the clinic). The height of the floors – unlike for the new buildings B and C – was adapted to match that of the original build-

ing A. The façade (even the colour of the plaster, the arrangement of the windows and their frames) was created in such a way that it corresponded with all the details of the demolished old building. (This was taken into account during the renovation of building A.) For the wall around the clinic building and its round and arch-shaped apertures the wrought-iron grids were reconstructed to reflect the historical record.

The final planning of the second building phase was resumed after an interval of two years (1992 until 1994), once H.-J. Möller had accepted the offer to become H. Hippius' successor on September 15, 1994. Following two years of plan-

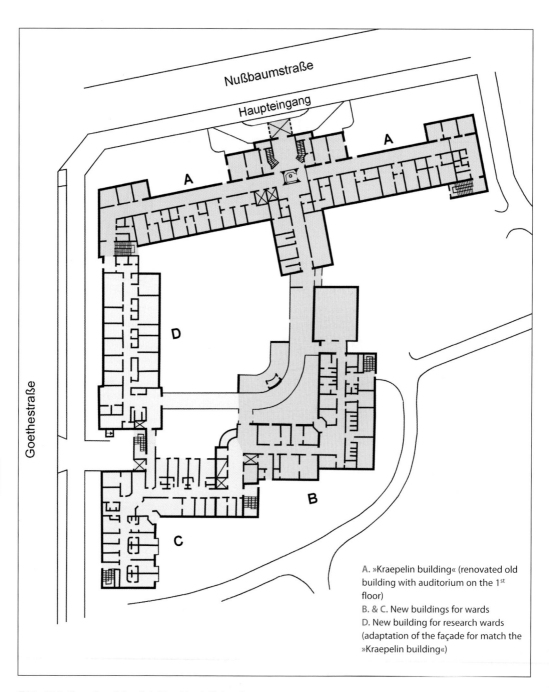

A. »Kraepelin building« (renovated old building with auditorium on the 1st floor)
B. & C. New buildings for wards
D. New building for research wards (adaptation of the façade for match the »Kraepelin building«)

◻ **Fig. 13.5.** Floor plan of the clinic (Graphics: J. Christan)

ning (1994–1996), the renovation and equipping of building A began. In 1998 all the building work was completed (▶ Chapter 15).

The Free State of Bavaria financed the project to re-build and extend the Psychiatric Clinic of the University with a total of DM 85 million.

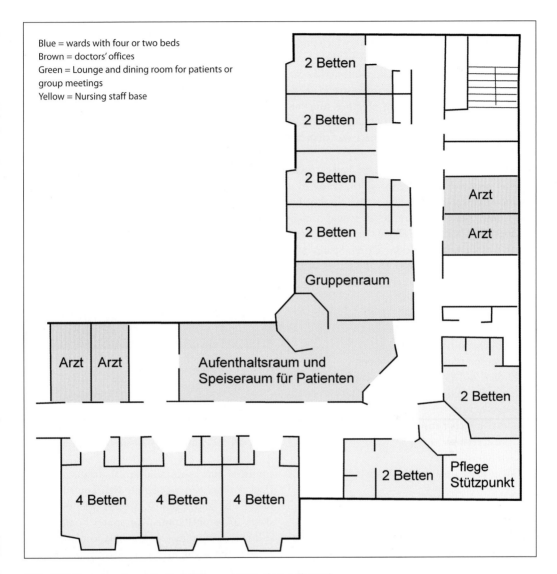

Blue = wards with four or two beds
Brown = doctors' offices
Green = Lounge and dining room for patients or
group meetings
Yellow = Nursing staff base

2 Betten

2 Betten

2 Betten

Arzt

2 Betten

Arzt

Gruppenraum

Arzt | Arzt

Aufenthaltsraum und
Speiseraum für Patienten

2 Betten

4 Betten | 4 Betten | 4 Betten

2 Betten

Pflege
Stützpunkt

◨ **Fig. 13.6.** Floor plan of a ward in the building part B (Graphics: J. Christan)

The Organizational Restructuring of the Hospital

The organizational problems caused by the change of the »clinic for nervous diseases« into a »Psychiatric Clinic« were quicker and easier to solve than the planning and realization of the re-building and extension.

Hippius had already presented his proposals and demands in an exposé during his negotiations with the Ministry at the end of 1969. The basic concept which had been agreed on by the Ministry and Deans of the Medical Faculty consisted of:

- Maintaining the clinic with a uniform structure and
- That the clinic director would be directly responsible for the »nucleus« of the clinic (with all the wards) and the out-patient clinic with the independent departments, integrated into the clinic as a whole, with their various specialist areas.

Until the end of 1970 only one function area existed at the »clinic for nervous diseases«, which pretty much corresponded to a department: the »x-ray department« headed by K. Decker. Nothing like the »EEG laboratory« of J. Kugler existed within »neuroradiology«. The monitoring of other function areas (clinical laboratory, department for expert opinions, psychological diagnostics) was done by the clinical senior consultants.

During negotiations the Ministry had accepted Hippius' proposal to set up (as of 1971) five to a maximum of six departments within the Psychiatric Clinic. The department heads would occupy H3 positions (later C3 professorships). The dean in office at the time, Professor Dr. W. Spann, and some clinic heads consulted on the duties of the future departments and defined them down as follows:

- Neuroradiology
- Forensic Psychiatry
- Neurochemistry
- Psychosomatics and Psychotherapy
- Clinical and Experimental Psychology
- Neurophysiology

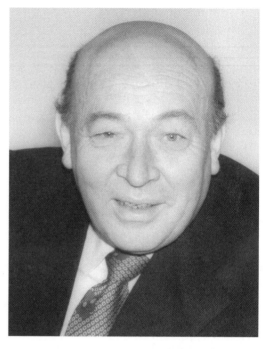

□ **Fig. 13.7.** Kurt Decker (1921–1985)

Two further departments, proposed by Hippius, were not agreed to:

- Gerontopsychiatry
- Social Psychiatry and Epidemiology

Department for Neuroradiology

The establishment and continuation of this department was a necessity, as it had already existed during Bumke's time in office and further developed by K. Decker (□ Fig. 13.7) to an important place for neuroradiological diagnostics and research in Germany, during Stertz and Kolle's time in office (▶ Chapter 10). On the separation of psychiatry from neurology, Decker had decided to stay at the Psychiatric Clinic, one of the deciding factors being the very good equipment in the department. After talks with the dean of the medical faculty and in agreement with the heads of the Clinics for Neurosurgery and Radiology (as of 1971) Decker could no longer perform neurosurgical operations and radiation therapy on patients with brain tumours in his department; the equipment, which

had been purchased in the fifties and sixties for this purpose, had to be handed over.

However, the department was further equipped for neuroradiological diagnostics and Decker remained a generally well-known neuroradiologist and scientist. Decker was originally skeptical about cranial computer tomography and »brain imaging«. Later plans to complement neuroradiological methods (mainly oriented to morphological media) by including biophysical-functional methods in a special department for brain-imaging in psychiatry did not materialice. Kurt Decker died unexpectedly in 1985 at the age of 63 years.

After Decker's death his co-workers managed the department, and negotiations with successors from Germany and Holland began. However, the negotiations were halted and the neurosurgical, radiological and neurological clinics in Grosshadern demanded the centralization of neuroradiological diagnostics in Grosshadern. Consequently, the neuroradiological tradition at the Psychiatric Clinic came to an end.

Department for Forensic Psychiatry

In the 19th century forensic-psychiatric expertise was one of psychiatry's roots. During this period psychiatric expertise developed independently from the field of psychiatric care evolving at the time. Later it was mainly the institution doctors (even the directors themselves) who took over expertise duties. And the situation was similar at the university clinics.

In Munich the first professor holding the chair of psychiatry, A. von Solbrig, became well-known for his expert opinion. Later A. Bumm wrote expert opinions together with his co-workers (in particular with W. Vocke). As clinic director Kraepelin made sure that his co-workers were competent in this field and held forensic-psychiatric seminars, demonstrating the problems of the experts' opinion with case studies. His first senior consultant R. Gaupp became a prominent assessor in Munich and even more so in Tubingen. Later the clinic's senior consultants, such as E. Kahn and in particular Max Mikorey, had a reputation as psychiatric experts in and outside Munich. Like in most of Germany's psychiatric clinics, at the Munich clinic too the senior consultants were responsible for expert opinions. These »expertise senior consultants« also held lectures on »Forensic Psychiatry« and instructed the assistants on all matters of assessing cases. At almost no psychiatric hospital the senior consultants had any direct subordinates to assist with assessments. During the seventies only a few faculties had such departments or institutes for forensic psychiatry. And unfortunately, these soon lost all necessary contact with clinical psychiatry.

By setting up a Department for Forensic Psychiatry, headed by a professor (H3 or C3 professor) with all the necessary staff (assistants, psychologists, social workers, secretaries) the disadvantages of the other systems could be avoided (the responsible senior consultant being overloaded with other duties or the department for forensic psychiatry being totally out of touch with the clinic).

Werner Mende (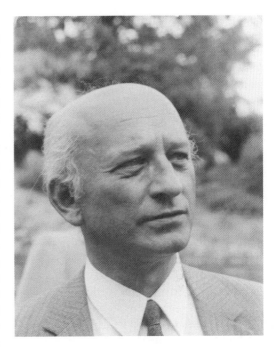 Fig. 13.8) was offered the position as head of the Department for Forensic Psychiatry.

W. Mende (1919–2003) had been scientific assistant at the clinic for nervous diseases at the university of Jena, headed by R. Lemke (1906–1957).

Fig. 13.8. Werner Mende (1919–2003)

In 1953 he had to leave the Democratic Republic of Germany and went to West Berlin. W. Schulte (1910–1972) took him from Berlin to become senior consultant at the Psychiatric Clinic of Westphalia in Gutersloh. Schulte knew Mende from his time at the clinic in Jena. When Schulte became successor to E. Kretschmer in Tubingen, Mende joined him as first senior consultant. In Tubingen Mende became particularly interested in problems of forensic psychiatry and continued the work he had begun in Berlin as psychiatric expert.

At the end of 1970 the Ministry for Social Welfare of the State of Baden Wurttemberg offered Mende the job of director of the district hospital for the mentally ill in Schussenried. Whilst negotiations were going on, he was offered the job at the Munich Hospital to set up and take over the new Department for Forensic Psychiatry. Mende accepted the offer from Munich and the Bavarian Ministry of Culture was responsible for negotiating Mende's release from any obligations and his move to Munich. W. Mende took up office in Munich on March 1, 1971.

Within a short period of time Mende managed to achieve a good reputation with his new department and it became a model for similar institutions at several psychiatric clinics in Germany. In an exposé on the situation of forensic psychiatry in Germany (Foerster, K.: Further education for forensic psychiatry in the Federal Republic of Germany in international comparison. Forensia, 1988; 9:257-261) it was stressed that the department at the Munich Psychiatric Clinic played an important role and should serve as a »model« for future developments. In this context Mende's insistence that forensic psychiatry not just be restricted to an expert opinion was crucial; apart from prognostic and therapeutic aspects, the contact to clinical psychiatry always had to be upheld.

All clinic assistants who were involved in further training, carried out and wrote expert opinions under Mende's guidance. Some assistant doctors either worked for a while (generally for one to two years) in the forensic department for further education purposes or in order to conclude their further education and training. Some of these assistants later resumed positions in the field of forensic psychiatry, e.g. within the penal system or in the medical service of district law courts.

Mende headed the Forensic-Psychiatric Department until he retired in 1984. Co-workers between 1971 and 1984 were I. Widerholt, D. Athen, N. Nedopil and the psychologist J. Weber. Athen and Nedopil qualified as university lecturers with theses on forensic-psychiatric topics.

Following Mende's retirement Nedopil continued to head the department ad interim, then until 1987 D. Athen took over, also provisionally.

On April 1, 1987 **Henning Sass** (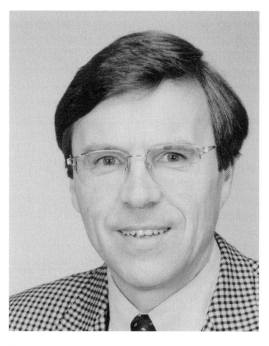 Fig. 13.9) took over the position as head of the Department for Forensic Psychiatry in Munich. H. Sass (born 1944) completed his clinical training at the Heidelberg Clinic under W. Janzarik. He qualified as university lecturer with a thesis on »Psychopathy – Sociopathy«. Immediately after receiving his qualifications, Sass left Heidelberg and joined the Forensic Psychiatric Department in Munich as department head. In order to remain in close contact with clinical psychiatry, he was also senior consultant in charge of the ward for addictive diseases. In 1990 H. Sass was offered the chair of psychiatry in Aachen, which he accepted.

Although Sass only spent a few years in Munich, he passed on the competence for expertise prob-

Fig. 13.9. Henning Sass (born 1944)

lems, which he had acquired in Heidelberg under Janzarik (based on the tradition of German psychopathology) to many co-workers at the Munich Clinic.

When Sass left for Aachen, his co-worker, P. Hoff (born 1956) headed the Forensic Psychiatric Department provisionally until N. Nedopil (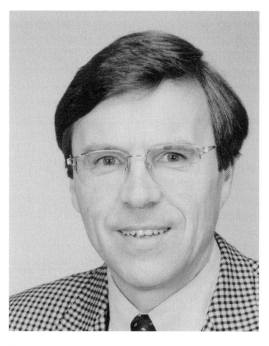 Fig. 13.10) arrived from the University of Wurzburg to become Sass' successor.

Norbert Nedopil (born 1947) had already worked at the Munich Clinic from 1977 until 1989. During this period he had worked a few years for Mende, received his lecturer qualifications in 1988, was co-worker to Sass and in 1989 he received a C3-professor title for Forensic Psychiatry in Wurzburg. Nedopil returned to the Munich Clinic in 1971 as Sass' successor.

On Nedopil's arrival in Munich, P. Hoff gave up the position as provisional head of the Forensic Psychiatric Department, became senior consultant at the clinic and received his qualifications as university lecturer in 1994. In 1996 Hoff was offered the position of a C3-professor and first senior consultant at the Psychiatric Clinic in Aachen under Sass. Since 2003 Hoff has been head physician of the department at the Psychiatric Clinic of the University of Zurich »Burghoelzli«, where W. Rossler holds the chair for Social Psychiatry.

Department of Neurochemistry

With the discovery of modern psychotropic drugs (antipsychotic drugs (1952) and antidepressants (1957)), biochemical research in psychiatry boomed. The clarification of the relevant, biological mechanisms responsible for the therapeutic efficacy of these drugs, opened a scientific gateway for research into the basic, biochemical mechanisms of psychiatric diseases (especially for schizophrenia and manic-depressive psychoses). Via these developments, psychopharmacological fundamental research and scientific clinical research became particularly promising research areas in biological psychiatry. Initially pharmaco-psychiatric research was a focal point of research at only a few German university clinics (Berlin, Erlangen, Mainz). Hippius had been one of the main instigators of this development in Berlin in 1953. It was therefore the natural course of things that this research direction would continue to be pursued and a close collabo-

ration be established, following Kraepelin's tradition at the Munich clinic, between biochemists and pharmaco-psychiatric research clinicians.

With this objective in mind, in summer 1971 a Department for Neurochemistry was set up. Head of this department was **Norbert Matussek** (◘ Fig. 13.11). He was responsible for the staff working in neurochemical research, as well as the routine laboratory diagnostics of the clinic.

Norbert Matussek (born 1922) studied medicine in Heidelberg, Munich and Tubingen where he worked together with the winner of the Nobel Prize, A. Butenandt. In 1956 he came to Munich and became co-worker of the neurochemist H. Jatzkewitz at the Max-Planck-Institute for Psychiatry. There he had been one of the first (after experiments on substance P and hallucinogenic drugs) to carry out studies on biogenic amines and the biochemical mode of action of modern psychotropic drugs. In 1961/1962 Matussek worked in the group of B. Brodie at the »National Institute of Mental Health« in Bethesda/USA. On returning to the Max-Planck-Institute for Psychiatry in Munich, he worked on the role of biogenic amines (nor-

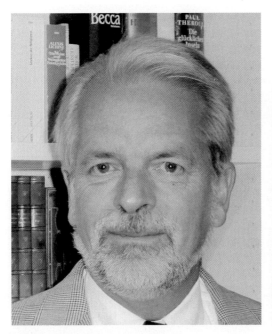

◘ **Fig. 13.10.** Norbert Nedopil (born 1947)

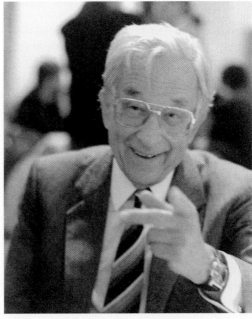

◘ **Fig. 13.11.** Norbert Matussek (born 1922)

adrenaline, serotonine) on the onset of depressive disorders and the mode of action of antidepressant medication. After qualifying as university lecturer for »Experimental Psychiatry« at the Munich medical faculty in 1967, Matussek took over the work group for psychopharmacology at the Max-Planck-Institute for Psychiatry.

Matussek had already decided to leave the Max-Planck-Institute in 1969 and to build up a neurobiological work group at the Munich Clinic. As he was not able to leave the Max-Planck-Institute until September 30, 1971, he encouraged one of his previous co-workers, Manfred Ackenheil, to move from Erlangen to Munich in summer 1971 and to make all necessary preparations (equipping, etc.) for work to start at the new department on October 1, 1971.

Matussek's enthusiasm for science at the Max-Planck-Institute had already attracted numerous young scientists, who have now become established researchers in fundamental, neurobiological science and are heading university institutes or departments (e.g. D. Weiss, Greifswald; P. Baumann, Lausanne; M. Ackenheil, Munich). When Matussek departed from the Max-Planck-Institute to the Munich hospital he was followed by several students and young assistants who qualified as university lecturers at the clinic, became senior consultants and later took over professorial chairs for psychiatry (O. Benkert, Mainz; H. Beckmann, Wurzburg; E. Rüther, Gottingen).

Matussek and his co-workers in the Neurochemical Department worked well with the clinical assistant doctors and a fruitful collaboration existed between both groups soon given the Munich clinic a good reputation as a successful research centre for biological psychiatry. The success of this arrangement was proved by the number of co-workers (other than those already mentioned), who received their university lecturer qualifications with theses on biological psychiatric topics, and who were also responsible for clinical psychiatric tasks (e.g. M. Albus, W. Greil, H. Klein, G. Laakmann, F. Müller-Spahn, D. Naber). The German Research Association (Deutsche Forschungsgemeinschaft (DFG)) supported the clinic's projects generously (e.g. long-term support within the DFG program on »Clinical Pharmacology«,

later within the DFG program on »Psychiatric Genetics«). The Sandoz Foundation for Therapeutic Research also generously supported the (initially meager number) of staff in the Neurochemical Department. An external sign of international recognition was given by the World Health Organization (WHO) naming the Munich Clinic a »National Collaborating Center for Biological Psychiatry« and an »International Reference Center for Psychotropic Drugs«.

On Matussek's retirement, Manfred Ackenheil (◘ Fig. 13.12) became head of the Neurochemical Department. Ackenheil continued Matussek's concept successfully and carried out scientific work on the basis of close collaboration between fundamental researchers and clinical doctors.

M. Ackenheil (1939–2006) left the psychopharmacology work group at the Max-Planck-Institute in 1970 and took over the laboratory at the district mental asylum in Erlangen, headed by W. W. Wieck. In 1971 he returned to Munich to work together with Matussek at the Psychiatric Clinic. He was Matussek's closest co-worker and in 1987 became his successor as head of the Neurochemical Department.

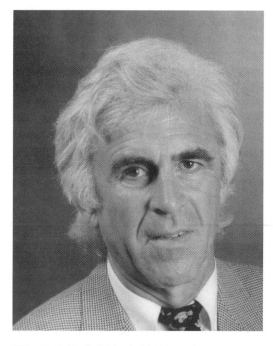

◘ **Fig. 13.12.** Manfred Ackenheil (1939–2006)

Ackenheil followed Matussek's research direction and also succeeded in founding a research group of international renown on psychiatric genetics. For the first time after the Second World War the Munich Clinic organized the »1st Munich Talks on Genetics« during the World Congress for Genetics in Berlin in 1987 on topics of psychiatric genetics. The »2nd Munich Talks on Genetics« took place in Prien (Upper Bavaria) in September 1991 in collaboration with the Collegium Internationale Neuropsychopharmacologicum (CINP).

The DFG program on »Psychiatric Genetics« which had been created by a specialist in genetics, P. Propping, and the Munich Clinic ,formed the basis for the revival of psychiatric genetic research in Germany. Various co-workers from the Neurochemical Department (e.g. B. Bondy and D. Wildenauer) were key to these developments. Further areas of interest were psychiatric stress research, psychoneuro-immunology (with N. Müller) and clinical pharmacology (e.g. drug monitoring).

With Mutussek and Ackenheil as department heads the concept of encouraging the exchange of opinions between fundamental researchers and clinicians was maintained and flourished, and it is also for this reason that numerous foreign guest scientists have spent time working in the Department for Neurochemistry (see below).

Department for Psychotherapy and Psychosomatics

Before and after the First World War psychoanalytical psychotherapy had been scarcely accepted in university psychiatry. During the Nazi regime psychoanalysis had been ostracized, but after the Second World War psychoanalysis experienced a revival. During this period the training and teaching of psychotherapy was taken over by predominantly independent institutes and academies. At some university clinics young co-workers began psychotherapeutical or psychoanalytical training, but hospital heads put up with it reluctantly.

At the time of the very liberal G. Stertz, some of his co-workers did a psychoanalytical training. Amongst others H. Stolze (born 1917) who had been voluntary doctor in 1946/47 and from 1948–1952 scientific assistant to Stertz. Through his connections to J.H. Schulz and G. Heye, Stolze became one of the co-founders of the »Lindau Psychotherapy Week«. The psychoanalyst, P. Matussek (1919–2003), also worked for Stertz as voluntary doctor and later became head of the Research Department for Psychopathology and Psychotherapy at the Max-Planck Association.

Under K. Kolle psychotherapy was not encouraged at the Munich clinic. Clinic assistants who had begun a psychotherapeutical training usually left the clinic after a couple of years.

However, W. Seitz (1905–1997), expert for internal medicine, who had been chosen for the professorial chair of internal medicine (medical out-patient clinic) in 1948, was an advocate for psychosomatics with in depth psychology orientation. During the fifties Th. Von Uexkull, W. Cremerius, M. Pflanz, W. Brautigam and many others had worked with him and later became prominent in the field of psychosomatics. In 1950 Seitz set up a »Psychosomatic Outreach Clinic« within the medical out-patient clinic; the first head of the outreach clinic was W. Cremerius. When Cremerius was offered the chair for psychosomatic medicine in Freiburg in 1965, Seitz offered the job to S. Elhardt who had been working for him until 1959.

In 1972 S. Elhardt became the first head of the Department for Psychotherapy and Psychosomatics at the Psychiatric Clinic.

Shortly after taking up office in Munich, Hippius had discussed the matter with W. Seitz and informed him of his idea to set up a department for psychotherapy and psychosomatics.

During their discussions Hippius and Seitz both expressed their hope that with the establishment of the department for psychotherapy and psychosomatics and by setting an example, other faculty clinics for somatics would follow and set up work groups or departments for integral psychosomatics. Unfortunately, these plans did not get very far, although some exceptions were made. The main concept was to establish a network from all departments and work groups for psychosomatics at various clinics connected to the Department for Psychotherapy at the Psychiatric Clinic, so that psychosomatics and psychotherapy would become established as a »cross-section« subject within the clinical disciplines. This concept had been developed in order to avoid that at the Munich faculty – contrary to the developments in most other medical faculties in Germany – only one institution be set up for psychosomatics responsible for the wide diversity of psychosomatics of all diseases in the many hospitals of the inner city and Grosshadern (with almost 3000 beds).

(It was fortunate that the sporadic efforts to take the Department for Psychotherapy and Psychosomatics out of the Psychiatric Clinic and to turn it into a completely autonomous department, and into an entirely self-sufficient institute for psychosomatics, were abandoned.)

During their discussions Seitz and Hippius realized that the working conditions for the future head of the Department for Psychotherapy and Psychosomatics at the Psychiatric Clinic were much better than as head of the Psychosomatic Outreach Clinic at the Medical Out-Patient Clinic. Consequently, Seitz and Hippius agreed to inform S. Elhardt of the situation and to leave the decision which position he would prefer up to him. Elhardt hesitated out of loyalty towards his tutor Seitz, but Seitz finally convinced Elhardt that the position at the Psychiatric Clinic offered better opportunities and would be a starting point for the development of psychotherapy within the Munich Medical Faculty.

Siegfried Elhardt (◘ Fig. 13.13) was born in Augsburg in 1922 and after graduation as doctor for internal medicine worked at the Medical Out-Patient Clinic with W. Seitz from 1948–1959. He then spent seven years as a specialist for internal medicine and psychoanalyst in his own practice. During this period he also gave instructions at the Munich »Academy for Psychoanalysis«. When Cremerius left the Out-Patient Clinic in 1965, Elhardt returned there and took over the Psychosomatic Outreach Clinic. In 1970 he qualified as university lecturer. At the end of 1971 he was offered the job as head of the newly founded Department for Psychotherapy and Psychosomatics at the Psychiatric Clinic.

Following negotiations, Elhardt accepted the offer and began work in the summer term of 1972. With Seitz's agreement some co-workers from the Medical Out-Patient Clinic (e.g. R. Pfizner and later O. Seidl, and the psychoanalysts Mrs. E. Zan-

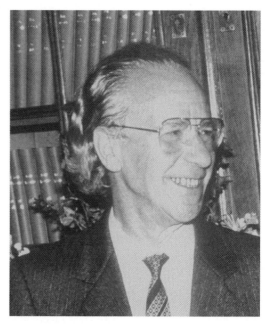

◘ **Fig. 13.13.** Siegfried Elhardt (1922–1990)

der and Mrs. D. Zagermann) joined Elhardt at the new department. Elhardt was departmental head from May 1, 1972 until March 31, 1984. For health reasons he took early retirement; he died in 1990.

Following graduation, Michael Ermann (born 1943 in Stettin) (◘ Fig. 13.14) was research assistant from 1970 to 1976 at the Psychotherapeutic Center in Stuttgart and completed his training as psychoanalyst there. In 1976 he became senior consultant at the Psychosomatic Clinic of the Central Institute for Mental Health in Mannheim at the Heidelberg Medical Faculty. In 1980 he qualified as professor for psychosomatic medicine and psychoanalysis at the Heidelberg University. In 1985 he became department head at the Department for Psychotherapy and Psychosomatics at the Munich Clinic.

Elhardt and later Ermann with co-workers represent the psychodynamic pole amongst the spectrum of therapeutic concepts at the clinic and supply an interface between psychodynamically based psychosomatics and psychiatry – in clinical practice, in research, in further education and student training. Apart from its involvement with the Psychiatric Clinic, the department has developed scientific projects with other clinics and in other

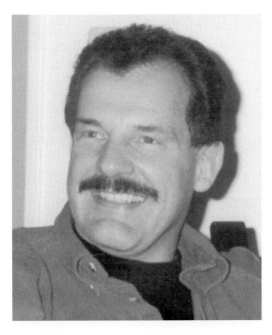

most important »auxiliary sciences« in psychiatric research (▶ Chapter 7).

In most psychiatric clinics potential contribution from psychological study methods in clinical psychiatry had been reduced to psychological tests within the diagnostic process. A revival of Kraepelin's approach took place at the beginning of the fifties. The introduction of modern psychotropic drugs led to Kraepelin's studies »On the influence of simple mental processes by some drugs« being acknowledged and accepted firstly by psychologists, but soon by psychiatrists as well. At some university institutes for psychology, »pharmaco-psychology« became an important research topic. At the same time, at several psychiatric hospitals, where scientific work was being done in the field of pharmaco-psychiatry, research groups included clinicians working closely with psychologists.

In connection with the psycho-pharmacological work in a national and international context (e.g. via the congresses of the »Collegium Internationale Neuropsychopharmacologicum (CINP)« and the »Arbeitsgemeinschaft für Neuropsychopharmakologie »(Work Alliance for Neuropsycho-Pharmacology) (AGNP), which Hippius had started already as an assistant doctor at the FU Berlin during the fifties) he had good contacts to psychologists (in particular G. A. Lienert; later amongst others also to W. Jahnke and P. Netter). Their research approaches gave impulses for clinical psychiatric research work and it was a matter of course that a Department for Clinical and Experimental Psychology be set up at the Munich Clinic.

fields. Generally, consiliary services are the basis for such project developments. In this manner and in cooperation with the Department for Haemostaseology at the Medical Hospital, an outreach clinic was set up for HIV patients. With federal financial support a research project (including an outreach clinic for female patients) was set up to study the psychosocial situation of HIV infected patients and those suffering from AIDS; the project was also involved with a similar set up for HIV sufferers at the Dermatological Clinic. At Grosshadern and in collaboration with one of the Medical Clinics, studies on the life quality and coping after stem cell transplants were carried out in the field of psycho-oncology. In collaboration with the Dental Clinic patients with oro-facial pain syndromes were studied with regard to the patients' attitude and motivation towards psychotherapy.

Hospital and Experimental Psychology

The establishment of this department followed up on Kraepelin's tradition. Under W. Wundt's influence Kraepelin considered psychology's empirically founded research methods to be one of the

Helmuth P. Huber, a pupil of G.A. Lienert, took on the task as departmental head.

Helmuth P. Huber (born 1937) (◘ Fig. 13.15) had studied psychology in Vienna, then studied medicine and became assistant at the Institute for the History of Medicine in Vienna. In 1964 G. A. Lienert (1920–2001) offered Huber a job at the Psychological Institute in Dusseldorf. Here, Huber worked on psychological diagnostics, test theory and test construction. He also set up a pharmacological laboratory where he studied the influence of various personality dimensions on the effect of psychotropic substances. In 1972 he qualified as professor with Lienert with a thesis on psychomet-

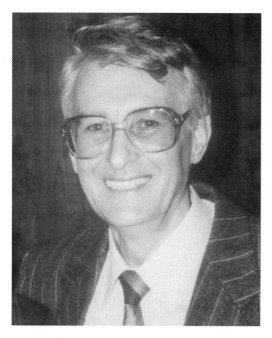

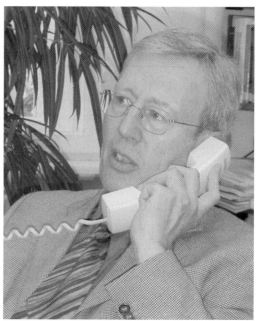

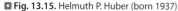

Fig. 13.15. Helmuth P. Huber (born 1937)

Fig. 13.16. Rolf Engel (born 1946)

ric, single case studies, a study which soon became known as standard work. In 1972 Huber took over the Department for Clinical and Experimental Psychology at the Munich Clinic. R. Engel, Huber's co-worker, arrived in Munich before Huber and started work at setting up the equipment and monitoring the necessary re-building work.

In 1973 Huber received an offer as ordinary professor to the chair of Clinical Psychology at the Hamburg University. He accepted the offer and began work in Hamburg during the winter term of 1974. In 1980 he moved to Graz to the professorial chair for Psychology at the University of Graz.

Huber's co-worker, Rolf Engel, became his successor.

Rolf Engel (**■** Fig. 13.16) was born in 1946 in Saarbrucken; he studied psychology in Saarbrucken, Tubingen, Marburg and Dusseldorf. As a student in Dusseldorf Engel already started work at G.A. Lienert's Institute and worked together with H. Huber. In 1972 Engel graduated at the Scientific Faculty in Dusseldorf with a experimental study on »Psychophysiology of dreams«. When Huber decided to move to Munich in 1972 and set up the Department for Clinical and Experimental Psy-

chology there, he suggested that Engel join him. As Huber could not leave the institute in Dusseldorf immediately, Engel moved to Munich before him and was responsible for the preparatory work there. When Huber left Munich again in 1974, Engel was given the position as provisional head of the department. In 1984 he qualified as professor for psychology at the Faculty for Psychology and Education at the Munich University. In 1985 he received his professor title as well as the position as Head of the Department for Clinical and Experimental Psychology at the Psychiatric Clinic.

Engel and co-workers from his department have influenced the scientific work in all areas of the clinic in many ways. For many of the scientifically working doctors at the clinic, Engel and his team of psychologists (e.g. N. Kathmann, now Professor for Keim's Psychology at the Humboldt University, Berlin) were often indispensable, selfless and helpful partners – from the test planning phase to the statistical evaluation of the findings. One of the first fields of interest for Engel and his co-workers were the diagnostic and treatment of sleep disorders. In the field of intelligence and personality diagnostics the development of computerized evaluation procedures (e.g. computerized evaluation and interpretation of the MMPI; construction of computerized capacity tests) was another focal point. In collaboration with the geronto-psychiatric research ward, methods for the diagnostics of dementia were developed. Further research programs included studies on the use of biofeedback in psychosomatic disorders and the effect of cognitive manipulation on event-correlated EEG potentials. In connection with pharmaco-psychiatric studies (e.g. on influencing anxiety syndromes) the effect of mental stress on vegetative and neurochemical variables was studied.

The meta-analyses of the effects and side-effects of psychotropic drugs, as initiated by Engel and followed by many other scientists, are particularly important. Engel's collaboration was exceptionally important and fruitful for the research projects »AMUEP« (Arzneimittelüberwachung in der Psychiatrie; 1979–1989 (Medicament Monitoring in Psychiatry)) and »AMSP« (Arzneimittelsicherheit in der Psychiatrie; since 1992 (Medicament Security in Psychiatry)); further participants in these studies are a large number of clinics in Germany, as well as Austria and Switzerland.

Department for Clinical Neurophysiology and EEG Diagnostics

With the separation of neurology from psychiatry at the beginning of 1971, J. Kugler and his EEG laboratory were allocated to the Neurological Clinic, but remained responsible for the EEG diagnostics of all in- and out-patients at the Psychiatric Clinic. This ruling remained in force until the Neurological Clinic was finally established in Grosshadern in 1976. In negotiations between the Ministry and the director of the Neurological Clinic (A. Schrader) it was agreed that Kugler and the staff in the EEG laboratory did not have to transfer to Grosshadern, but that they would be taken over in 1976 together with the staff inventory of the Psychiatric Clinic. Based on this arrangement, Kugler became head of the »Department for Clinical (Psychiatric) Neurophysiology and EEG Diagnostics« of the Psychiatric Clinic.

Johannes Kugler (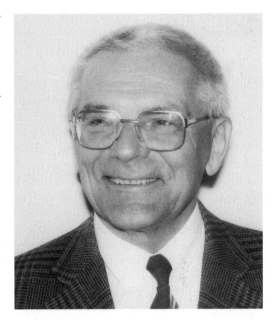 Fig. 13.17) was born in Vienna in 1923. He began studying medicine in 1941, but being wounded and hospitalized could

Fig. 13.17. Johannes Kugler (born 1923)

only complete his training in Munich and Vienna after military service. After graduation he worked as a general practitioner, spent long study periods in France (amongst others with H. Gastaut) and worked from 1953 until 1956 at a clinic for neurosurgery in Austria.

In 1956 K. Kolle offered him a job as assistant doctor at the Munich Clinic for Nervous Diseases, with the intention that on R. Weber's resignation, he take over the EEG laboratory at the clinic. Kugler turned the EEG laboratory into a renowned research and training center. Many psychiatrists and neurologists, and in particular many technical assistants from the surgical, neurosurgical and anesthesiology departments spent time training in Kugler's EEG laboratory. In 1967 Kugler started giving annual, one-week courses on »Further Education on EEGs«, intended for doctors and technical staff, which became a main event in the field of neurophysiology in Germany. With his good international connections, Kugler was able to invite well-known speakers for these events.

Together with his co-worker R. Spatz, Kugler set up the first out-patient unit in Germany for patients with epilepsy; the unit continued its work after Kugler's retirement in 1988.

Developments in Training and Further Education

After the Second World War the **training** and study plans for the medical students had not been changed or adapted for many years. In 1971, during the last term before graduation, the students were only offered tuition in a one-term series of lectures entitled »Psychiatry and Neurology« with a total of five hours a week. As most of the students had already prepared themselves for the exams during the last term, they considered »Psychiatry and Neurology« to be less important than all of the other subjects. For the overall exam marking system results in »Psychiatry and Neurology« were of less significance: To calculate the overall mark, the marks scored for the so-called »standard subjects« (internal medicine, surgery and gynaecology) were multiplied by a point-value of 6, whilst psychiatry and neurology were only multiplied by 1. As more and more faculties were separating tuition in psychiatry and neurology and were also giving separate exams on these subjects, it was a matter of course that each subject had the significance of half a point and thus had landed at the end of the scale of relevance!

It was not until the study and examination guidelines and the licensure to practice medicine were changed, that psychiatry's position as a »tail light« improved. In general, the entire material on nervous diseases became more important during the seventies. Instead of the usual five hours of lecture a week in a main lecture, in 1971 these were replaced by separate courses for psychiatry and neurology and in the following years a number of different events were arranged (lectures, courses, practical work, seminars). Consequently, psychiatry (together with psychosomatics and psychotherapy) was positioned next to the »grand old subjects«.

Once the students had heard lectures and done courses on medical psychology and medical sociology during the pre-clinical terms, they followed up in a second clinical phase during three subsequent terms with on-going tuition on psychiatry, psychosomatics and psychotherapy. In this manner the students visited compulsory courses for a relatively long period and, with practical exercises in compulsory lectures, were confronted with all areas of psychiatry, psychotherapy and psychosomatics.

Although these fundamental changes in student training for psychiatry/psychotherapy and psychosomatics were necessary and welcome, they made great demands on the Munich clinic: Training had to be organized for 250 to 300 students. The size of the course groups could not exceed a maximum of 15 to 20 students. However, this was taken care of by capable staff on all the wards together with experienced doctors and nursing staff.

The patients also played an important role in the training: The predominant majority of patients agreed to be explored at one of the larger lectures or during the student group sessions.

Previous clinic co-workers who took over senior positions at district mental asylums near Munich, and also others who had habilitated at the faculty started giving »one to two week« blocks of practical study at their clinics (e.g. Kaufbeuren, Gabersee, Haar), thus relieving the work load of the doctors and nursing staff at the Munich clinic. Students were and still are particularly fond of these blocks of practical study.

In connection with the introduction of the practical year of study during the third clinical phase (the so-called internship), it was arranged that a limited number of students would spend a vocational period in psychiatry (at the university clinic and/or in a hospital officially recognized by the Ministry as an academic hospital). Student, who took advantage of this choice during the clinical studies, and therefore were integrated into the daily work of a psychiatric clinic for several months, often chose later to become psychiatrists or psychotherapists.

The **further education** for the clinic's assistant doctors, up until qualification as specialist doctor, was improved step-by-step at the Munich clinic.

Originally, the qualification as specialist doctor was certified by the district medical association, once the clinic director, responsible for further education, had confirmed this in an attestation and once the period of specialist education had been formally fulfilled. At the beginning of the seventies it was at the discretion of the senior doctors who organized the staffing of the wards, and to the initiative of the assistant doctors themselves, to choose which areas (male/female wards; open/closed wards) they would complete their specialist training in. According to a procedure adhered to at the clinic in Berlin, in 1971 the »further education booklet« was introduced. All sectors worked in during the years of further education and all courses attended (clinical case presentations; seminars given by the Department for Psychotherapy and Psychosomatics; Balint groups; EEG diagnostics; neuro-radiological demonstrations; forensic-psychiatric seminars; scientific seminars in the Department for Clinical and Experimental Psychology – e.g. on psychological test diagnostics; seminars by the Department of Neurochemistry – e.g. on psycho-pharmacology;) were noted and attested in this booklet. Such attempts to have tighter control of further education were abandoned once resolutions passed at the German Medical Days (Deutsche Ärztetage) with respect to further education, set down precise rules and introduced examinations for specialist qualifications.

On the whole, the rules laid down with respect to specialist qualifications for psychiatry and the necessary neurological training could be handled by exchanging jobs with assistants from the Neurological Clinic in Grosshadern for the majority of assistants. In the case of large psychiatric institutions arrangements were made with other district hospitals in Upper Bavaria and Swabia.

Unfortunately, an agreement with the health authorities of the city of Munich, whereby clinic assistants could work in a job offered by the health authorities, or for example at an outreach clinic for addicts, lasted only until the mid eighties. The work in the city of Munich gave excellent opportunities to see special areas of psychiatry, for example by visiting psychiatric patients in their everyday living environment.

At most of the psychiatric university clinics teaching of the usual training for nursing staff, social services, physiotherapy and occupational therapy was entrusted to experienced assistant doctors. In 1988, in co-operation with the Academy of Arts, the Ministry of Science agreed that art therapy also be taught as a new subject.

One of the generally important further steps was the establishment of a **training venue for psy-chiatric nursing staff**. This development actually originated from a recommendation made by the »Evaluation Commission« and was set up in collaboration with the Psychiatric Clinic of the TU Munich and the Clinic of the Max-Planck-Institute for Psychiatry (1978).

This institution (20 positions) was run according to guidelines set down by the German Hospital Association. Male and female nurses who had passed the main nursing exams and worked for at least one year at a psychiatric clinic, could complete a two-year training course to become »Specialist Psychiatric Nurses«. This training and qualification was initially only possible at a few German university clinics probably contributing to the fact that even in times of serious nursing staff deficit (at the end of the eighties) the Munich clinic hardly ever had a problem finding sufficient nursing staff.

The heads of the clinic's nursing corps were also instrumental in employing well-trained male and female nurses from 1971 onwards.

From the opening of the clinic in 1904 until the mid seventies the senior nun was always a central figure with respect to the entire nursing staff; all wards were headed by nuns. In 1976, a very responsible and deserving matron (Sister M. Klarella Sailer) who had worked at the clinic since the end of the Second World War, left the clinic and was succeeded by Sister M. Tabitha Goetschl. During her time in office (1976–1986) changes in the distribution of responsibilities were introduced step by step. The wards were headed by male or female nurses as opposed to nuns. The head of the nursing staff (M. Spaeth) was involved wherever nursing matters were concerned. Together with dedicated nurses on the wards (e.g. senior nurses on the research wards), the senior nun and head of the nursing staff continuously attracted very experienced, but also young and motivated nurses to the clinic.

Development of the Hospital and Research

Until the opening of the hospital on the Nussbaumstrasse in 1904, the Upper Bavarian district mental hospitals (Haar, Eglfing, Gabersee and some smaller private clinics) had been responsible for the in-patient care of psychiatric patients. As of

1904 the clinic made a tremendous contribution to psychiatric care: Already in its first year the clinic treated 1,600 in-patients. In the following years – until the Psychiatric Clinic was changed into a Clinic for Nervous Diseases – an average of 2000 in-patients were admitted annually. After 1926 the number rose to 3,400 per year. During the years after the Second World War the clinic was constantly overcrowded; for example, in 1950 all together 5,500 psychiatric and neurological patients were given in-patient care. During the first years the clinic was changed into a Psychiatric Clinic, 2,900 patients were treated annually. This figure could be reduced in the following years. The previous practice of admitting patients with the first appearance of a disease and immediately referring those, who had been ill several times, to the district clinics, was changed: If former clinic patients – regardless of diagnosis or whatever – were referred for treatment, they were admitted and treated. Further transfer to the district clinics for continuation of therapy was

only done if improvement could not be expected after several weeks (or even months) of treatment, but the need for in-patient care remained. After 1971 the number of such therapy-resistant cases sank to less than 10 patients a year!

Several factors contributed to this development: Treatment with **psychotropic drugs** became the defining element for treatment and clinical research. For each patient a comprehensive **treatment schedule** was set down, taking into account all individually ascertained somatic, psycho- and social elements; if there was an indication for treatment with psychotropic drugs, these were prescribed according to differential therapeutic aspects. If the patient agreed, then the course of treatment was observed for research purposes and registered systematically by the AMDP system. In co-operation with co-workers from the Departments of Neurochemistry, Clinical Neurophysiology and Clinical Psychology the observations were expanded into scientific studies. In this manner the clinical action pattern of the »classical« antipsychotic drugs, drugs for episode prophylaxis, new kinds of antidepressants (SSRI), anxiolytic drugs and later also anti-dementia drugs and substances influencing the addictive behaviour (craving) of alcoholics were studied. The fundamental scientific and clinical studies on clozapine played an important role in this context. The »re-discovery « of clozapine in the USA at the end of the eighties (initiated by the first descriptions of a clinical mode of action of clozapine at the end of the sixties) and the world-wide breakthrough of the so-called »atypical neuroleptics« (2nd generation antipsychotic drugs) are connected with the work done at the Munich clinic on the further development of **psychiatric pharmaco-therapy**.

The Munich Clinic's work and standing was also influenced by the fact that Hippius and one of his senior consultants, H. Dilling, were asked in 1971 to become members of the »Evaluation Commission« set up by the German government to draft the report on »The State of Psychiatry in the Federal Republic of Germany«. And it was a matter of course that work on the evaluation (1971–1975) would involve the clinic in problems of psychiatric care from a scientific and practical point of view.

Psychiatrische Klinik und Poliklinik

		Gebäude	Geschoß
Direktor der Klinik:	Prof. Dr. H. Hippius	A	2
Oberärzte:	Prof. Dr. G. Laakmann	Zahnklinik	
„	(Ltd. OA)	Goethestr. 70	
„	Prof. Dr. F. Müller-Spahn	A	3
„	(Ltd. OA)		
„	Dr. P. Buchheim	B	0
„	(Leiter der Poliklinik)		
„	PD Dr. W. Greil	A	2
„	Dr. Dr. P. Hoff	E	1
„	Dr. H. Kapfhammer	B	3
„	Frau Dr. G. Kurtz	B	1
„	Frau PD Dr. I. Meller	A	2
„	Dr. N. Müller	B	2
„	PD Dr. D. Naber	B	3
Neurochemische Abt.:	Prof. Dr. M. Ackenheil	E	0
Forschungsbereich Genetik:	Frau PD Dr. Bondy	E	0
Klinisch - experimentelle	Prof. Dr. R. Engel	A	3
Psychologie und Psychophysiologie:			
EEG	Dr. R. Spatz	A	3
Abt. für Psychotherapie		Zahnklinik	
und Psychosomatik:	Prof. Dr. M. Ermann	Goethestr. 70	
Abteilung für			
Forensische Psychiatrie:	Prof. Dr. N. Nedopil	E	1
Allgem. Psychopathologie:	Prof. Dr. R. Meyendorf	E	1
Gerontopsychiatrie:	Prof. Dr. F. Müller-Spahn	A	3
Münchner			
Hochbetagten-Studie:	Frau PD Dr. I. Meller	A	2
Psychiatr. Epidemiologie:	Prof. Dr. M. Fichter	G	0
Pflegedienstleitung	M. Späth	A	0
Weiterbildungsstätte für psychiatrische Fachkrankenpflege, Zahnklinik			
	Fr. M. Thiede	Goethestr. 70	
Institut für Kinder- und Jugendpsychiatrie			
Direktor	Prof. Dr. J. Martinius	F	0
Konsiliardienst			

Besuchszeiten täglich von 14.00 - 19.00 Uhr

Zutritt nur für Patienten, Angehörige und Personal

◨ **Fig. 13.18.** Information board at the clinic entrance (1992)

The logistics of the clinic changed as of 1971 when the out-patient clinic received an independent status. Up until 1971 one or two assistant doctors were responsible for patients who came to the out-patient clinic; the assistants showed the patients which they had examined in the morning to one of the clinical senior consultants. In 1971 a position was made for a senior consultant at the out-patient clinic, which was occupied by M. von Cranach, P. Buchheim and H.-P. Kapfhammer in chronological order.

The senior consultant of the out-patient clinic was responsible for the department all day together with 3 to 4 assistant doctors, a social worker and one to two nurses. Later, one of the assistants, according to the Swiss system, had the function of a »triage« doctor; after an informative initial exploration the assistant decided whether detailed out-patient examinations should be conducted, whether the patient be transferred to a practicing psychiatrist or other specialist doctors (e.g. general practicioner) or whether the patient needed in-patient treatment. Throughout the day and together with a nurse the »day-time« doctors at the out-patient clinic also took care of transfers and telephone registration of patients for in-patient treatment coming from practicing specialists or hospitals; they also took care of acute and emergency cases from the emergency services or those brought directly to the clinic by the police. The »day-time« doctors at the out-patient clinic (and at the end of the day, the doctors on duty) were always kept up to date on ward beds being vacated or possible admissions; in this manner they had the function of a »central admission doctor« and could control the patient admissions. By establishing a »central admission« function, it was possible to achieve a 95 % occupancy (sometimes, with discharges and admissions on the same day, even 100 %).

In connection with scientific projects, the out-patient clinic maintained special out-patient units (e.g. for patients treated long-term with antipsychotic drugs or lithium, a sleep unit, a memory unit, units for alcoholics and other addicts, for HIV-patients, for methadone substitution and for anxiety patients).

The restructuring of the out-patient clinic, with respect to its effect on the »outside«, was implemented in the context of Hippius' and Dilling's work for the »Evaluation Commission«. Similarly, »patient clubs« were founded for out-patients and for discharged in-patients as part of the post-care concept; a workshop for the handicapped and – temporarily – a home was set up for vagrants. The head of the out-patient clinic was responsible for monitoring and supervising these activities and he was supported in this task by doctors, social workers and nurses, who often did the work voluntarily in their free time.

Based on the guideline framework of the Evaluation Report, the Munich clinic tried to complement the principles of in-patient treatment with a part in-patient unit.

> Inspired by experiences from a study sojourn in Montreal, Canada, Hippius set up a Psychiatric Day and Night Clinic (House Phoenix) during his work at the FU in Berlin and in collaboration with the local section of the German Red Cross. Berlin had such a part in-patient unit and so did Frankfurt/Main already before a recommendation could be made by the Evaluation Commission.

As of 1973 Dilling and Hippius tried to set up a day clinic as part of the Munich out-patient clinic and a small night clinic as part of the Munich in-patient clinic. For various reasons negotiations got drawn out and an attempt was made to follow the Berlin model and to set up a day clinic together with the local section of the Bavarian Red Cross. After initial reservation by the Bavarian Red Cross, a site was found in 1980, close to the clinic and easily accessible by public transport, with 25 places. The Bavarian Red Cross became sponsor to the »Day Clinic of the Bavarian Red Cross on the Lindwurmstrasse«. According to the agreements, the day clinic was closely attached to the University Clinic since its founding.

For a long time the day-clinic treatment (group therapy, occupational therapy) had only provisional rooms at its disposal. With the plans for a new building it was possible to make adequate space available and thus combine these activities for the in-patients and day-clinic patients.

All of these efforts to extend the care functions and logistics of the clinic beyond the in-patient treatment, meant that in-patient care had to change as well. The traditional structure of the clinic into the »male side« and the »female side« with its respective »closed« and »open« wards was soon abandoned; as soon as the space and sanitary conditions permitted it, the open wards became »mixed« wards for both sexes. Certain individual wards became »specialist« wards. Already prior to moving eight wards from the old building (A) to the newly built parts of the clinic (B and C), a ward for addiction patients was set up. When the Neurological Clinic moved out in 1976, a **research ward** with 12 beds was put in the available space. Headed by a senior consultant, the doctors working on this ward were supported by qualified technical and nursing staff and dealt with constantly changing scientific topics. In this context, one of the first sleep laboratories was set by E. Rüther for research into sleep and sleep disorders. Once the new buildings had been prepared, the research ward with its 12 beds was moved into new rooms in building section D. A second research ward was set up by F. Müller-Spahn with a further 12 beds for research into dementia and geronto-psychiatry. The two research wards were well-staffed and equipped and the research direction could be defined by the senior consultants in charge (e.g. sleep research; geronto-psychiatry; psycho-neuroendocrinology; clinical psycho-pharmacology).

For the clinic's activities and care offer in the regions of Munich and Upper Bavaria it was advantageous that soon after 1971 good and effective co-operation with other clinics, authorities of the district of Upper Bavaria and the City of Munich, but also with free agencies, e.g. the Bavarian Red Cross (BRK) and private clinic agencies (the Schön group of companies), was initiated and came into effect. As of the beginning of the seventies, it was important for the clinic to be supported in all possible aspects by all possible instances. In this context it should be mentioned that the consultants from the various state ministries, from the local government and local MPs were involved, also particular reference must be made to the President of the Upper Bavarian government, Georg Klimm.

It is thanks to G. Klimm (1913–2000) and negotiations with the Ministry of Culture, the university, the medical faculty and the local government, that the ordinary chair for child psychiatry was established. J. Martinius (born 1932) was offered the job and took over the District Clinic for Child Psychiatry (Heckscher Clinic) thus having a large, renowned clinic at his disposal. G. Klimm also arranged for collaboration with the district of Upper Bavaria to allow for one or two assistants from the clinic to be employed by the district at Haar (Director: Chr. Schulz) and Gabersee (Director: H. Kroiss) in order to gather experience for their specialist training. At a later stage the District Mental Hospital in Haar was the first institution– and for a long time the only one – to be given the status of a »Psychiatric Training Hospital« as proposed by the Medical Faculty and agreed to by the State Ministry for Education and Culture. Also in collaboration with the district of Upper Bavaria a catalogue was made of all existing care institutions – from practicing psychiatrists to clinical institutions – in Munich and Upper Bavaria which could be used as the basis for planning and improving future co-operation.

An agreement was made with the health authorities of the City of Munich to employ a clinic assistant for three to six months at the Psychiatric Service of the Municipal Health Authorities and a further assistant for six to twelve months at the outreach clinic for addicts.

The main objective of such agreements on the delegation of staff was to improve the situation for the patients, but also to expand the training of clinic assistants into areas previously neglected at psychiatric university clinics. (The delegation of a clinic assistant as head of the Outreach Clinic for Addicts of the City of Munich ended after a co-worker, who had spent several years working in the Addiction Department of the Maudsley Hospital in London, returned to Munich and took on the job permanently. This was R. Wille.)

As of 1971 the organizational restructuring of the clinic led to many young doctors applying for jobs, not just to complete their further training, but to work scientifically. This objective was accommodated in particular by the nursing staff at the Munich clinic – for all intents and purposes contrary to the situation at some other universities – who did not impede scientific work on the wards, but supported it with enthusiasm. The nursing staff considered it an honour to work on one of the research wards.

This open and **research-oriented atmosphere** was a contributing factor to the number of clinic co-workers (27), who achieved their postdoctoral lecturer qualifications between 1971 and 1994 (theses on psychiatry, forensic psychiatry, experimental psychiatry and – in collaboration with the faculty for psychology and teaching – on psychology).

The **theses for qualification as university lecturer** and the topics chosen were often the starting point for the further scientific and professional development of their authors, as shown in a brief overview of some of the topics between 1971 and 1994:

1975   R. Meyendorf (born 1934)
»Mental and neurological disorders from coronary surgery«

1976   O. Benkert (born 1940)
»Neuroendocrinological and pharmacotherapeutical studies of patients with sexual impotence«
Benkert took over the chair of psychiatry at the University of Mainz in 1981.

1976   H. Dilling (born 1933)
»Psychiatric epidemiological studies on the care facilities in a provincial area in Upper Bavaria«
Dilling took over the chair of psychiatry at the University of Lubeck in 1978.

1978   H. Beckmann (1940–2006)
»On the classification of depressive syndromes. Studies on differing traits and prognostic factors for responsiveness to somatic therapy procedures«
Beckmann became first senior consultant at the Central Institute for Mental Heath in Mannheim in 1978 and took over the chair of psychiatry at the University of Wurzburg in 1985.

1980   M. Ackenheil (1939–2006)
»Clinical and animal-experimental biochemical effects of clozapine; studies on the mode of action with regard to the importance of the dopamine hypothesis in schizophrenia«

1983   D. Athen (born 1937)
»Psychopathological status of acute alcohol intoxication – clinical and forensic relevance«

Athen became director of the District Psychiatric Hospital in Ansbach in 1985.

1983   W. Bender (born 1941)
»Insight into one's condition and feeling of illness in psychiatric patients«
Bender became director of the District Psychiatric Hospital in Haar in 1987.

1984   M. Fichter (born 1944)
»Annorexia: empirical studies on the epidemiology, symptomatology, nosology and course of illness«
Fichter became director of the Psychosomatic-Medical Clinic Roseneck/Prien in 1985. He was offered the chair for psychiatry at the Humboldt University Berlin (Charité), but turned the offer down.

1984   R. Engel (1946)
»Activation and emotion. Psychophysiological experiments on the structure of reaction patterns under mental stress«

1985   E. Rüther (born 1940)
»Course of efficacy of neuroleptic therapy. Course studies of antipsychotic therapy with haloperidol and clozapine«
After turning down the professorial chair for psychiatry in Lausanne, Rüther took over the chair of psychiatry in Gottingen in 1986.

1986   G. Laakmann (born 1944)
»Psychotropic drugs, anterior pituitary hormone secretion and depression research«

1987   H. Klein (born 1945)
»Psychopathological and neuroendocrinological findings in affective disorders«
Klein became director of the District Psychiatric Clinic in Regensburg in 1984 and took over the chair for psychiatry at the University of Regensburg in 1996.

1987   D. Naber (born 1947)
»Studies on the etiology and therapeutic importance of endorphins in endogenous psychoses«
Naber took over the chair for psychiatry at the University of Hamburg in 1994.

1987   R. Steinberg (born 1946)
»Music psychopathology: Musical expression and mental disease«
Steinberg became director of the Palatinate Clinic in Klingenmunster in 1987.

1988   W. Günther (born 1949)
»Psychometric and neurophysiological studies of disturbed voluntomotoricity in endogenous psychoses«
Günther became the director of the Psychiatric Clinic in Bamberg in 1991.

1988   N. Nedopil (born 1947)
»Standardized psychopathological recording of mentally ill criminals with aggression offences«
Nedopil became head of Department for
Forensic Psychiatry at the Psychiatric Clinic
of Wurzburg in 1989. In 1992 he returned
to the Psychiatric Clinic of the Munich University and became department head there
for Forensic Psychiatry.

1988   F. Müller-Spahn (born 1950)
»Neuroendocrinological studies on the stimulation of dopaminergic and alpha-adre-
nergic receptors in schizophrenic patients«
Müller-Spahn became head of the Department for Gerontopsychiatry at the University of Gottingen in 1990. In 1991 he returned
to Munich and took over the chair of psychiatry at the University of Basle in 1994.

1989   W. Greil (born 1942)
»Withdrawal trials with lithium prophyla-
xis«
Greil became director of the Psychiatric
Clinic in Kilchberg, Zurich, in 1992.

1990   Margot Albus (born 1951)
»Specificity of physiological and biochemi-
cal reaction patterns in psychiatric diseases«
M. Albus has been Head Doctor at the
District Psychiatric Hospital in Haar since
1989.

1990   M. Schmauss (born 1951)
»Epidemiology of suicide in East Bavaria
and Swabia: Identification of risk factors«
Schmauss has been director of the District
Psychiatric Hospital in Augsburg since 1989.

1991   Brigitta Bondy (born 1948)
»3H-spiperone binding to lymphocytes as
potential vulnerability markers for schizophrenic psychoses«

1991   Ingeborg Meller (born 1952)
»Disease behaviour in the entire population
– usage of psychiatric and medical services.

Results of an epidemiological longitudinal
study«

1993   P. Buchheim (born 1937)
»Multidimensional diagnostics in patients
with anxiety disorders. Results of multi-
method diagnostics on the level of clinical
syndromes, personality and inter-personal
relationships«
Buchheim became professor at the Clinic for Psychotherapy and Psychosomatics
at the Technical University of Munich in
1995.

1993   H.-P. Kapfhammer (born 1952)
»On the psychosocial development and
problems of young adulthood. Empirical
comparison studies on psychiatric patients
and mentally healthy probands«
Kapfhammer took over the chair for psychiatry at the University of Graz in 2002.

1993   N. Müller (born 1949)
»Psychoneuro-immunological studies on
patients with endogenous psychoses and
controls«

1994   P. Hoff (born 1956)
»Emil Kraepelin and psychiatry as a science
– a contribution to the self-conception of
psychiatric research«
in 1997 Hoff became first senior consultant
at the Psychiatric Clinic of the Technical
University of Aachen. In 2003 he became
head physician at the Cantonal Hospital
»Burghoelzli« at the Psychiatric Clinic of
the University of Zurich.

1994   M. Soyka (born 1959)
»Addictive diseases in schizophrenia«

(Fig. 13.19–45)

During Hippius' term in office not only clinic members, but also co-workers from the Max-Planck-
Institute for Psychiatry achieved their postdoctoral
lecturer qualifications or qualified for different subjects (E. Zerbin-Rüdin, H. Emrich, W. Mombour,
F. Strian, A. Steiger, I. Heuser). In 1987 H.-L.
Bischof (born 1930), head of the District Mental
Hospital Gabersee, qualified as a university lecturer
for forensic psychiatry.

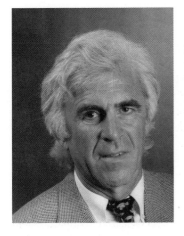

Fig. 13.19. M. Ackenheil (1939–2006)

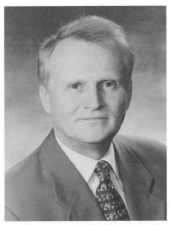

Fig. 13.22. H. Beckmann (1940–2006)

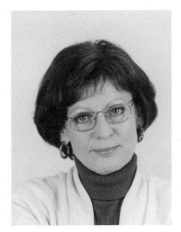

Fig. 13.25. Brigitta Bondy (born 1948)

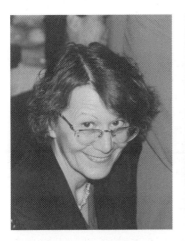

Fig. 13.20. Margot Albus (born 1951)

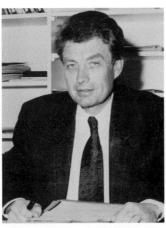

Fig. 13.23. O. Benkert (born 1940)

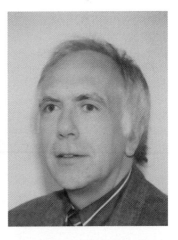

Fig. 13.26. P. Buchheim (born 1937)

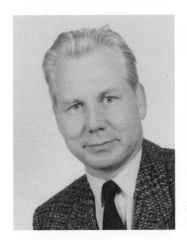

Fig. 13.21. D. Athen (born 1937)

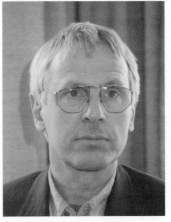

Fig. 13.24. W. Bender (born 1941)

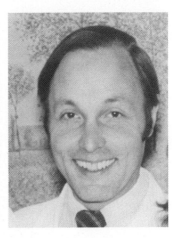

Fig. 13.27. H. Dilling (born 1933)

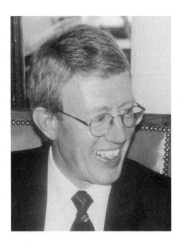

■ **Fig. 13.28.** R. Engel (born 1946)

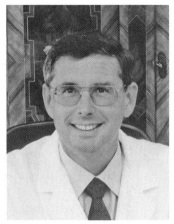

■ **Fig. 13.31.** W. Günther (born 1949)

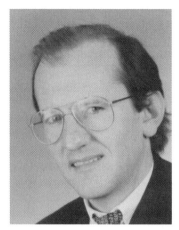

■ **Fig. 13.34.** H. Klein (born 1945)

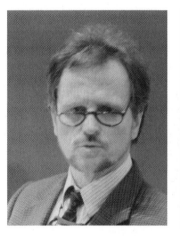

■ **Fig. 13.29.** M. Fichter (born 1944)

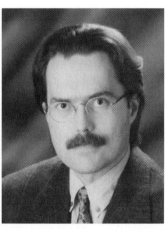

■ **Fig. 13.32.** P. Hoff (born 1956)

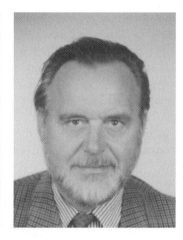

■ **Fig. 13.35.** G. Laakmann (born 1944)

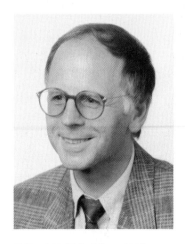

■ Fig. 13.30. W. Greil (born 1942)

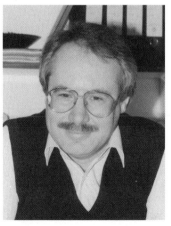

■ **Fig. 13.33.** H.-P. Kapfhammer (born 1952)

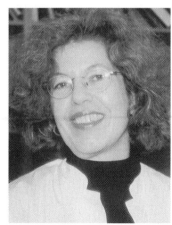

■ **Fig. 13.36.** Ingeborg Meller (born 1952)

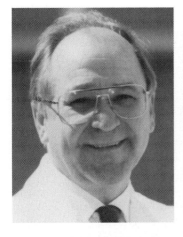

Fig. 13.37. R. Meyendorf (born 1934)

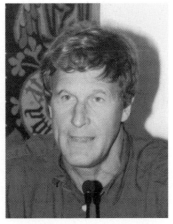

Fig. 13.40. D. Naber (born 1947)

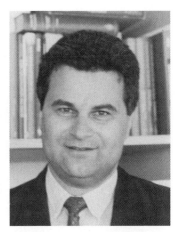

Fig. 13.43. M. Schmauss (born 1951)

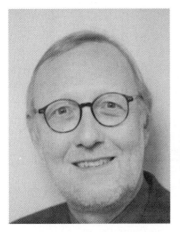

Fig. 13.38. N. Müller (born 1949)

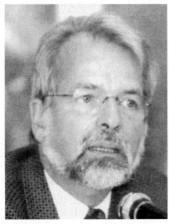

Fig. 13.41. N. Nedopil (born 1947)

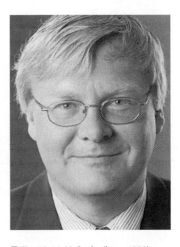

Fig. 13.44. M. Soyka (born 1959)

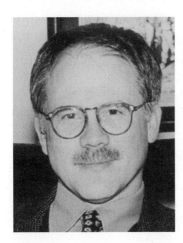

Fig. 13.39. F. Müller-Spahn (born 1950)

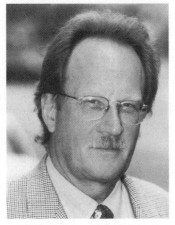

Fig. 13.42. E. Rüther (born 1940)

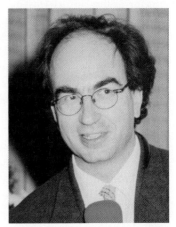

Fig. 13.45. R. Steinberg (born 1946)

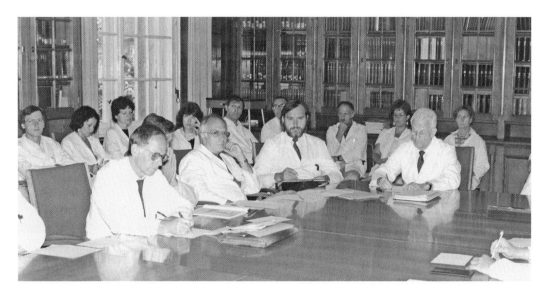

◨ Fig. 13.46. Morning conference in the library (1988)

G. Jungkunz (born 1946), assistant from 1975–1986 and later senior consultant at the Munich clinic, qualified as university lecturer at the Medical Faculty of the University of Wurzburg. Jungkunz left the Munich clinic to become director of the District Mental Hospital Lohr/Main.

Other co-workers also left the clinic to take over jobs as directors of Bavarian District Mental Hospitals. M. v. Cranach (born 1942) became director of the Psychiatric Hospital of the District of Swabia in Kaufbeuren in 1980; H. Schulz (born 1939) became director of the District Hospital in Wollershof in Upper Palatinate in 1978. In the New Laender R. Lehle (born 1957) took over the Saxon Hospital Hochweitzschen in 1993; N. Sassim (born 1958), who joined W. Greil as senior consultant at the Psychiatric Clinic in Kilchberg in 1992, has been head of a psychiatric clinic in Dresden since 1998.

In comparison F. Holsboer (born 1945) only worked at the Munich clinic for a short period of time (1979–1981). He and W. Maier (born 1949) left the clinic in 1981 to join O. Benkert in Mainz. In 1987 Holsboer was offered the chair for psychiatry in Freiburg and has been director of the Max-Planck-Institute for Psychiatry in Munich since 1990. Maier has been director of the Psychiatric University Clinic in Bonn since 1995.

Chr. Hock (born 1961) left the clinic in 1994 and become senior consultant at the University Clinic in Basle with F. Müller-Spahn; since 1999 he has been head of the Department for Psychiatric Research and head physician at the Psychiatric Clinic »Burghoelzli« of the Zurich University.

Renate Grohmann (born 1952) worked at the clinic from 1977 until 1988; since 1988 she is responsible (together with E. Rüther and R. Engel) for Drug Monitoring Programmes (AMUEP and AMSP) evaluating data on »drug safety« in psychiatric clinics and hospitals in Germany and Switzerland.

Other former co-workers from the clinic took over important positions in neighbouring subjects: Karl M. Einhäupl (born 1947), assistant at the clinic from 1981 to 1982, was offered the chair for neurology at Berlin's Humboldt University and has since been director of the Neurological Clinic of the Charité. F.-J. Freisleder (born 1956) worked at the clinic from 1984 until 1986, he then changed to child psychiatry and since 1997 has been director of the Heckscher Clinic of the District of Upper Bavaria.

The scientific atmosphere at the clinic was often enriched by clinic co-workers receiving grants from the DFG (German Research Association) and DAAD (German Academic Exchange Service) to

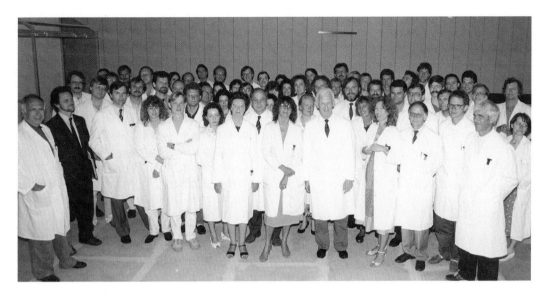

Fig. 13.47. H. Hippius with his co-workers (1988)

visit and work at research centres abroad (e.g. at the National Institute of Mental Health in Bethesda/MD, at the New York Medical College in New York, at the Maudsley Hospital in London, at the Hôpital Val de Grâce in Paris, at the Karolinska Institute in Stockholm).

It was also beneficial for the clinic's research activities that co-workers had the opportunity to work with guest doctors and research scholars from abroad. The research scholars (from other psychiatric university clinics in Germany, Austria and Switzerland as well as many other countries) had a small daily, clinical workload and therefore had time to work closely with clinical staff and in particular with the staff of the Department for Neurochemistry. Once they had returned home, the foreign guest scientists (e.g. scholars of the Alexander von Humboldt Foundation, the DAAD or foreign governments) could use the concepts they had worked on in Munich as basis for further scientific study. Many of them worked at the clinic long-term (e.g. M.R. Louza Neto, Brazil; R. Schilkrut, Chile; P. Douillet, France; E.S. Markianos, Greece; O. Chandra, India; A. O. Ige, M. Nakagawara, W. Omata, Y. Saito, T. Sato, Japan; M.P. Deva, Malaysia; G. Heinze, Mexico; M. Harrer, G. Langer, B. Pakesch, Austria; B. Wasilewski, Poland; M. Trixler, Hungary).

In 1992 G. Heinze became Director of the National Psychiatric Research Institute in Mexico. M. Trixler became professor for psychiatry and took over the chair for psychiatry at the University of Pecs in 1993.

The scientific work at the clinic was greatly supported by practicing psychiatrists and neurologists in and outside Munich, who had completed their specialist training after the war. The good co-operation with former clinic employees and many other practicing colleagues was a necessary requirement for the success of research projects, as was the case for the DFG project on psychiatric epidemiology in Upper Bavaria (catchment area of Gabersee), initiated by H. Dilling and S. Weyerer (born 1947) and later continued by M. Fichter, and similarly for the pharmaco-psychiatric out-patient studies run by G. Laakmann.

To promote exchange between clinic doctors and practising psychiatrists with respect to specialist subjects, together with F. Marguth and O. Stochdorph (also supported by J. Kugler and in the style of Kraepelin), in 1972 Hippius started the »Munich Colloquium for Psychiatrists and Neurologists« in 1972. The 300th colloquium was held on the clinic's anniversary. The events are usually held in the clinic's auditorium and on special occasions, celebrations and academic ceremonial e have taken place, of which three are mentioned here:

- In 1976 in remembrance of Kraepelin's 50th day of death: On this occasion an academic celebration was organized together with the Max-Planck-Institute for Psychiatry and the golden Kraepelin Medal was awarded to
  W. v. Baeyer
  M. Bleuler
  E. Strömgren

- In 1979, the clinic's 75th birthday was celebrated with the President of the World Psychiatric Association (WPA), Pierre Pichot, who was given an honorary doctorate to the Medical Faculty of the University of Munich.

- In 1986 in remembrance of Bernhard von Gudden's 100th day of death: Following a scientific symposium in the clinic's auditorium, all participants were invited to Neuschwanstein Castle, where – in the presence of His Royal Highness Franz of Bavaria – the members of the Bavarian Doctor's Orchestra, conducted by R. Steinberg, played Richard Wagner's »Siegfried Idyll« in the Singer's Hall.

Important national and international congresses have also been held in Munich (e.g. Congress of the German Society for Psychiatry and Neurology (DGPPN), 1972; International Congress for Neuropsycho-Pharmacology (CINP), 1988).

Many other events, unrelated to psychiatry, took place in the clinic; A.-U. Walther (clinic assistant) was responsible for art exhibitions. In the meantime these have become a tradition under H.-J. Möller and are taking place in the gallery on the third floor; similarly »Musical Soirees in the Nussbaumstrasse« have also become a tradition.

Financial means for the »Art on Buildings«, as part of the building project, led to parts of the clinic (such as the wards, the staircases, the glass corridor at the cafeteria and the interior gardens) being designed artistically, thus allowing the architecture to convey less of a typical hospital impression.

At the end of Hippius' term in office G. Klinge and F.J. Schön donated a bronze sculpture, designed by the Munich sculptor Erich Koch: it is a statue of St. Christopher standing in the interior garden of the inner city clinics, by the wall of the nuns' house, facing the psychiatric clinic where the wards are located (◻ Fig. 13.48).

Although the entire building and renovation activities of the Psychiatric Clinic were not finished when H. Hippius handed over directorship to H.-J. Möller, the dates on the four sides of the key, made by clinic craftsmen in 1989, show the planning and completion phases of the re-construction and extension work on the clinic from 1971 to 1998 (◻ Fig. 13.49).

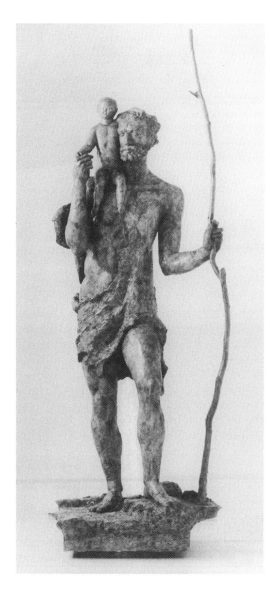

◻ **Fig. 13.48.** St. Christopher (by E. Koch, 1994)

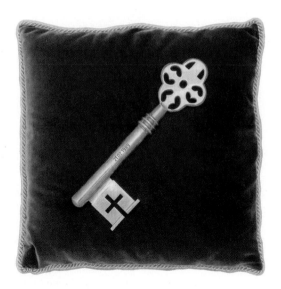

■ **Fig. 13.49.** Symbolic clinic key

January 1, 1971
H. Hippius takes over the clinic

February 21, 1989
Official handing over of the clinic after completion of the first building phase

September 15, 1994
H.-J. Möller becomes clinic director

May 11, 1998
Official handing over of the clinic on completion
of the entire construction work

The Re-Opening of the Historical Old Building

For the re-opening celebration of the historical old building, originating from 1904 and officially opened by E. Kraepelin, a week of festivities was organized from Monday, May 11 to Saturday, May 16, 1998. The completion of the »Kraepelin Building« was the crowning finale of the reconstruction and renovation work. The historical old building had actually already been opened in April 1998. The diagnostic and research areas are located here, as well as out-patient departments and also the administration, the senior consultants and the management. The departments and research areas could finally be re-united under one roof (▶ Chapter 14).

The prelude to the week of festivities was the official hand-over of the key by the Bavarian Minister for Education, Culture, Science and Art, Dr. Hans Zehetmair (◼ Fig. 14.1).

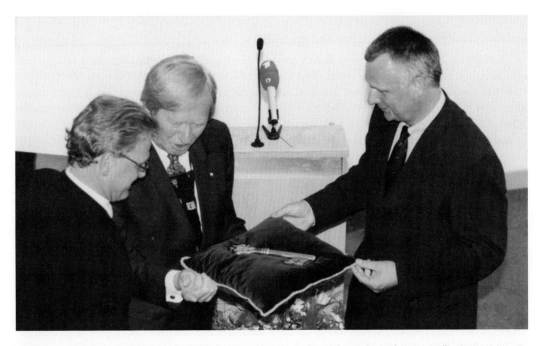

◼ **Fig. 14.1.** Handing over of the key by State Minister, Dr. H. Zehetmair; from left to right: Prof. Dr. H.J. Möller, State Minister, Dr. H. Zehetmair, Building Director P. Pfab (Photo J. Motzet)

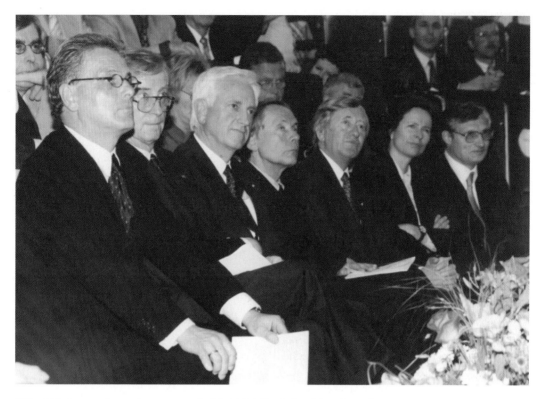

◻ Fig. 14.2. Guests at the opening ceremony: Prof. Dr. H.-J. Möller, Prof. Dr. P.C. Scriba, Prof. Dr. K. Peter (Dean), Prof. Dr. A. Heldrich (Rector), State Minister, Dr. H. Zehetmair, Princess Beatrix and Prince Luitpold of Bavaria (Photo J. Motzet)

Not only the elite of the university, faculty and clinical center, represented by the rector, Andreas Heldrich, the dean Klaus Peter, and the medical director of the clinical center Peter C. Scriba, contributed to the celebratory opening with speeches and salutations, but also representatives from international and national psychiatric associations (◻ Fig. 14.2). Representatives from the catholic and evangelical church inaugurated the building with an ecumenical service. The celebration concluded with musical accompaniment.

The opening celebrations were a worthy platform for the award of three psychiatric prizes for science.

The international »Alois Alzheimer Award«, endowed with US-dollars 20,000.- was given to Bengt Winblad from Stockholm by the Chairman of the Board of Trustees Hanns Hippius (◻ Fig. 14.3).

The »Emil Kraepelin Prize« was awarded to Bernhard Bogerts, Director of the Psychiatric Clin-

ic in Magdeburg and the »Bernhard von Gudden Prize«, which was awarded for the first time to a young psychiatric researcher, was halved between Elisabeth Friess from the Max-Planck-Institute for Psychiatry Munich, and Harald Hampel from the Psychiatric Clinic in the Nussbaumstrasse. The awards were handed over by Hans-Jürgen Möller. The chairmen of the Prize Board of Trustees were all from the Nussbaumstrasse, because the eponyms had worked at the clinic in Munich.

The academic opening celebrations were followed by the scientific program. In line with the international character of the scientific symposia and in order that the international guests could participate in the discussions, the language of the day was English.

The topics of the symposia – schizophrenia, dementia and affective disorders – dealt with the clinic's traditional research areas. The scientific program began with two half-day symposia on the

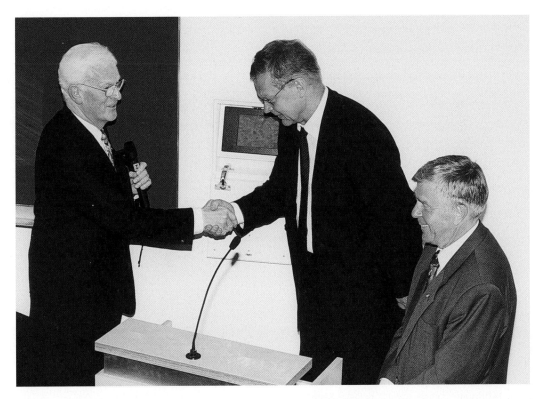

Fig. 14.3. Bestowing the Alois-Alzheimer Award: from left to right: Prof. Dr. H. Hippius, Prof. Dr. B. Winblad, Prof. Dr. C.G. Gottfries (Photo J. Motzet)

topic »Schizophrenia: Basic research and therapeutical implications«.

Presided over by H.-J. Möller, talks were given by the prize-winner B. Bogerts, H. Häfner from Mannheim, as well as S. Kasper (Vienna) and A. Carlsson from Gothenburg, the latter being one of the pioneers of biological research in psychiatry and founder of the dopamine hypothesis in schizophrenia, representing an important milestone in psychiatric theories (A. Carlsson won the Nobel Prize in 2002). During the second part of this symposium on Tuesday morning, current therapeutic developments were discussed. With P. Pichot, Paris, and H. Beckmann, Wurzburg, as chairmen, talks were given by H.Y. Meltzer (Cleveland/Ohio), W. McCarley (Brockton/Massachusetts), H.J. Möller (Munich), as well as K. Hahlweg (Brunswick).

On Tuesday afternoon two half-day symposia started on the topic »Dementia: Present approaches

and future perspectives« (Fig. 14.4). Wednesday afternoon and Thursday morning were dedicated to »Molecular and Clinical Aspects of Affective Disorders«, presided over by H. Hippius, H. Holsboer, M. Ackenheil and O. Benkert.

In a special way a symposium on neuromorphology and neuropathology rounded off the scientific tradition of the Munich clinic: on Thursday afternoon international participants joined in discussions on »The Munich School of neuropathology: Implications for modern research«. Contributions from G. Kreutzberg, Munich, and P. Mehrain, Munich, described the development of the historical Munich School of neuropathology to present day molecular genetics, with a re-analysis of original section slides from A. Alzheimer using modern molecular-biological methods.

The scientific part of the re-opening celebration week was closed with an all-day »Research Festival« on Friday, where clinic staff could present

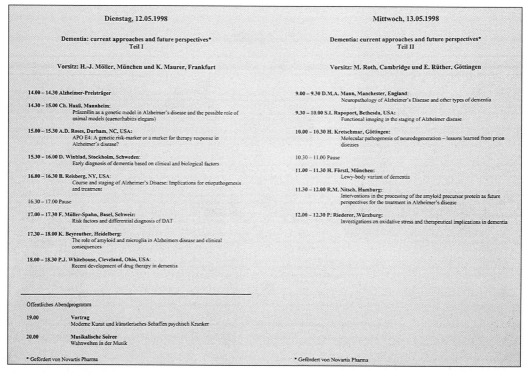

Dienstag, 12.05.1998	Mittwoch, 13.05.1998
Dementia: current approaches and future perspectives* Teil I	Dementia: current approaches and future perspectives* Teil II
Vorsitz: H.-J. Möller, München und K. Maurer, Frankfurt	Vorsitz: M. Roth, Cambridge und E. Rüther, Göttingen
14.00 – 14.30 Alzheimer-Preisträger	9.00 – 9.30 D.M.A. Mann, Manchester, England: Neuropathology of Alzheimer's Disease and other types of dementia
14.30 – 15.00 Ch. Haaß, Mannheim: Präsenilin as a genetic model in Alzheimer's disease and the possible role of animal models (caenorhabitis elegans)	9.30 – 10.00 S.I. Rapoport, Bethesda, USA: Functional imaging in the staging of Alzheimer disease
15.00 – 15.30 A.D. Roses, Durham, NC, USA: APO E4: A genetic risk-marker or a marker for therapy response in Alzheimer's disease?	10.00 – 10.30 H. Kretschmar, Göttingen: Molecular pathogenesis of neurodegeneration – lessons learned from prion diseases
15.30 – 16.00 D. Winblad, Stockholm, Schweden: Early diagnosis of dementia based on clinical and biological factors	10.30 – 11.00 Pause
16.00 – 16.30 B. Reisberg, NY, USA: Course and staging of Alzheimer's Disaese: Implications for etiopathogenesis and treatment	11.00 – 11.30 H. Förstl, München: Lewy-body variant of dementia
16.30 – 17.00 Pause	11.30 – 12.00 R.M. Nitsch, Hamburg: Interventions in the processing of the amyloid precursor protein as future perspectives for the treatment in Alzheimer's disease
17.00 – 17.30 F. Müller-Spahn, Basel, Schweiz: Risk factors and differential diagnosis of DAT	12.00 – 12.30 P. Riederer, Würzburg: Investigations on oxidative stress and therapeutical implications in dementia
17.30 – 18.00 K. Beyreuther, Heidelberg: The role of amyloid and microglia in Alzheimers disease and clinical consequences	
18.00 – 18.30 P.J. Whitehouse, Cleveland, Ohio, USA: Recent development of drug therapy in dementia	

Öffentliches Abendprogramm

| 19.00 | Vortrag Moderne Kunst und künstlerisches Schaffen psychisch Kranker |
| 20.00 | Musikalische Soiree Wahnwelten in der Musik |

* Gefördert von Novartis Pharma   * Gefördert von Novartis Pharma

Fig. 14.4. Excerpt from the scientific program: Dementia Symposium

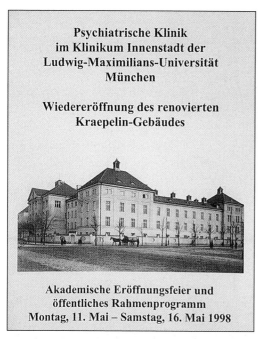

Fig. 14.5. Title page of the official social program

their own research results with lectures and scientific posters.

Presided over by former clinic co-workers (H.E. Klein, Regensburg; H. Dilling, Lubeck; P. Hoff, Aachen) together with Munich clinic co-workers (N. Müller, R. Engel, B. Bondy, G. Laakmann) the program included more than 20 lectures and almost 100 scientific posters. Contributions were made in the following areas: Affective psychoses, alcoholism and addictive diseases, anxiety, imaging processes in psychiatry, dementia, epidemiology, experimental psychology, forensic psychiatry, neurochemistry, neuroendocrinology, neurophysiology and EEG diagnostics, psychiatric genetics, psycho-neuroimmunology, psychopharmacology, psychosomatics and psychotherapy, schizophrenia, sleep research, tick diseases and Tourette syndrome, transcranial magnetic stimulation and compulsive-obsessive disorders.

Apart from the scientific part of the celebrations, there was also an official social program (**Fig. 14.5**), aimed at showing the public views

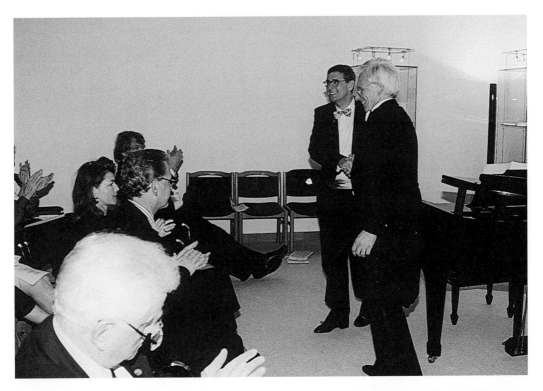

Fig. 14.6. Musical soiree: W. Günther (grand piano) and W. Heldwein (baritone, standing in front), front left: W. Poeldinger (presenter); (Photo: J. Motzet)

and problems in psychiatry, at reducing prejudice and fears, as well as demonstrating diagnosis and therapy procedures.

Public lectures were given in the evening, dealing with various aspects of psychiatric diseases and their therapy, on the topics »Understanding the diseases and modern therapeutic possibilities in psychiatry« (H.-J. Möller), »Art by the mentally ill and their importance for modern art« (W. Schmied, former director of the Academy of Art in Munich), »Changes experienced by the mentally ill in music« (R. Steinberg) and »The role of psychotherapy in psychiatry« (H. Kapfhammer). In a special way the »King Ludwig Evening« followed up on the clinic's tradition. Controversial views were shown by H.-J. Möller in his lecture on »King Ludwig the Second – On the doctor-patient relationship in psychiatry« and by the film director Ch. Rischer in his semi-documentary film »Ocean of Longing« illustrati a somewhat anti-psychiatry point of view.

There were three musical soirees dealing also with psychiatric themes: Mourning, melancholy and death wish in music (moderated by H.-J. Möller); illusion, dream and delusion in music (moderated by W. Pöldinger); between creativity and transgression: from the musical production of Robert Schumann (moderated by R. Steinberg). These soirees, held in the Alois Alzheimer laboratory for microscopy, revived a clinic tradition and were appreciated by the public (**Fig. 14.6).

Art work was exhibited in the corridors of the old building grouped according to varying psychiatric perspectives: A.U. Walther had organized an exhibition by contemporary Munich artists who suffer from a psychiatric disease (Günther Neupel, Sabine Henning), as well as art by Konrad Balder Schäuffelen, who works as psychiatrist and psychotherapist. Historical photographs from the Psychiatric Clinic and selected objects from the occupational and work therapy groups rounded off the exhibition.

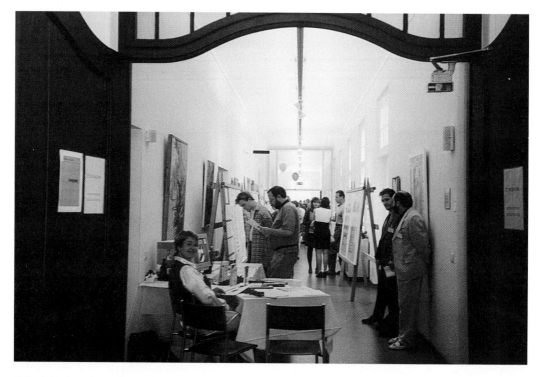

■ **Fig. 14.7.** Open day: A glimpse along the corridors of the KRAEPELIN building

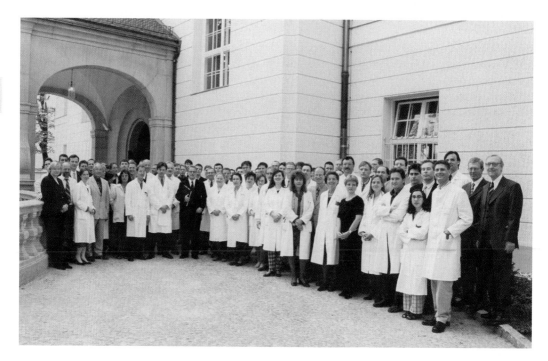

■ **Fig. 14.8.** Clinic co-workers of Prof. Dr. H.-J. Moeller (Photo: J. Motzet)

With the support of H. Hippius and N. Müller, G. Neundörfer-Kohl's historical psychiatry exhibition was on show in Alois Alzheimer's microscopy laboratory. Documents and things of interest were exhibited in eleven showcases, illustrating the development of psychiatry based on the example of the Munich clinic and its important representatives. The exhibition was opened officially on May 12, 1998 with a small inauguration celebration. A copy of the original case history from Frankfurt, in which A. Alzheimer described the first case of Alzheimer's disease, was integrated into the exhibition.

At the end of the week of festivities an open day was organized (◘ Fig. 14.7); for the first time in history the public was allowed to gather information on-site.

All clinic areas which included (special) outpatient units, the day clinic, the nursing staff, ergotherapy, the art and music therapy, physiotherapy, social services and the departments for EEG, psychology, psychosomatics and neurochemistry, as well as epidemiology and forensic psychiatry departments, participated actively in the festivities. Photos and posters illustrated the work done, flyers and information material was available for all interested.

From 9:30 a.m. to 5 p.m. films and lectures could be enjoyed simultaneously in two rooms, giving information about psychiatric diseases and care, diagnostics, available therapies and research projects. Guided tours were given through the wards and the day clinic every hour. Everyone rushed to the information stands on the ground floor of the old and new buildings and research departments. From ergotherapy to physiotherapy, those keenly interested were offered the chance to get to know and understand these departments' work by trying things out themselves. Patients' work was on sale at the bazaar held by the department for ergotherapy; the public could surf on the internet site of the clinic.

The celebration was a great success. (◘ Fig. 14.8).

The Psychiatric Hospital since 1994

On 15th September 1994, Professor Hans-Jürgen Möller took over the chair for psychiatry of the University of Munich (Ludwig-Maximilians University, LMU) and was appointed medical director of the Department of Psychiatry.

Professor Möller was trained mainly at the Max Planck Institute for Psychiatry in Munich. In 1979, he transferred to the newly-founded Psychiatric Hospital of the Technical University of Munich

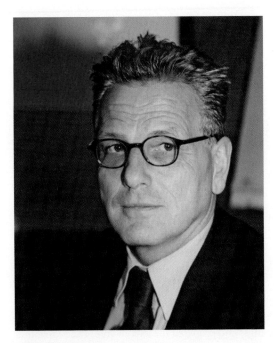

◻ **Fig. 15.1.** Hans-Jürgen Möller (born 1945)

(TU) as a senior registrar where he achieved his postdoctoral qualification (Habilitation) in 1980 based on data from a large case control study that he had performed at the Max Planck Institute for Psychiatry on patients with endogenous psychoses. Shortly afterwards he took on a position as C3 professor for psychiatry (1980) at the TU Munich. In 1988, he was offered the chair for psychiatry at Bonn University and held the position of medical director of the Department of Psychiatry until he was offered the chair in Munich in 1994. His main scientific interests include clinical psychopharmacology and research on the course of psychiatric disorders, with special focus on the relevant methodological questions.

The psychiatric hospital currently treats approximately 2,000 inpatients a year, whereby the largest group of patients is suffering from schizophrenic and affective disorders. Patients stay in hospital for an average of 40 days. Important features of the psychiatric hospital out-patient clinic are a 24-hour service for all psychiatric crises and low-level, long-term out-patient treatment for severely ill psychiatric patients and for patients with psychiatric co-morbidity. Additionally, the consultation service for the Munich Central Municipal Hospital (Klinikum Innenstadt) (1,250 beds) is linked to the out-patient clinic. Furthermore, several specialised out-patient departments offering disorder-specific diagnosis, psychopharmacotherapy and psychotherapy are integrated into the out-patient clinic. The psychiatric consultation service at the Munich Grosshadern hospital is responsible for 14

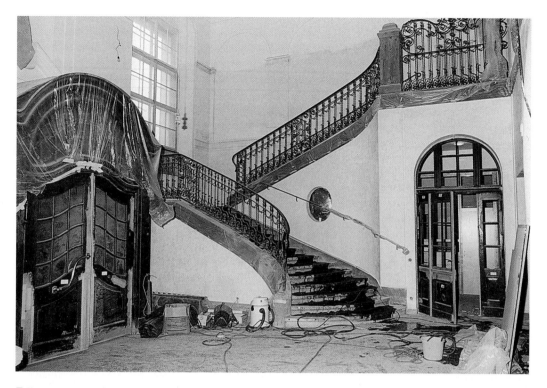

◘ Fig. 15.2. Entrance hall with staircase during renovation

somatic-medical hospitals with a total capacity of 1,600 beds.

All hospital personnel with a postdoctoral qualification as well as all house officers, are involved in teaching psychiatry to approx. 450 students annually. The main part of the psychiatric teaching traditionally consists of propedeutics, the main psychiatric lectures, a psychiatric placement and a lecture for advanced students. In addition, numerous lectures and seminars are on offer in diverse specialist areas. The introduction of the »MECUM« programme a few years ago, has changed the teaching for medical students considerably. Teaching has become more interactive, interdisciplinary and problem-oriented. Nowadays, psychiatry is mainly part of the interdisciplinary »Module 4« which unites psychiatry, neurology, psychosomatics, ophthalmology, dermatology, pharmacology and otorinolaryngology. Elements of this course are – apart from a daily plenary lecture – seminars, tutorials and bedside teaching in small groups. Further details of the MECUM programme are given in ▶ subchapter 15.23 below.

From an architectural point of view, the renovation of the old hospital building (Building A), the Kraepelin Building, was extremely important. Work began in 1995, following a long period of planning by H. Hippius and after the Bavarian parliament had given financial approval as part of the agreement made with H.-J. Möller when he was appointed chairman of the Department of Psychiatry. The firm of architects responsible for planning the new building was also commissioned to plan the difficult refurbishment of the Kraepelin Building. The architects GA Roemmich and A Zehentner meanwhile had left the firm responsible for the first stage of construction; HJ Ott was now head of the company together, with H Geiselbrecht, A Beeg and partners, taking over the planning of the renovation and refurbishment. From 1996 to 1998 the Kraepelin Building was refurbished for approx. 35 million German Marks (considering regulations for the protection of historic buildings) and prepared for its new role. The renovation was completed in 1998, and the reopening of the

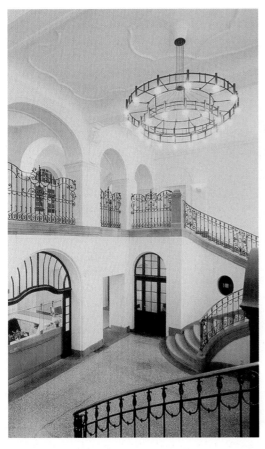

◘ **Fig. 15.3.** Entrance hall of the renovated Emil Kraepelin building

Kraepelin building was celebrated on the May 11, 1998.

The Kraepelin building is now home to the following departments:

- Hospital directorship
- All outpatient facilities (outpatient clinic with specialised departments and the outpatient branch of the psychosomatic department)
- The departments of
  - Neurochemistry
  - Clinical and experimental psychology
  - Neurophysiology
  - Forensic psychiatry
  - Several research groups
- library (Emil Kraepelin library)

- A large conference and seminar room (Alois Alzheimer Room), which also accommodates the collection of historical psychiatric documents.

A decisive event for the psychiatric hospital was its administrative 'integration' in the City Centre Hospital of the Ludwig-Maximilians University; in 1999, the City Centre Hospital was united with the Großhadern Hospital to form the Hospital of the LMU. The (formerly completely self-sufficient) psychiatric hospital thereby lost its own administration and workmen, and the nursing director responsible for the entire hospital took over responsibility for the nursing staff. This information alone is enough to convey that this loss of autarky was a crucial event for the hospital which formerly had been run in a rather family-like manner, similar to a medium-sized firm. This change in organisation had far-reaching (as far as the psychiatric hospital was concerned) mostly disadvantageous consequences for the familial atmosphere and the complexity of individual decision-making processes and procedures. However, despite this gloomy view, it is true that advantages may have resulted from this structural change, for example in the sense of greater economic efficiency, especially in times when the financial situation of hospitals is under great pressure due to structural health system reforms and increasing restriction of public finances (including health insurances).

There are currently plans to accommodate a Department for Paediatric and Adolescent Psychiatry in the East Wing of the psychiatric hospital, an annex to the Kraepelin Building that was built in the 1920s and which has not yet been refurbished. This would allow a closer working relationship between the care- and research-related areas of adult, paediatric and adolescent psychiatry. Although this appears to make sense from a planning perspective, regrettably this will significantly encroach upon the future planning of the Department of Psychiatry. Part of the agreement made with H.-J. Möller when he was appointed chairman of the Department of Psychiatry was that after refurbishment of the East Wing its rooms would be available for use by the Department of Psychiatry.

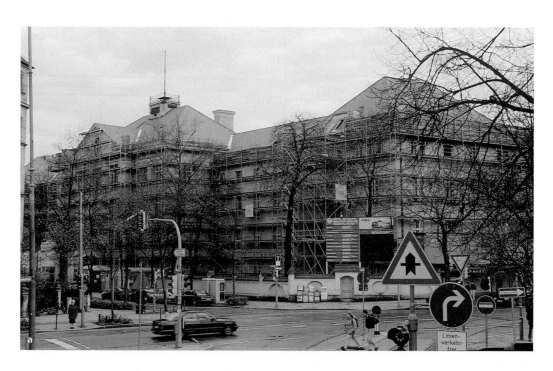

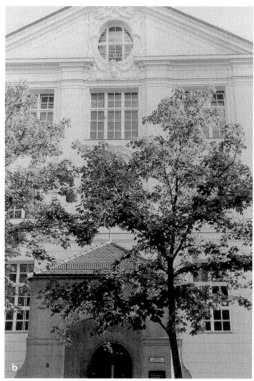

Fig. 15.4a,b. Exterior facade of the clinic shortly before completion of renovation work (1997)

The previous concept of patient care has been maintained to a large extent. However, some changes have been made, in order to keep up with the development of treatment approaches in psychiatry and, amongst other things, the new concept of a specialist doctor in this field (specialist for psychiatry and psychotherapy). These changes have led to the idea of integrating special psychotherapeutic procedures to a greater degree into everyday care, in addition to offering an extremely high-quality psychopharmacotherapy following the very latest standards of knowledge and the most recent relevant developments in drug treatment. In particular, behavioural therapeutic approaches on the basis of single and, above all, group therapy were included in the overall therapeutic concept for in- and outpatient treatment. In addition to the psychologists, who mainly took on this work, it was attempted to entrust doctors and nursing staff with this behavioural therapy task, according to their level of knowledge and experience. This concept is being applied on three wards, the depression ward, the schizophrenia ward and the anxiety ward in order to examine the degree to which psychopharmacotherapy and behavioural therapy complement each other. Family-related care concepts were also given

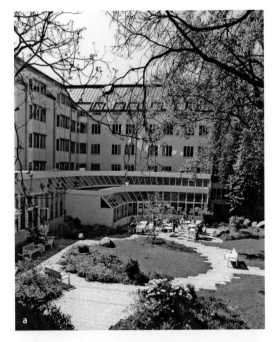

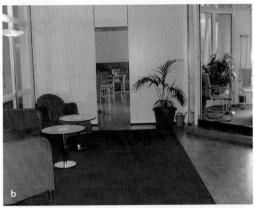

☐ **Fig. 15.5a,b.** a. External view of the new hospital building
b. Sitting room in one of the wards

not successful enough, for example patients with borderline disorders. As one would expect from a university hospital, these psychotherapeutic activities are not only on offer to the patients but also analysed as to their degree of success.

With the newly-founded specialised wards, the principle of specialisation which had begun with the establishment of the addiction ward by Professor Hippius, was continued. A further specialisation in the area of inpatient care appeared sensible when considering the relatively large number of beds in the hospital (200), in order to achieve the most competent diagnosis and treatment possible for the various patient groups, and simultaneously to also stimulate interested personnel to perform relevant, hospital-orientated research. In addition to the traditional addiction ward, the hospital currently has a depression ward, schizophrenia ward and a ward for anxiety disorders. As well as these primarily treatment-orientated specialised wards, there are two »research wards«, one for dementia disorders and one for depressive disorders. An important step in the further development of the wards was the decision, reached after careful discussion and consideration, to turn the two »closed« wards into mixed wards, and to no longer separate men and women. Experience has shown that is improves the atmosphere on the wards, as well as the behaviour of the patients.

The out-patient clinic was also specialised with respect to treatment and research. Various specialist departments were established in addition to the traditional out-patient clinic: for anxiety disorders, compulsive disorders, prevention of relapse in affective disorders, pregnancy/postpartum psychoses, phototherapy, for HIV patients and for psychosomatic patients. The activities of the »memory clinic« were continued and expanded further.

In addition to its extensive teaching and research tasks, the psychiatric hospital has always been intensively involved in the care population of the city of Munich and surrounding areas. This responsibility gained further importance when in 2003 the psychiatric hospital, at the suggestion of the district of Upper Bavaria, became responsible for caring for the sector Munich-South; a total of approx. 60 beds are available for this task.

more consideration than before. On another ward (ward for psychoanalytically-oriented treatment), a stronger link between psychopharmacotherapy and psychotherapy (in this case psychoanalytically-orientated psychotherapy) was introduced. This ward is mainly for patients who are suffering from severe disorders but who do not have a functional psychosis in the classical sense, and for whom pharmacotherapeutic concepts of care are

The departmental structure of the psychiatric hospital has essentially remained unchanged. The only exception is the neurophysiological department which has been removed from its association with experimental clinical psychology and turned into a self-sufficient department. This decision was based on the fact that clinical neurophysiology has re-gained its importance for psychiatry, especially in recent years, through the development of better technical facilities, above all improved methods of evaluation. Since the completion of the refurbishment of the hospital, all departments are housed under one roof in the Kraepelin Building. This has put an end to the temporary fragmentation caused by the various departments being housed in different buildings, and the associated complications in internal communication. All other scientific research groups are now housed in the Kraepelin Building.

15.1   Department of Neurochemistry

**Head from 1990 to 2006:
Manfred Ackenheil**

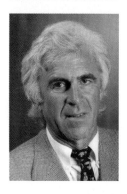

Under the leadership of Professor Manfred Ackenheil, the technically distinguished Neurochemistry Department developed to cover both clinical routine laboratory diagnostics in psychiatric patients and in research, in close collaboration with all clinical science research groups.

Key aspects of clinical diagnostics do not only cover routine laboratory parameters, such as clinical chemistry or the haemogram, but also more specialized investigations for psychiatry such as the screening for addictive drugs, the therapeutic

drug monitoring, or the investigation of Tau-proteins and ß-amyloid in the cerebrospinal fluid to improve the diagnostics of Alzheimer's Disease.

Most prominent among the research activities of the Neurochemistry Department were not only neurochemical investigations of neurotransmitters, their metabolites and the determination of neurotransmitter receptors in peripheral models, but also, and most intensively, the introduction of molecular genetics with its multiple modern extensions – pharmacogenetics, genotyping and phenotyping, genomics and proteomics.

After the retirement of Professor Ackenheil from his official position in 2004, the department was compartmentalized into three different sections in order to cover the increased requirements of excellent scientific research and of specialized psychiatric diagnostics.

15.1.1   Section for Psychiatric Genetics and Neurochemistry

Head: Brigitta Bondy

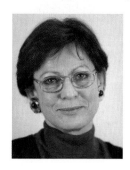

Scientific member: Peter Zill

Although numerous studies have shown the important role of hereditary factors in psychiatric disorders, the exact mechanism of the genetic transmission and the related disease-causing mechanisms remain unclear to date. A major challenge of psychiatric genetics is the identification of susceptibility genes, respectively genetic risk factors or profiles for the development (molecular genetics) and therapy of the disorder (pharmacogenetics).

Therefore, the main scientific research area of the Section for Psychiatric Genetics and Neurochemistry is not only the field of molecular genetics and pharmacogenetics, but also functional genomic and proteomic studies of psychiatric disorders.

Additionally, specialized diagnostic investigations for inpatients and ambulatory psychiatric patients are carried out by this section. The cerebrospinal fluid is routinely investigated in order to exclude organic alterations within the brain, such as inflammatory or degenerative processes like Alzheimer's Disease. Patients undergoing treatment for addictive behavior are routinely screened for addictive drugs.

The Section for Psychiatric Genetics and Neurochemistry is continuously carrying out numerous scientific projects on the genetic basis of depression, schizophrenia, addiction and suicidal behavior either independently, or in cooperation with other groups or departments of the Psychiatric Hospital Munich, or within national or international cooperations.

Molecular genetics and pharmacogenetics

Although both psychiatric disorders and the response to treatment (or the development of adverse drug effects) are complex by nature, there is no doubt that genetic factors play an important role as susceptibility factors. Molecular genetic investigations have therefore been widely used in psychiatry since their introduction a decade ago.

Various laboratory and statistical techniques for molecular genetic and pharmacogenetic studies have been established by Brigitta Bondy and Peter Zill. In collaboration with special research groups of the Psychiatric Clinic or other national or international institutions, clinically well-defined and characterized patient groups and/or homogeneous subgroups have been recruited. Many genetic association studies with candidate genes for the pathophysiology of the disease or the response to treatment (especially with depressive patients) have been carried out and published by this group. Apart from the identification of genes being relevant as pathophysiological contributing factors, a major interest of recent investigations has been interdisciplinary research. One such study investigated a common (genetic) basis underlying depression and cardiovascular

disorders, as some of the association studies gave evidence that a gene coding for the angiotensin converting enzyme (was already associated with cardiovascular disease) might also be important in depression. Another important field is to unravel the genetic contribution in the development of serious physical adverse effects during treatment, such as the metabolic syndrome, which may develop under treatment with atypical antipsychotics.

Furthermore, since 2006 the Section for Psychiatric Genetics and Neurochemistry serves as a reference laboratory in Germany for the AmpliChip CYP450 GeneChip technology by Roche Diagnostics (Roche Diagnostics). AmpliChip CYP450 is a microarray hybridization method for the determination of genetic variants in the cytochromes CYP2D6 and CYP2C19 genes. Cytochrome P450 enzymes (CYP) are the main metabolizers of lipophilic drugs and thus responsible for their degradation and excretion. Genetic variabilities within CYPs with functional consequences on enzyme activity may thus affect the pharmacokinetics of many psychotropic which finally could lead to adverse effects and disturbances in response.

Functional Genomics and Proteomics

Among the identification of susceptibility genes for psychiatric disorders and the response to psychotropic treatment, the Section for Psychiatric Genetics and Neurochemistry uses the investigation of gene and protein expression patterns in peripheral blood cells, in cell culture and in human post mortem brain tissue (in collaboration with the Institute for Legal Medicine of the University Munich) to identify further susceptibility or predisposing genes. Thus, evidence could be provided for the existence of the second, brain specific isoform of the tryptophan hydroxylase in the human brain. Several techniques and methods have been established to analyze the mRNA and/or protein expression differences in patient tissues compared to healthy controls (quantitative RT-PCR, cDNA- and antibody microarrays, 2-dimensional electrophoresis). A further approach is the application of peripheral cell models to study pharmacological effects as possible mechanisms of antidepressant or antipsychotic efficacy. These investigations allow the analysis of molecular biological mechanisms starting from altered receptor densities and/or activities over changes in signal transduction pathways up to genomic level. All these investigations will lead to a better understanding of the pathogenesis of development and treatment of psychiatric disorders and will also finally provide a better knowledge of the interaction with environmental factors.

15.1.2 Section for PsychoNeuro-Immunology and Therapeutic Drug Monitoring

Head: Markus J. Schwarz

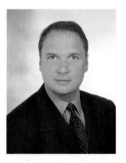

This laboratory section is specialized in neurobiochemical and pharmacological methods focussing on two major fields of interest: The functional relationship between nervous system and immune system with its special role in psychiatric disorders, and the determination of neuropsychotropic drugs and their major metabolites in psychiatric and neurological patients.

Psychoneuroimmunology

Recent research has overcome the old paradigms of the brain as an immunologically privileged organ and the exclusive role of neurotransmitters and neuropeptides as signal transducers in the central nervous system. Growing evidence suggests that the signal proteins of the immune system – the cytokines – are also involved in modulation of behaviour and induction of psychiatric symptoms. One immunological model in psychiatric research is the induction of depression by therapeutic administration of Interferon-α. Together with a group at the Charité (Berlin), we have investigated the predictive value of immune alterations for the occurrence of depression as a side effect of Interferon administration. Those findings may be highly relevant for major depression. In fact, we and other groups have found a marked increase of pro-inflammatory cytokines in patients suffering from major depression.

In addition to the direct effect of cytokines on mood and behaviour, a functional link between cytokines and the production of the neurotransmitter serotonin may also contribute to the immunological basis of psychiatric disorders: The essential amino acid tryptophan is not only the precursor of the neurotransmitter serotonin, but also of several neuro-active intermediates of the so-called kynurenine pathway. The key enzyme of the kynurenine pathway is markedly regulated by cytokines: Pro-inflammatory cytokines are strong inducers, while anti-inflammatory cytokines are potent inhibitors of this enzyme. Since the central nervous availability of tryptophan was shown to be the limiting factor in serotonin synthesis, the kynurenine arm of the tryptophan metabolism appears to be directly related to the synthesis of serotonin. Together with national and international groups, our laboratory section is working on these mechanisms.

Though this is a promising field, there are several other important aspects of the kynurenine pathway. Two of its intermediates, 3-hydroxykynurenine and quinolinic acid, are potent neurotoxic agents. Several lines of evidence point to the important role of these intermediates in the neurodegenerative process observed in Alzheimer's disease. Without going into further details, it should be noted that we were able to demonstrate a markedly enhanced production of 3-hydroxykynurenine in Alzheimer's disease patients. Further investigations have to confirm whether this finding may have consequences for diagnosis and therapy of Alzheimer's disease.

In recent years, the main focus of psychoneuroimmunological research of our laboratory section was on schizophrenia. A large body of evidence points to the involvement of an immune process in the pathophysiology of schizophrenia. Although there is a controversial discussion regarding the type of immune activation (autoimmune as in rheumatoid arthritis versus Th2 dominant, allergy-like), a mild chronic immune process in the CNS may be related to the repeatedly reported progressive reduction of brain volume in schizophrenia. In close collaboration with Norbert Müller and Michael Riedel, our laboratory section has significantly contributed to the immunologic research in schizophrenia. Our findings strongly indicate a predominance of the Th2 system of the specific immune system, while the monocytic system seems to be also markedly activated. We are currently interested in the possible involvement of the endogenous NMDA receptor antagonist kynurenic acid and its relationship to astrocytic function.

Besides these psychoneuroimmunological studies, we have participated in several other studies on classical neurotransmitter systems, e.g. in collaboration with Alexander Neumeister's group at Yale University.

Therapeutic Drug Monitoring

Therapeutic Drug Monitoring (TDM) is not only restricted to drugs showing a strong relationship between serum levels and therapeutic effect or toxic side effects. The risks related to pharmacogenetic factors, drug-drug interactions, and last but not least problems concerning patients' compliance are sometimes even stronger indications for TDM. Our laboratory section is one of the best established laboratories in the field of TDM in psychiatry. We provide a wide range of classical and new antidepressants, antipsychotics, anticonvulsants and benzodiazepines. Measuring not only the parent drugs, but also their major metabolites enables us to estimate both compliance and metabolism rate. We thus contribute to the efficacy and safety of modern psychopharmacologic therapy. Among the routinely performed TDM, we are also investigating the relationship between blood levels of new antipsychotic and antidepressant drugs and their therapeutic effect or occurrence of side effects.

15.1.3 Section of Molecular and Clinical Neurobiology

Head: Dan Rujescu

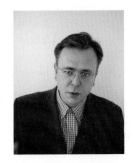

Scientific members:
Ina Giegling, Annette Hartmann,
Just Genius, Jens Benninghoff

The Section emerged 2004 form the Molecular and Clinical Neurobiology Group, which was founded in 1997. It consists of a multidisciplinary team with several areas of expertise: Ina Giegling has a major interest in human genetics and intermediate phenotypes, Annette Hartmann is specialized in genetics and molecular neurobiology, Just Genius is focused on cellular neurobiology and histology, and Jens Benninghoff's interest is in adult stem cell biology. Additionally, Hans-Joachim Kuss is conducting HPLC-based studies. The Section follows a multidimensional translational approach to neuropsychiatric diseases and behavioral phenotypes at genetic, molecular, cellular, structural, functional, cognitive and behavioral levels, and also integrates animal and cellular models. It is involved in extensive academic and industrial national and international genome and post-genome efforts on neuropsychiatric diseases and behavioral phenotypes. A variety of neurobiological methods has been established including high-throughput genotyping, allele-specific RNA expression analysis, microarray-based RNA expression techniques, protein quantification, neuronal and stem cell cultures including a variety of assays for cell viability, proliferation, differentiation, migration, apoptosis, reactive oxygen species, Ca^{2+} fluxes, as well as post mortem and behavioral studies in rodents.

The major focus is on the genetics and neurobiology of neuropsychiatric diseases and behavioral phenotypes, especially of schizophrenia, cognition, aggression, suicide and addiction. A multidimensional translational approach which involves recruitment and extensive phenotyping of large samples, high throughput genotyping, and cellular and animal models is implied.

Dan Rujescu is also co-director of the Genetics Research Centre (GRC), a joint biotech initiative between LMU and GSK which provides high-throughput genotyping for SNP validation and association studies employing both pooled and individual DNA samples.

Genetics of Schizophrenia and Intermediate Phenotypes

There is evidence for a strong genetic component in the etiology of schizophrenia, as demonstrated by family, twin and adoption studies. The risk of developing the disease increases exponentially with the genetic relatedness to an individual suffering from the disorder. In comparison to the 1% risk for schizophrenia in the general population, third-degree relatives carry an approximate 2% chance of developing schizophrenia, and the risk increases to 9% in first-degree relatives. Moreover, in identical (MZ) twins the concordance rate is approximately 50%. Adoption studies provide strong evidence that the familial aggregation is not the result of shared environmental factors, as individuals adopted into families containing an affected individual do not suffer an increased risk of developing schizophrenia, whereas the existence of a biological relative with schizophrenia does lead to an increased risk in adoptees. The relative contribution of genetic factors in the etiology of schizophrenia has been estimated to be approximately 80%. The mode of inheritance is complex and non-Mendelian, involving the combined action of several genes, each of which might account for only a small increase or decrease in susceptibility to the disorder. To identify schizophrenia susceptibility genes, we recruited a large number of extensively phenotyped schizophrenic patients, relatives and healthy controls for linkage-, genetic case-control-, and whole genome association studies.

A complementary approach to the genetics of schizophrenia is to use endophenotypes. The rationale for their use in gene discovery is that endophenotypes associated with a psychiatric disorder are more elementary compared to clinical phenotypes. This also implies that the number of genes required to produce variations in these traits may be fewer than those involved in producing a psychiatric diagnostic entity. Our endophenotype project includes a broad range of schizophrenia endophenotypes. These comprise, among others neuropsychological parameters (e.g. working memory, attention/vigilance, verbal learning and memory, visual learning and memory, speed of processing, reasoning, problem solving and antisaccades). Extensive academic and industrial national and international genome and post-genome collaborations have been initiated to understand the genetics and pathophysiology of schizophrenia and intermediate phenotypes.

Molecular and Cellular Neurobiology

We established NMDA receptor antagonist animal model which mimics several aspects of psychosis to identify further candidate genes which can be used in our human studies. In our model, chronic, low-dose treatment with MK801 alters the expression of NMDA receptor subunits in a pattern similar to schizophrenia on the molecular level. On a cellular level, the number of parvalbumin-positive interneurons was decreased, a finding which parallels observations in post mortem brains from schizophrenic patients. On a functional level, recurrent inhibition of pyramidal cells was altered, as postulated in histological findings. Finally, on a behavioral level these animals showed cognitive deficits like disturbed working memory, which again parallels findings in schizophrenia. We used a functional genomic approach for the identification of hippocampal candidate genes for psychosis-related traits and identified several differentially expressed genes and pathways. Furthermore, genetically manipulated mice are used to further characterize disease-related genes. A variety of neurobiological methods is established including allele-specific RNA expression analysis, microarray-based RNA expression techniques, protein quantification, adult stem and neuronal cell cultures including assays for cell viability, proliferation, differentiation, migration, apoptosis, reactive oxygen species, Ca^{2+} fluxes, as well as behavioral studies in rodents. These techniques have been extensively used to e.g. understand the physiology of adult stem cells in health and disease and to elucidate the role of glutamatergic neurotransmission and oxidative stress in schizophrenia.

Pharmacogenetics

Apart from genetics, endophenotypes and neurobiology, pharmacogenetics and pharmacogenomics of antipsychotics are another focus. A large pharmacogenetic study on response to antipsychotics was conducted. The fact that dopamine receptors are the primary targets of current antipsychotics prompted the investigation of genes involved in dopamine neurotransmission in response to treatment. Furthermore, this ongoing study investigates the association of response to antipsychotics with a high number of microsatellites and SNPs in various genes selected, based on their role in neurotransmission and differential gene expression in animal models.

Genetics of Suicidal Behavior and Personality Traits

Suicidal behavior is a major health problem worldwide. The risk of suicide-related behavior is supposed to be determined by a complex interplay of sociocultural factors, traumatic life experiences, psychiatric history, personality traits, and genetic vulnerability. This view is supported by adoption and family studies indicating that suicidal acts have a genetic contribution which is independent of the heritability of Axis I and II psychopathology. The heritability for serious suicide attempts was estimated to be 55%. The Section conducted a series of molecular genetic studies on suicidal behavior and personality traits (i.e. aggression, impulsivity, neuroticism) as risk factors for suicidal behavior. Microarray- and qPCR-based RNA expression studies were conducted to identify differentially expressed genes in the orbitofrontal cortex of suicide victims which were used in genetic association studies.

15.2 Department of Clinical Neurophysiology

Heads: Oliver Pogarell
(Clinical Neurophysiology Branch)

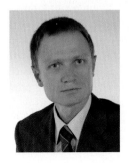

Christoph Mulert
(Functional Brain Imaging Branch)

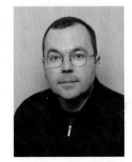

Current scientific members: Susanne Karch, Gregor Leicht, Nadine Schaaff.

Former scientific members:
Ulrich Hegerl (head of the department from 1994 to 2006), Georg Juckel, Roland Mergl

Clinical Neurophysiology

The Department of Clinical Neurophysiology and Functional Brain Imaging is excellently equipped and performs all neurophysiological routine diagnostics (EEG, event related potentials) for inpatients as well as out-patients. Each year more than 4,000 measurements are digitally recorded and evaluated. Furthermore, this department performs the ECG recordings for the entire clinic (more than 3,000 per year).

In addition to clinical routine tasks, the department of Clinical Neurophysiology is strongly engaged in scientific research. The Research group on brain function is interested in several EEG features and ERP components with a focus on psychiatric diseases. In this context, a number of innovative and analytical procedures are being employed (for ex. dipole source analysis, Low Resolution Electromagnetic Tomography Analysis). One focus is the investigation of the Loudness Dependence of the Auditory Evoked Potential. It is being used to indicate serotonergic functions of patients with depressive and obsessive-compulsive disorders.

Functional Brain Imaging

A major focus is the combination of EEG with Brain Imaging techniques like Functional Magnetic Resonance Imaging, Positron Emission Tomography (PET) and Single Photon Emission Computed Tomography (SPECT). In cooperation with the Dept. of Radiology at the LMU Munich Klinikum Grosshadern, Christoph Mulert has established one of the first recording units in Europe where it is possible to investigate EEG/ERP and fMRI simultaneously. This is a visionary approach because these two research tools complement each other. EEG and ERP provide immediate information about neuronal activity with the high temporal resolution that is crucial for the analysis of brain correlates of cognitive functions. The fMRI only shows indirectly neuronal activities, however, it has a high spatial resolution. Consequently, the combination of EEG and fMRI allows a deeper understanding of brain functions. This will be especially helpful regarding psychiatric diseases. Using the simultaneous EEG and fMRI approach, the research group on brain function is investigating different cognitive functions like for example attention and decision making processes. Patients suffering from schizophrenia experience an impairment of these cognitive functions. This methodological approach can contribute significantly to a deeper understanding of the basic brain functions leading to these restrictions.

Radioimaging techniques, studied by Oliver Pogarell in cooperation with the Dept. of Nuclear Medicine, allow a comprehensive investigation of brain neurochemistry. PET or SPECT with dopaminergic or serotonergic radioligands provide the basis to characterise and differentiate central monoaminergic systems of the human brain.

A wide range of PET and SPECT studies in patients with neuropsychiatric disorders (such as schizophrenia, depression, obsessive-compulsive disorder, personality disorders, movement disorders) have been launched and contributed to the understanding of the pathomechanisms of these conditions.

The combination of neurophysiological and nuclear medicine tools allows us to detect monoaminergic properties of brain electric activity. This approach provides multiple insights into the pathophysiology of central neurotransmission and leads to a differentiated view of the neurobiological background of distinct neuropsychiatric disorders.

Analysis of motor function: hand and facial movements

Hand-motor analysis using digitising graphic tablets is an additional neurophysiological investigation tool recording the signals of natural hand movements with a high spatial and temporal resolution. In order to obtain data for the evaluation of motor performance, special software is being employed for analyses of hand movements while writing or drawing: speed, acceleration and automation parameters can be calculated this way. Roland Mergl has shown that this method allows objective registration of subtle motor disturbances in schizophrenic, depressive and demented patients, and also the differentiation between those motor disturbances that are caused by disease and those caused by medication.

Another important area of research, set up by Georg Juckel, is the facial analysis, an objective registration method offering a high degree of spatial and temporal resolution. With this method it is possible to record facial movements of psychiatric patients showing different dynamic, qualitative and quantitative aspects. Facial movement analysis allows conclusions regarding affective disorders which are mainly expressed through involuntary, emotional and intuitive movements. It can be helpful to separate disorders caused by disease from disorders caused by side-effects from neuroleptics. These investigations are taking place at the laboratory for analysis of facial movements at the Department of Psychiatry; the controls are being filmed with a video camera while watching a funny film including their involuntary facial movements; special markers fixed to the face are emitting ultrasonic signals and with the aid of a measurement device these are being recorded. The results are then being transformed into positional curves by computer.

15.3 Department of Neuropsychology

Head: Rolf R. Engel

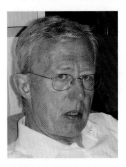

Current scientific member: Kristina Fast

Former scientific member: Norbert Kathmann

Research in the Neuropsychological Section is focused on three main areas:

Neuropsychological behavioral studies and functional imaging studies

This line of research was founded by Professor Norbert Kathmann (now at the Humboldt-University in Berlin). Current work is coordinated and led by Dr. Kristina Fast.

This research is concerned with the explanation and prediction of normal and disordered human behavior and experience. It takes a multi-method approach, and includes neuropsychological measures of cognitive functioning, emotional experiencing, expressive behavior, autonomic physiological responses, and brain activation. For example, functional magnetic resonance imaging (fMRI) allows for the »observation« of brain processes involved in specific psychological operations (e.g. memory encoding and retrieval). This interdisciplinary research and educational field could be termed »Cognitive Neuroscience« or »Cognitive Neuropsychology« in psychiatry. It aims to understand mental illness and psychopathology in terms of models of normal psychological functions. It is also a way of uncovering normal psychological processes by studying the effect of their change or impairment. It is derived from the fields of cognitive neuropsychology, cognitive neuroscience, and psychiatry. These three related disciplines play important interactive and slightly different roles in brain-behavior studies.

Neuropsychological and experimental studies

The objective of the current research program is to gain an understanding of the processes and brain mechanisms mediating memory, attention and perception as well as the interaction of emotion and cognition.

The principal focus of research is determining processes of memory encoding, associative learning and retrieval in healthy people and in patients with a wide range of psychiatric disorders. To deliver insight into our research some exemplary studies are given here:

First, studies on associative verbal and non-verbal learning in PTSD, depression, bipolar disorder and herpes encephalitis as well as on threat related perception, memory and attention in PTSD and BPD were implemented. Secondly, remote memory (episodic and semantic) in patients with organic and psychogenic amnesia as well as in healthy people and patients with progredient diseases is being examined. Moreover, different parameters of visual attention in e.g. ADHD or schizophrenia are estimated by the *Theory of Visual Attention*, as collaborative study with the department of experimental psychology, LMU. Finally, behavioral and cognitive changes following transcranial magnetic stimulation in the Gilles de la Tourette syndrome are investigated.

Functional neuroimaging of cognition

An ongoing challenge in the exploration of human cognition is developing and applying methods that can link underlying neuronal activitiy with cognitive operations. Functional imaging provides a means of measuring local changes in brain activity. Imaging can be done in normal and in compromised brains. One aim is to analyse functional imaging data to identify interactions among brain regions with the underlying idea that cognitive processes result from such interactions.

We are interested in the examination of the interaction of emotion and cognition, especially in patients with PTSD and BPD, adopting an emotional version of a directed forgetting paradigm, a stroop task and a cognitive regulation paradigm.

Recent research efforts in our lab are directed towards the neurofunctional mechanisms underlying memory processes, emotional modulation of cognitive functions and inhibitory functions in different populations. We are conducting fMRI studies in collaboration with the institute of radiology on brain activity of self-related episodic memory and suppressing the memory retrieval in healthy people and patients with organic and psychogenic amnesia. Other experimental studies mainly focus on neural correlates of associative learning and its active manipulation as a function of aging, psychiatric or neurological disorders (PTSD, herpes encephalitis).

Furthermore, age related changes in episodic and semantic memory in healthy elderly people and in patients with mild cognitive impairment as well as dementia compared to youngsters are additional topics of interest.

A line of basic research studies on gender difference in cortical networks of higher cognitive functioning (e.g. working memory) and secondary emotions (e.g. embarrassment) are partly realized together with Maudsley Hospital, London, Great Britain.

Basic and applied research in (neuro)psychological assessment

Neuropsychological assessments in research evaluate the following functions:

Aspects of cognitive functioning that are assessed typically include *new-learning/memory, executive-control/self-awareness, visuoperception, attention, intelligence, language, and affective perception/regulation, expression, interaction of emotion and cognition* in patients with psychiatric disorders (e.g. depression, bipolar disorder, obsessive-compulsive disorder, post-traumatic stress disorder [PTSD], schizophrenia, dementia) and personality disorders (e.g. borderline personality disorder [BPD]) as well as with other diagnoses (e.g. Gilles de la Tourette, attention-deficit-hyperactivity disorder [ADHD], herpes encephalitis, amnesia).

Within the clinical routine work about 500 patients each year are assessed with a broad spectrum of neuropsychological tests. All psychologists of the department take part in the routine work. A large part of the assessments concerns neuropsychological questions (dementia, schizophrenia, bipolar patients, ADHS, substance abuse, and others). From a technical point of view, all data are stored in a database system, with graphical test profiles and written reports produced within the database system. Around 600 patients are assessed with the MMPI-2 using a fax-based system designed in the hospital and now distributed by the publisher »Verlag Hans Huber«.

Basic test construction research centers on the possibilities and restrictions of adaptive tests based on item-response-theory, with internet-based testing as a form of data collection. Applied work has led to the development of a German computer version of the Halstead Category Test (Fast and Engel), a German version of the Famous Faces Test (Fast, Fujiwara und Markowitsch), and a German inventory for assessing autobiographical memory (Fast, Fujiwara, Schröder, Markowitsch). Diagnostic issues of Attention Deficit / Hyperactivity Disorder (ADHS) in adults are targeted with the construction of a self rating questionnaire assessing the longitudinal aspect of changing symptoms across the life cycle and with the analysis of neuropsychological functions in these patients (Engel and Fast, formerly C. Schöchlin). Following many years of research with the MMPI-2, we currently adapt and standardise a possible competitor, the Personality Assessment Inventory, for its clinical use in German (Engel and Groves).

Basic methodological work

In the psychological section of the hospital various lines of methodological research have been conducted in the past. Currently, there is a focus on meta-analyses of drug treatment in schizophrenia and other areas (together with Stefan Leucht, TU Munich). A general theme here is to derive methods to improve our insight in the clinical significance of experimental results.

15.4   Department of Psychotherapy and Psychosomatics

Head: Michael Ermann

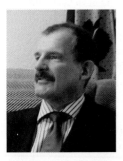

Scientific members: Eckhardt Frick, Christian Kinzel, Claudia Rupp, Otmar Seidl

The department was established in 1972 after the special field »Psychosomatic Medicine and Psychotherapy« was introduced as compulsory subject into the curriculum of medical studies. Since then it has gained an important and undeniable place in the hospital as psychoanalytically oriented pole within the scope of approaches and methods in patients' supply, research and medical training. It is situated in the upper floor of the old building of the hospital, covering a considerable number of rooms, including a representative seminar room, a small library and a modern dream laboratory.

At present there are seven academic employees, two of them specialists of Psychosomatic Medicine and Psychotherapy, and one psychiatrist. Five of them are established psychoanalysts. Additionally, four specially trained nurses as well as special therapists are involved in the inpatient therapy: four psychoanalytic trainees, an art therapist, a music therapist, a social worker. In addition, academic guests are involved in research programmes.

The department runs an outpatient clinic section and a special inpatient ward with 12 places for psychodynamic psychotherapy. The scope of indications includes acute crises, chronic neurotic and somatisation disorders, posttraumatic stress disorders and personality disorders. The ward was opened in 2000. Also, the department maintains a consultation service for psychodynamic diagnostics and indications for psychiatrists, including a psychosomatic consulting service.

The medical training includes Psychosomatic Medicine and Psychotherapy in two different versions. In the beginning of the clinical training the students are introduced into the bio-psycho-social approach to patients in general medicine. Thereafter, in the middle part of the clinical training, they are taught diagnostics and therapy methods of psychogenic disorders. Teaching is held mostly in small groups which are embedded in lectures and seminars.

In the research area, the main topics cover coping processes under psychodynamic aspects, dream remembrance and trauma representation:

- Psychosocial HIV studies: The government sponsored project managed by Otmar Seidl was run from 1988 to 1992 and dealt with coping processes in respect to HIV infection and AIDS in the pre antiviral medication period. It was found that coping processes are closely related to identity, social and psychodynamic protective factors and – above all – to the state of the illnesses. The biographical reconstruction of identity appears to be most significant in the support of HIV patients.
- Dream research: Since 1995 several laboratory studies guided by Michael Ermann et al. have investigated dream generation in patients with different diagnoses, especially with sleep disorders. Currently, the mentalization hypothesis of dream generation is being evaluated in a study comparing borderline and higher level neurotic patients.
- Psychooncological studies: From 1999 to 2006, Eckhard Frick and his group run an interdisciplinary study sponsored by the Carreras Foundation on patients after hematopoietic stem cell

transplantation (HSCT). They found out that life quality is fundamentally improved by psychodynamic based imaginary psychotherapy and supporting short term psychotherapy and that psychotherapy more efficient if set up early after surgery.

- The Munich Children of the War Project, managed by Michael Ermann since 2003, is studying the long term outcome of psychic traumatisation of the 2nd World War children (born 1936–1945). The first statistic result is that the data document a high degree of trauma exposure during war childhood. Comparing to other studies on PTSD in war children, there is a persisting high prevalence of war-associated PTSD-symptoms in this sample. The qualitative evaluation of interviews is under way.

15.5 Department of Forensic Psychiatry

Head: Norbert Nedopil

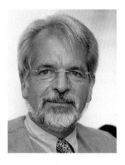

Current scientific members:
Cornelis Stadtland, Susanne Stübner, Joachim Weber, Elena Hutwelker

Former scientific members:
Martin Krupinski, Matthias Hollweg

Assessment

The Department of Forensic Psychiatry offers psychiatric expertise to courts and administrations concerning the culpability and risk of offenders, the competency of mentally disordered individuals and the compensation needs and requirements of invalidity due to mental illness. More than 400 written statements are provided by the staff of the department each year. The main focus, both in practice and research, lies in the psychiatric assessment of complex criminal cases, exploring the personality and psychopathology of violent offenders and their risk for re-offence.

Teaching and Training

The Department has a long tradition of being one of the foremost teaching institutions in Germany, with seminars dating back to E. Kraepelin, and still practiced in similar albeit modern forms. Most lectures are presented interdisciplinary by law professionals and staff members of the department. The traditional interdisciplinary lecture, in which current criminal cases examined in the department are presented by Professor Schöch, a criminologist, Dr. Weber, a psychologist, and the head of the department, still attracts large audiences. The training seminars for young professionals, which are organised by the department, are attended by psychiatrists and psychologists from all over Germany. The newest development is a seminar together with police officers, in which experiences from crime scene analysis and psychiatric assessments are evaluated for the benefit of both professions. Treatment in forensic settings, ethical questions in psychiatry and psychological assessment for forensic evaluations are further topics of the seminars offered by the members of the department.

Research

A number of studies are carried out by the different members of the department:

- Long-term outcome of offenders after assessment (Stadtland).
- Evaluation of current instruments for risk assessment and improvement of risk assessment methods (Stadtland).
- Risk management in forensic outpatient settings (Stübner).
- Assessment and prevention of inpatient violence in forensic and clinical settings (Mohr).
- Development of new psychological assessment instruments for sex offenders and violent offenders on the basis of an Implicit Association Paradigma (Hutwelker).
- Evaluation of the outcome of invalidity claims after assessment (Stadtland).

- Quality assurance of forensic assessments in criminal cases (Nedopil).
- Evaluation of supervision of released sexual offenders by police and probation (Nedopil).
- Evaluation of competence in special situations (mental illness, research with psychiatric patients, pre-suicide situation, natural dying) (Nedopil).

15.6 Alzheimer Memorial Centre & Geriatric Psychiatry Research Branch

(including Clinical Research Unit D2, Memory Clinic, Dementia Day Clinic, and Dementia Neurochemistry-, Genetic-, & Neuroimaging Research Groups)

Head: Harald Hampel

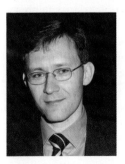

Current scientific members:
Katharina Bürger, Stefan Teipel,
Arun Bokde, Michael Ewers, Muamer Omerovic,
Djyldyz Sydykova

Former scientific members:
Frank Padberg, Susanne Stübner, Frank Faltraco,
Jens Prüssner, Andreas Haslinger,
Andreas Scheloske, Thomas Fuchsberger,
Hans-Ulrich Kötter

The vision of linking research tradition with innovation and the dedicated support of Professor Hanns Hippius and Professor Hans-Jürgen Möller as subsequent chairmen of the department of Psychiatry and Psychotherapy, laid the substantial groundwork for the strategic development of an inter-

nationally leading Alzheimer Memorial Research Centre (in memoriam of Alois Alzheimer who established his seminal neuropathological findings in our department exactly 100 years ago). On this basis, first pioneering work was done by Professor Franz Müller-Spahn in the beginning of the 1990s when he recruited a clinical research team (including Professors Hampel and Hock) focussed on dementia research and designed the newly opened Clinical Dementia Research Unit D2.

The state-of-the-art in neuroscientific research over the past decade has evolved rapidly, and ambitious research programmes such as the Alzheimer Memorial Centre, integrating these different approaches, were able to build successfully on this progress. As a consequence, the outlines of 21st century integrated neuroscience focussed on major mental health threats (such as AD) are starting to become visible, and this new science will be quite different in character to what preceded it. A 21st century approach to a particular brain function or disorder will have access to a full genomic profile of the human research participants within the study; the cognitive or other processes of interest will be described in terms of the brain systems that subserve it; the molecular and electrophysiological events underlying these cognitive processes will be described in detail, and the intervention focus at molecular, cognitive and other levels will be predicated on a full understanding of these prior factors. Discovery programmes in translational neuroscience will therefore depend on the capacity to effectively integrate approaches from differing backgrounds, using and developing supporting and underpinning technologies (such as brain imaging or deep-brain stimulation), in the context of particular brain diseases (such as AD), disorders or syndromes (such as dementia), such as brain ageing, brain repair, or depression, among other things. In other words, personalised medicine is pending.

Modern epidemiological research has shown, in light of significant world-wide demographic changes, that the number of patients suffering from AD will substantially increase during the next few decades. To reduce the expected dramatic increase of socioeconomic burden and patient suffering, biological, i.e. neurochemical and neuroimaging markers of AD are urgently needed to improve early and differential diagnosis, map disease progression, monitor effects of disease modifying treatment, and predict AD in subjects at risk at a pre-dementia/pre-clinical stage of the disease.

The pathophysiologic process leading to neurodegeneration in AD is thought to begin long before clinical symptoms develop. Existing treatments for AD improve symptoms, but increasing efforts are being directed toward the development of therapies to impede the pathologic progression of the disease. Although these medications must ultimately demonstrate efficacy, there is a critical need for biomarkers that will stratify pre-clinical and clinical patient populations for trials and indicate whether a candidate disease-modifying therapeutic agent is actually altering the underlying degenerative process.

During the last decade, promising biomarker candidates for prediction and diagnosis of AD have been identified. In particular, in cerebrospinal fluid (CSF) candidate markers were studied, validated and established, such as total tau protein, marker of neurodegeneration, hyperphosphorylated tau-protein (p-tau), as a surrogate measure of neurofibrillary tangles, ß-Amyloid-peptide1-42 (Aß42), as a measure of Aß burden, level and activity of beta secretase (BACE), a key-enzyme in the development of the pathological amyloid cascade, as well as inflammatory markers derived from the acute-phase interleukin-6-receptor complex (IL-6RC). Phase II research (i.e. study of the biomarkers in selected samples) has demonstrated high sensitivity and specificity for the detection of AD, suggesting that measures related to core disease neuropathology provide promising targets towards establishing AD-specific biomarkers. Increased research efforts, however, are necessary in patients with AD, relevant differential diagnoses, and healthy controls to further study and validate these markers, before they can be implemented in a clinical routine. Currently, they are world leaders in the development of blood-based biomarkers for AD as well.

In the clinical research studies, the utility of CSF- and blood-based biomarkers for the prediction of AD in at-risk groups, such as predementia MCI, is evaluated. Longitudinal studies are conducted in order to examine changes in biomarker levels during the progression of AD. This is of pivotal importance in order to assess whether biomarkers reflect progression and disease severity. Moreover, utility of neurochemical based biomarkers for monitoring treatment effects are evaluated. Since the biomarkers, such as Aß42, BACE, and p-tau, are thought to reflect pathophysiological mechanisms in the brain, those markers could potentially provide useful measures of disease-modifying effects of novel and innovative pharmacological treatment.

At present, there is no single genetic marker available for sporadic AD, but ApoE å4-genotype is associated with earlier onset of dementia. Also, the ApoE genotype might influence particular biomarker levels. Therefore, patients and populations at risk are stratified for the evaluation of biomarkers according to known or newly established genetic risk markers of AD.

In the field of computer-based structural and functional neuroimaging research, Prof. Hampel, together with his long-term key imaging research associates Priv.-Doz. Dr. Stefan J. Teipel, Dr. Arun W. Bokde, and Dr. Michael Ewers, have accomplished a large number of internationally competitive peer-reviewed neuroimaging publications, substantial funding, as well as key coordinating positions in large-scale international multi-centre networks and research initiatives, such as the role of national reference centre for morphometric imaging in the German Competence Network in Dementia.

AD is associated with a distinct pattern of neurodegeneration affecting specific brain areas such as medial temporal lobes, neocortical association areas and cholinergic nuclei. Loss of synaptic density and neurons in these specific predilection sites leads to functional uncoupling of brain regions, loss of fiber connectivity and cognitive impairment. Prof. Hampel and his team, particularly supported by Priv.-Doz. Dr. Teipel and Dr. Bokde, have used recent advances in MRI imaging to detect the functional and morphological consequences of AD pathology in the living human brain. Together they found significant atrophy of allocortical and neocortical brain areas in patients at risk for AD before onset of clinical dementia and demonstrated for the first time in vivo atrophy of cholinergic nuclei in AD patients. They developed MRI based markers of regional atrophy as markers to predict AD in non-demented, at risk patients and with particular support of Dr. Ewers investigated the diagnostic use of these markers in a network approach compromising MRI scans obtained from 14 universities across Germany. Diffusion tensor imaging (DTI), a recent development of MR technology, can be used to determine the integrity of fiber connections between brain areas. Using this technique together with a newly developed network detection algorithm, they found decreased integrity of intracortical projecting fiber systems and preserved integrity of extracortical projecting fiber systems in AD. Decline of fiber tract integrity in AD was associated with atrophy of corresponding areas of the cortical grey matter. Corresponding to the loss of fiber connectivity, they found a decline of functional coupling between brain regions in functional MRI studies during activation of the visual system and memory related networks. Using FDG-PET, the neruoimaging research team demonstrated a decline of cortical glucose metabolism as surrogate marker of synaptic transmission in AD patients. The pattern of decline was associated with a distinct pattern of cognitive decline and could be used to determine effects of cholinergic treatment on cortical activation.

15.7 Research group Anxiety and Depression Neuropsycho-pharmacology (Including clinical research unit D1)

Head: Rainer Rupprecht

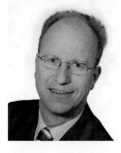

Current scientific members:
Thomas Baghai, Cornelius Schüle,
Daniela Eser, Caroline Nothdurfter,
Sibylle Häfner, Christoph Born,
Gregor Leicht, Anna Länger, Katrin Henes

Former scientific members: Peter Zwanzger, Katrin Mainka, Stefan Wenninger, Brigitte Eisensamer

Modern neuropsychopharmacological research requires exact clinical assessments for diagnosis and treatment course as well as neurobiological characterization of endophenotypes, for example by neuroendocrinological means, functional neuroimaging, etc.

The research department D-1 is dedicated to anxiety and depression research and provides a unique opportunity to combine neurobiological clinical research with high throughput genetics and basic neuroscience. The research concept is dedicated to translational medicine in the sense of research from bench to bed and back.

This research department is engaged in the following research programs:

Genetics, endophenotypes and neuroendocrinology in major depression

It is well known that major depression has a strong genetic impact. Moreover, a dysregulation of the hypothalamic-pituitary adrenal system is one of the most consistent abnormalities found in major depressive disorder.

Our research group (principal investigator: Thomas Baghai) was able to show that neuroendocrinological abnormalities in major depression are linked to genetic polymorphims, e.g. in the angiotensine converting enzyme (ACE) gene. Moreover, the ACE-gene appears to be an important determinant for the response to various additive present treatment strategies including both pharmacological and non-pharmacological methods such as sleep-deprivation, repetitive transcranial magnetic stimulation and electroconvulsive therapy. Relevant single nucleotid polymorphisms within regulatory regions of the ACE gene, have recently been identified by our group by means of high throughput genotyping of two independent samples of depressed patients in collaboration with the Max-Planck-Institute of Psychiatry in Munich. This collaboration has also contributed to the first genome wide screen in depressed patients and the identification of novel genes that may be related to antidepressant treatment response. Moreover, refined neuroendocrinological tests (principal investigator: Cornelius Schüle) provided a tool for a function probe for psychopharmacological agents both in patients but also in healthy volunteers to further unravel mechanisms of action of psychopharmacological drugs. Currently, we are investigating to what extent polymorphisms in the ACE-gene and neuroendocrinological alterations provide a link between depression und cardiovascular disease.

Mechanisms determining the efficacy of electroconvulsive therapy

Currently, electroconvulsive therapy is still the most effective treatment intervention in severe depression. Our group is studying neurobiological mechanisms (principal investigator: Thomas Baghai) underlying efficacy of this non-pharmacological treatment procedure in depression. Moreover, we are investigating clinical determinants of treatment efficacy such as anesthesia parameters, ictal parameters, impact of concomitant medication etc. These studies aim to optimize treatment regiments of electroconvulsive therapy in major depression.

Neuropsychopharmacology of neuroactive steroids

Neuroactive steroids are endogenous metabolites of progesterone which are important regulators of mood and behaviour such as sleep and anxiety. We previously demonstrated that such neuroactive steroids play an important role as endogenous modulators of depression and anxiety. Moreover, we could show that such neuroactive steroids may contribute to the pathophysiology of depression and anxiety disorders and to the mechanisms of action of antidepressant drugs. Neuroactive steroids are quantified by means of a highly sensitive and specific gas/chromatography/mass-spectometry method in collaboration with the group of Prof. Elena Romeo in Rome. Moreover, the impact of antidepressants on neurosteroidogenic enzymes is examined in heterologous expression systems in collaboration with Doncho Uzunov, Novartis, Basel. So far, our results indicate that neuroactive steroids contribute to the pharmacological action of antidepressants but not to that of non-pharmacological treatment procedures such as sleep deprivation, repetitive transcranial magnetic stimulation, or electroconvulsive therapy.

Nevertheless, neuroactive steroids might play an important role for the anxiolytic action of antidepressants in depression and anxiety disorders. In addition, we could demonstrate a differential role for various neuroactive steroids in modulating anxiety and stress responses during challenge procedures, which indicates that these molecules may be interesting targets for novel anxiolytics.

Novel treatment approaches in anxiety disorders

There is considerable need for novel fast acting anxiolytic drugs in view of the unwarranted side effect profile of benzodiazepines and the latency to onset of action of antidepressants in anxiety disorders. The challenge of treating with anxiety symptoms by pharmacological means, e.g. by cholecystokinin tetrapeptide (CCK-4), offers the unique opportunity to investigate the leading symptoms such as panic and anxiety in healthy volunteers. By means of this challenge paradigm, we could reconfirm the anxiolytic profile of anxiolytic drugs such as benzodiazepines but also demonstrate for the first time the anxiolytic potential of other GABAergic compounds such as vigabatrin and tiagabine with a different mechanism of action. Meanwhile, tiagabine has entered clinical development as an anxiolytic drug. Moreover, in co-operation with Novartis, Basle, we performed two proof-of-concept studies for novel anxiolytic compounds. These proof-of-concept studies were considered go/no go-milestones for further clinical development. It should be emphasized that these proof-of-concept studies provide a good example for successful cooperation between academic institutions and industry during early stages of drug development in psychiatry in Germany. Current research (principal investigator: Daniela Eser) focuses on the functional neuroanatomy of induced anxiety attacks by neuroimaging methods such as functional MRI. This research line aims to provide a basis for the use of such challenge paradigms in further proof-of-concept studies for the development of novel anxiolytic compounds.

Modulation of ligand-gated ion channels by psychopharmacological drugs

Indirectly through the generation of neuroactive steroids antidepressants may modulate ligand-gated ion channels such as GABA$_A$-receptors. However, we could show in electrophysiological patch clamp studies that antidepressants and antipsychotics may also exert direct effects at ligand-gated ion channels, such as endogenous and recombinant 5-HT$_3$ receptors. The functional antagonism at this ligand-gated ion channel is conferred in a non-competitive manner as shown by binding assays. In collaboration with the Max-Planck-Institute of Psychiatry in Munich we could show that an enrichment of psychopharmacological drugs in so-called lipid rafts is determinant for the ability to modulate such ligand-gated ion channels. Currently, we are investigating (principal investigator: Caroline Nothdurfter) whether the localization of ligand-gated ion channels in lipid rafts is a general principle for their allosteric modulation. This allosteric modulation of ligand-gated ion channels by psychopharmacological drugs constitutes a widely unrecognized pharmacological principle of psychopharmacological drugs and offers the possibility to design novel agents primarily acting at such modulatory sites.

15.8   Research group Neuroimaging

Head:
Eva M. Meisenzahl, Hans-Jürgen Möller

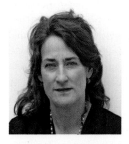

Current scientific members:
Gisela Schmitt, Thomas Frodl, Thomas Zetzsche, Nikolaos Koutsouleris, Hanna Scheurerecker, Dörthe Seifert, Sandra Ufer, Bernhard Burgermeister

Former scientific members:
Tobias Rüther, Thomas Mühlbauer, Eduard Kraft, Alain Marcuse, Torsten Mager

Since Hans-Jürgen Möller took over as chairman, imaging techniques have become an important focus of the hospital's research strategies. Up to now, the main conceptual focuses have been basic scientific and clinical research to clarify the pathogenesis of schizophrenic and affective disorders. One of the main strategies of the neuroimaging group is the successful approach of investigating scientific hypotheses and comparing study results from large samples of schizophrenic patients with those from cohorts of patients with depressive disorders and personality disorders of the borderline type. The group's research is strategically aimed at the stringent examination of different levels of the disorders:

On the first level imaging procedures to investigate disturbed connectivity in the CNS. Our activities focus on the search for abnormal structures and disturbed functions in the CNS of patients with the disorders mentioned above. This approach only makes sense when closely interlaced with psychopathological-epidemiological research approaches (epidemiological cross-sectional and follow-up research). This association is necessary since it can be assumed that the current diagnostic entities may possibly differ from the actual illness groups. Again, the research group has a comparative approach in attempting to compare the various diagnostic illness entities with respect to the specificity of their biological markers, such as brain structure or function.

Due to the pathogenesis (as yet unclear) of the named central psychiatric disorders, intensive work is carried out on a different level to link various biological markers such as those from imaging procedures with those obtained from genetics (»Imaging Genomics«) and neurophysiology.

On level three, the research group advances current receptor research on the animal experimental level using AnimalSPET; this work is performed in close cooperation with the department for nuclear medicine.

A broad spectrum of imaging procedures is being applied. In the past decade of brain research, the technique of magnetic resonance spectroscopy has taken up central position in the research activities of the scientific community. From the beginning, the research group has used structural magnetic resonance imaging intensively in order to evaluate the neuroplastic changes of macro-structures in the CNS in affective disorders and schizophrenia. The additional use of diffusion tensor imaging has been strongly developed since 2004 and applied by the research group in pilot studies to investigate the fibre systems of the CNS and their disturbed connectivity, for example to validate the therapeutic approach of electroconvulsive therapy in treatment-refractory depression.

In the psychiatric hospital of the LMU Munich, the application of functional magnetic resonance tomography plays a central role in the evaluation of affective and cognitive processes in healthy subjects and patients. Extensive projects are performed to validate models of disturbances of cerebral networks. An additional important focus is the validation of psychopharmacological and psychotherapeutic strategies using measurement instruments such as fMRT.

For years, the research group has evaluated and measured these data independently with a large degree of know-how. The group has extensive equipment at its disposal to perform these tasks, including linux computers and software tools to analyse brain structure and function (SPM, VBM, BRAINS, ANALYZE).

Apart from the evaluation of macrostructures and functional connectivity in the CNS, receptor research with SPECT and PET is the third method required to investigate pathogenetic causes of affective and schizophrenic disorders. Over the last few years, the research group has worked intensively using single photon emission tomography to evaluate receptors in patients who have never been treated. A further central aspect is the validation of current receptor targets of different psychopharmacological strategies in order to obtain a clearer understanding of the efficacy and tolerability of psychopharmacological interventions. The application of increasingly specific ligands for the complex regulatory systems of pre- and postsynaptic receptors of the various transmitter substances is a high priority of the research group. Furthermore, as mentioned above, the research group has a great interest in linking of in vivo imaging with basic scientific research in affective disorders with the

animal experimental MicroSPECT implemented in cooperation with the department of nuclear medicine.

In schizophrenic neuroimaging research with its focus on possible structural brain changes and the timing of these changes over the course of the disease, clear results were achieved from cross-sectional as well as longitudinal studies. In large samples of patients compared to healthy control subjects, there was a highly significant reduction of gray matter density and volume in befrontal-bitemoral areas, and this from the onset of the disease. Furthermore, the cross-sectional design already shows dynamic structural brain changes: patients with first manifestations show noticeable structural brain changes, in particular a reduction of the frontal lobes and hippocampus and an enlargement of the lateral ventricles, which increases significantly in relapsing disorders. These cerebral changes, such as reduction of hippocampal volume, can also be observed in depressive disorders and personality disorders of the borderline type. The clear increase of the size of the reduction when healthy, depressive and schizophrenic subjects are compared is noteworthy: from the healthy controls through the depressive first manifestations and relapsing disorders, to the schizophrenic disorders, where relapsing disorders exhibit the largest amount of hippocampal reduction.

The subsequent longitudinal imaging studies clearly show a disease-specific reduction of bifronto-temporal brain structures in schizophrenic patients beyond expectations at the age concerned. This is especially clear in the first year of illness, but also in the 2nd and 3rd and up to the 12th year, which is the longest time covered by the research group's follow-up studies so far.

The specific relevance of these structural changes for the schizophrenic disorder and its dynamics are being further investigated in ongoing follow-up studies in depressive and borderline patients. Up to now, these ongoing projects have demonstrated that after one year – depending on the course of their disease – depressive patients show a hippocampal reduction, and after three years there is a further reduction of brain structures in the whole group of depressive patients, depending on the clinical outcome of these patients.

The research results of the working group in the sector of functional imaging with investigations of neuropsychological deficits support the structural changes, particularly in the frontal cortex. In unmedicated schizophrenic patients they show a clear deficit in executive functions accompanied by reduced activations in the prefrontal cortex. It is noteworthy that these patients show improved executive performance and at least a slight increase in brain activation in the prefrontal cortex after psychopharmacological treatment with an atypical neuroleptic such as quetiapine.

The group's research strategy deals with comprehensive investigations into the cause of these structural-functional deficits in schizophrenic patients by investigating the disturbance of the dopamine system in patients never treated. In studies of large samples it became obvious that compared to healthy controls these patients have a significant reduction of postsynaptic striatal D2/D3 receptors for the ligands. In addition, there is a significant relationship with the degree of positive symptoms: the more positive symptoms are present, the lower the degree of D2/D3 receptor availability. This result clearly points to the dopaminergic overstimulation that is definitely present in the psychotic state. The investigation of the relationship between dopamine, its interactions with other messenger substances, glutamate and the structural-functional changes have been the focus of extensive research activities in animals for the past year.

In the evaluation of the underlying mechanisms of psychopharmacological strategies, extensive standardised evaluations show that also atypical antipsychotics (such as amisulpride, olanzapine and risperidone) can sometimes achieve very high D2 receptor blockade profiles, even though clinically they show significantly better tolerability and a lower rate of extrapyramidal side effects. This supports hypotheses that the better tolerability of atypical neuroleptics is explained by either limbic selectivity in the CNS or faster dissociation of these drugs from striatal D2 receptors. Finally, in the area of Imaging Genomics research, yielded fascinating and promising results.

Finally, the impact of genes involved in neuronal development, migration, neuroplasticity and apopthosis on brain structures of healthy control subjects, and specifically on altered brain structures of schizophrenic, depressed patients or patients with a personality disorder, was shown extensively by the research group. Especially polymorphisms of genes like the Prion Protein, the interleukin 1ß, or the BDNF polymorphism show a clear impact on brain structures and may provide a better understanding of the concept of vulnerability for psychiatric diseases in human subjects in the future.

15.9 Research group Clinical Psychopharmacology

Head: Michael Riedel, Hans-Jürgen Möller

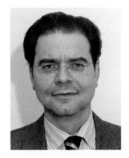

Current scientific member: Ilja Spellmann

The activities of the research group on clinical psychopharmacology cover four main areas. One of these areas consists of the evaluation of the safety and tolerability of new drugs or therapeutic approaches, mostly in schizophrenia, depression, dementia and anxiety disorders. Most of these studies are being performed to collect data necessary for a licensing application allowing the collection of information about the efficacy and side effect spectrum at an early stage. In this way, knowledge is gained about almost all antipsychotics, including amisulpride, aripiprazole, iloperidone, quetiapine, olanzapine, risperidone, long-acting risperidone, sertindole (ziprasidone), zotepine, and substances currently going through the licensing process. The situation is similar to that of antidepressants and studies have been performed with agomelatine, duloxetine, milnazipram, mirtazapine, nefazodone, reboxetine, sertraline and others.

Schizophrenia is another area of research, whereby in recent years the focus was on cognition, psychopharmacokinetics and genetics. Cognitive impairments can have a lasting, negative impact on occupational and social reintegration of schizophrenic patients, and also their compliance, resulting in its rather unfavourable long-term course. Hence, studies were performed to assess the extent to which improvement of symptoms can be achieved with psychopharmacological interventions, and to investigate the respective differences in the efficacy of the newer antipsychotics. Attempts are also being made to assess the predictive value of cognitive disorders for the long-term course of clinical variables.

The degree of association between disorders of sleep architecture and cognitive impairments is currently being investigated in a double-blind, parallel-group, randomised study. In explorative studies, the atypical antipsychotics being investigated were efficacious in the treatment of cognitive impairments. Furthermore, the results of these studies suggest that the different receptor profiles of the atypical antipsychotics are associated with their differential effects on areas of cognitive functioning. It was also shown that the severity of cognitive impairment in individual areas at the start of treatment, has a predictive value for the entire course of psychopathological features.

Pharmacokinetic investigations of various antipsychotics showed that treatment-resistant schizophrenic patients often have higher serum-plasma levels than treatment responders, although treated with the same dose. In cases of non-response to medication, the dose is often increased in the further course of treatment ('dose escalation'), although patients already have raised plasma levels. This underlines the importance of therapeutic drug monitoring. Pharmacokinetic investigations of a possible relationship between the occurrence of adverse drug reactions and possible polymorphisms of metabolising enzymes are another focus of interest, as well as studies of dopamine and serotonin receptors and glycoprotein P. Further studies showed, for example, that polymorphisms of the beta-adreno receptors caused a significantly greater weight gain in homozygous allele carriers than in the control group. Cognitive disorders are also a focus of interest in the context of bipolar disorders. Studies are being performed to investigate the relationship in euthymic bipolar patients between functional outcome and cognitive impairment, as well as between homocystein levels and cognitive impairment. In addition, it was shown that increased homocystein levels are associated with negative effects on patients' cognitive performance. The efficacy of cognitive psychoeducative group interventions are also being studied.

Studies being performed as part of the competency network on schizophrenia and depression form the fourth focus of the research group on clinical psychopharmacology. The most important network studies are the so-called basic studies, which are performed of a naturalistic design, and the controlled, double-blind, randomised studies, including the so-called 'acute study'. As part of the investigations in depressed patients, data from over 1,000 patients are being collected to investigate the occurrence rate of atypical depression, and how often the administration of antidepressants has resulted in the occurrence or worsening of suicidality, among other things. Data from the basic study on schizophrenia were used to assess whether there are differences in the psychopathological characteristics and treatment response of patients with a first episode of schizophrenia and those with multiple episodes. The results are compatible with the hypothesis that treatment response becomes less favourable during the course of schizophrenic illness. An 8-week, double-blind, randomised study ('Acute study') was performed under the leadership of Prof. Möller to compare risperidone and haloperidol in the treatment of 289 first-episode schizophrenic patients. The dose range for both substances was 2 to 8 mg/day whereby the average dose over the course of the study was 3.8 mg for risperidone and 3.7mg for haloperidol. The study results show that psychopathological features improved to a similar degree with both substances, but that in the risperidone group there were significantly fewer extrapyramidal-motor side effects and significantly fewer patients discontinued treatment prematurely.

15.10   Research Group on Clinical and Applied Psychology

Head: Annette Schaub

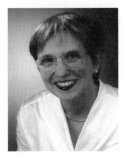

Current scientific member:
Iris Liwowsky, Britta Bernhard

Former scientific members:
Susanne Amann, Marketa Charypar,
Ulrich Goldmann, Petra Kümmler,
Nicole Neubauer, Elisabeth Roth, Brigitte Wolf

Cognitive Behavioural and Psychoeducational Interventions in Severe Psychiatric Illness

Implementation and research on illness management programmes and their integration into standard treatment

One year after Hans-Jürgen Möller took over as chairman, illness management programmes including psychoeducational as well as cognitive-behavioural strategies became an important focus of the hospital's treatment strategies. Specialised treatment units for schizophrenia as well as depression were established integrating pharmacological and cognitive-behavioural strategies. Three different group programmes covering schizophrenia, depression and bipolar disorder were implemented, aimed at improving treatment adherence, coping with symptoms and stressors, modifying dysfunctional beliefs about the illness and the self, developing relapse prevention skills, strengthening social support and developing a lifestyle promoting health. Psychoeducational groups for relatives are also provided if needed. The primary goals of these programmes are to enhance the patients' and relatives' ability to manage their

illness and to improve its outcome. They are based on stress-vulnerability-coping and transtheoretical models. The first model highlights the interactions between biological vulnerability, stressors and protective factors. The latter proposes that the motivation to change develops over a series of stages; should therefore be performed as early as possible to help clients identify and pursue their personal goals and to explore how improved illness management can help them achieve these goals. All illness management programs last for 12 to 14 sessions (twice a week for 60–90 minutes), and published treatment manuals for therapists, handouts for the patients as well as supervision at a regular basis are provided. Deficits in neuropsychological functioning accentuate the importance of sound didactic and behavioural principles in illness management programs for severe psychiatric illness.

All programs proved to be clinically feasible in studies, including 98 patients with schizophrenia, 279 patients with major depression and 86 patients with bipolar disorder. The patients were very satisfied with their treatment and the increased knowledge about their illness. In 1997 and in 2000 randomised controlled trials were started to evaluate two programmes. The first study including 197 patients with schizophrenia compared the coping-oriented (BOT) with a supportive group (SUP). Patients in the first programme were significantly better informed about psychosis and gained more knowledge from pre- to post treatment. At a one-year follow-up they showed less dysfunctional illness models than their counterparts. There were no significant differences between psychopathological symptoms in total (BPRS-E), however, patients in the BOT had significant lower scores in depression and avolition/apathy (SANS). Patients with severe negative symptoms did benefit more from the BOT than the SUP. There were no significant differences in relapse at a one and two year follow-up. In the second study including 177 patients with depression, three treatment options were studied: a) clinical management (CM), b) combined with the illness management group programme (VOG), c) the latter in combination with individual sessions (VOG+). At post-assessment, patients in the VOG claimed high satisfaction with the programme.

There were no significant differences between the treatment options with regard to gains in knowledge, psychopathological symptoms, dysfunctional attitudes, locus of control, coping strategies and self-concept. In a secondary analysis symptom severity was taken into account. Patients with severe depression (Median HAMD>21) who participated in the illness management programmes showed significantly higher gains in self-confidence and problem solving than the control group. At one year follow-up these results were confirmed. High scores in self-confidence and problem solving correlated significantly with lower numbers of readmission. For five years the study was supported by the Federal Ministry of Education and Research within the competence-network »depression, suicidality«, and further analyses are in planning. With regard to the illness management programme in bipolar disorder, there only have been naturalistic studies so far. 52 participating patients with bipolar disorder were very satisfied with it and their knowledge about the illness, and psychosocial functioning significantly increased from pre- to post assessment. Looking at the one and two year outcome 25%, respectively 30% of the patients had been rehospitalised. The number of previous hospitalisations and male sex were significant predictors for relapse. One study including 49 relatives of bipolar patients who participated in distinct psychoeducational groups for relatives showed no significant reductions in High Expressed Emotion and burden at post-assessment, however, at one year follow-up. These results suggest that educating patients about their illness, training self-management skills, instilling hope and enhancing self-esteem as well as strengthening the patient's social network can be valuable components of a comprehensive approach to the treatment of inpatients.

The programmes described were integrated into standard treatment. Usually four group programmes, including two for depressive disorders and one each for schizophrenia and bipolar disorder are offered at the same time. Every four months, groups for relatives are offered for relatives facing the results side-effects of mood disorders or schizophrenia. Supervision is provided on a regular basis to guarantee treatment competence and fidelity. There are pre- and post-assessments including psychopathological (Brief Psychiatric Rating Scale Expanded) and subjective scales (Beck Depression Inventory, satisfaction with treatment) for the patients, as well as questionnaires about burden and satisfaction with treatment for the relatives in order to guarantee quality assurance.

Basic Research

Studies on neuropsychological functioning in patients with first episodes in depression or schizophrenia show heterogeneous results. 75 first-episode patients with depression and 38 patients with schizophrenia were assessed with the aid of a comprehensive test battery. Despite comparable psychopathological symptoms (BPRS-E, GAF), patients with depression showed significantly better results in verbal memory and fluency, visual-motor concentration and vigilance than patients with schizophrenia. Neuropsychological functioning plays an important role in psychiatry studies focusing on rate limiting factors for psychosocial interventions in schizophrenia as well as depression. Up to now but not education seems to be a predictor in some, but not all analyses. Another focus was on cognitive functioning (WCST, AVLM) and neuroimaging in 34 depressive inpatients and 34 healthy control subjects. Hippocampal volumes and frontal lobe volumes were significantly smaller in patients, compared to the control group and lower hippocampal volumes were correlated with poorer performance in the WCST. Further studies will explore whether these volumes are related to lower responsiveness to psychotherapy. Recently, quality of life has gained more importance in the evaluation of treatment outcome. 96 psychiatric inpatients with the diagnosis of schizophrenia, depressive disorders, substance use disorders or personality disorders were recruited and assessed with the Lancashire Quality of Life Profile. Patients suffering from schizophrenia were more satisfied with their life and inpatient treatment than patients with substance use disorders, depressive disorders or personality disorders. Quality of life showed close connections with self-assessed anxiety and coping behaviour, but only modest or no correlations with psychopathological symptoms or psychosocial functioning.

Training in Cognitive Behavioural Therapy and in Psychiatry

In 1997 a close collaboration was set up with Dr. Kraemer (TU) and the psychosomatic clinic Roseneck (Professor Fichter) to guarantee a high standard in training physicians and psychologists in cognitive behaviour therapy and in psychiatry. The acceptance as supervisor by the Bavarian State Medical Association and in all institutes at Munich (BAP, CIP, IFT, VFKV, DGVT) laid the basis for training psychologists in CBT at this department. Until today, 103 psychotherapists in training participated in this programme. Lecturing in clinical psychology and psychiatry (e.g., assessing psychopathological symptoms) as well as training in management programmes were also provided for students or at institutes and conferences. In 2006 the German Association for Psychoeducation was established and the board includes Dr. Bäuml, Dr. Pitschel-Walz, Professor Luderer, Professor Sadre Chirazi-Stark and Dr. Schaub. This association exists to foster the implementation and evaluation of illness management programmes in psychiatric illness in Germany and abroad.

15.11   Research group Psychoneuroimmunology

Heads: Norbert Müller, Markus J. Schwarz

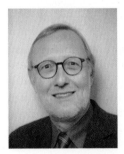

Current scientific members:
Michael Riedel, Anja Cerovecki, Sandra Dehning, Anette Douhet, Larissa de la Fontaine, Richard Musil, Ilja Spellmann,

Former scientific member: Martin Strassnig

The study group psychoneuroimmunology is exploring the role of the immune system during psychological processes and in psychiatric disorders. Schizophrenia, depressive disorders, anxiety disorders, tic disorders and Tourette syndrome are of main interest. The influence of infectious processes and – latent – chronic inflammatory processes in certain regions of the central nervous system (CNS) are in the focus of our research.

The investigations of the study group include basic research, e.g. the interaction of catecholamines and immune cells, and the role of the blood brain barrier. Also, clinical research including clinical pharmacological trials are being performed. Estimations of the cytokines, the transmitters of the immune system, in the peripheral blood and the cerebrospinal fluid of patients has led to the hypothesis that a dysbalance between the type-1 immune response (TH-1 response) and the type-2 immune response (TH-2 response) is essential for the pathogenesis of psychiatric disorders. In schizophrenia, an overweight of the TH-2 response and a lack in the activation of the TH-1 response plays a role. In depression, however, an overweight of the pro-inflammatory (cellular type-1 related immune response) can be observed, at least in distinct subgroups. In addition, in schizophrenia and in depression different courses and clinical types of the disorder are associated with different patterns of immune activation. This can be found especially in melancholic depression and in schizophrenia with marked negative symptoms. Moreover, during the last few years, the relationship between the immune system, the tryptophan-kynurenine metabolism and the glutamatergic neurotransmission has gained increasing interest. The interaction between neuroactive kynurenine metabolites and the glutamatergic NMDA receptors, but also the alpha-7-nicotinic receptors seems to play a crucial role in the pathogenesis of psychiatric disorders. This interaction is cytokine-driven. Additionally, the effects of psychotropic drugs to the cellular and humoral system and the influences to the blood brain barrier are an important field of the study group. The immunogenetic determination of the immune response by the HLA-system but also by polymorphic genes of cytokines and adhesion molecules is an important topic of studies using molecular-biological examinations.

Beside the »classical« immunological investigations in the peripheral blood by ELISA, ELI-Spot, and laser-flow-cytometry (FACS), one- and two-dimensional electrophoresis, studies of the cerebrospinal fluid and of post-mortem CNS-tissue, but also of cell cultures are being performed.

A further important topic of the study group during the last few years have been clinical studies on the influence of an immunomodulatory treatment in patients with psychiatric disorders. The therapeutic effects of antibiotics, i.v. immunoglobuline and plasmapheresis are studied in patients with tic-disorders and Tourette syndrome. In schizophrenia and depression, the use and the effects of cyclo-oxygenase-2 (COX-2) inhibitors are an important field of interest. We could describe therapeutic effects of these anti-inflammatory substances in schizophrenia (administered in the first years after onset) and in major depression. So far, COX-2 inhibitors represent a promising new anti-inflammatory, therapeutic approach in the treatment of psychiatric disorders. In the meanwhile, our results were replicated by several other groups.

15.12   Research Group Transcranial Brain Stimulation and Neuroplasticity

Head: Frank Padberg

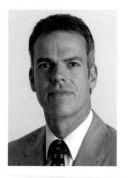

Current scientific members:
Till Krauseneck, Ulrich Palm, Andrea Sterr, Nicola Großheinrich, Olivia Krähenmann, Daniel Keeser

Former scientific members:
Peter Zwanzger, Robin Ella

Background

Based on findings in functional neuroimaging studies, numerous psychiatric disorders can be characterized by reversible changes in regional brain function, i.e. changes in regional cerebral blood flow and a regional glucose metabolism. These findings have a strong impact on the current understanding of the pathophysiology of these conditions, e.g. major depression is currently regarded as a system level disorder affecting numerous cortical and subcortical, limbic and paralimbic neuronal circuits. In addition, these findings are the background for the recent interest in brain stimulation approaches, targetting these circuits in order to improve function and to restore the integrity of these networks. Beside invasive stimulation approaches like deep brain stimulation (DBS) and vagus nerve stimulation (VNS), less invasive transcranial brain stimulation approaches, i.e. repetitive transcranial magnetic stimulation (rTMS), theta burst stimulation (TBS) and transcranial direct current stimulation (tDCS) have recently been discussed as promising new avenues for the treatment of psychiatric disorders.

Focus of research

The Laboratory of Transcranial Brain Stimulation was founded in 1998 at the Department of Psychiatry and Psychotherapy of the Ludwig-Maximilians University of Munich (F. Padberg, H.J. Möller). The laboratory focuses on these less invasive transcranial brain stimulation approaches, initially only on rTMS, and, more recently, on two novel methods: TBS and tDCS.

From the beginning, two independent research tracks have been established, one in healthy subjects and one in patients with major depressive episodes. In healthy volunteers, prefrontal rTMS has been investigated regarding the effects on mood and emotional regulation as well as hypothalamic pituitary adrenal (HPA) axis function (R. Ella, P. Zwanzger, F. Padberg). More recently, the effects of prefrontal rTMS on event related potentials and resting EEG have been studied in order to establish paradigms for further testing different stimulation conditions. The second research line consists of sequential clinical trials in patients suffering from major depressive episodes (F. Padberg, P. Zwanzger). These trials were supported by the Competence Network (BMBF) and later the German Research Foundation (DFG). In the framework of these studies, promising treatment parameters have been identified and high frequency prefrontal rTMS were found to be effective in therapy resistant major depressive episodes. These findings led to a large multicenter trial in Germany investigating rTMS as early treatment together with antidepressant pharmacotherapy. Moreover, very simular stimulation parameters have recently been used in a large US multicenter trial of rTMS in therapy resistant depression.

In general, the efficacy of therapeutic rTMS in depression has been found to be moderate and mechanisms of action appear to differ from other antidepressant interventions like pharmacotherapy and sleep deprivation. For instance, rTMS has little effect on HPA dysfunction as measured by the combined dexamethasone/suppression-CRH-test (P. Zwanzger). In contrast, prefrontal rTMS leads to a significant dopamine release in mesolimbic and mesostriatal regions in animal models and healthy volunteers, as well as to striatal dopamine release in depressed subjects. Remarkably, a single session of rTMS increases striatal dopamine release to the same degree as a single dose of 0.3 mg/kg d-amphetamine (O. Pogarell, Clinical Neurophysiology Section in collaboration with K. Tatsch, P. Bartenstein, Department of Nuclear Medicine).

Most recently, the spectrum of rTMS applications has been extended to other neuropsychiatric disorders, e.g. chronic tinnitus and Tourette syndrome. Target regions in chronic tinnitus are the temporal parietal junction close to the primary auditory cortex, and in Tourette syndrome the supplementary motor area (J. Nürnberger, in collaboration with N. Müller). Moreover, TBS, a promising rTMS protocol, has been established in the laboratory and is now being tested on healthy subjects and Tourette patients (N. Grossheinrich). TBS has been developed from stimulation protocols used in cellular neurophysiology for inducing long-term potention (LTP) and long-term depression (LTP) and is hypothesized to exert more robust effects on cortical excitability than standard rTMS. Thus, this approach is currently regarded as a powerful promising stimulation approach, possibly superior to conventional rTMS. Another pilot trial is investigating tDCS in therapy resistant depression combining tDCS with EEG par-

adigms (U. Palm, D. Keeser, in collaboration with C. Mulert, Functional Neuroimaging Section). In contrast to rTMS, which leads to a direct stimulation of cortical and intracortical excitatory or inhibitory circuits and networks based on the depolarisation of neurons, tDCS is a novel intervention shifting base line excitability in stimulated brain regions towards or away from the excitatory state. Thus, this approach may be particularly effective when combined with a second supra-threshold intervention like rTMS, but also pharmacotherapy and other non-pharmacological interventions.

Another more recent research focus of our group is the clinical course following psychological trauma, i.e. acute stress reactions and the development of posttraumatic stress disorder. In close collaboration with the Institute for Anaesthesiology (G. Schelling) we are conducting research on the consequences of intensive medical treatment, e.g. in patients undergoing cardiac surgery (T. Krauseneck). Additionally, we are conducting a study on trauma-induced brain plasticity using current MRI techniques (diffusion tensor imaging and voxel-based morphometry) in public transport drivers involved in severe accidents (e.g. due to suicide) and patients experiencing occupational or traffic accidents (T. Krauseneck, O. Krähenmann). In the same study, we are investigating functional changes within the HPA system in the acute aftermath of trauma using the low dexamethasone suppression test.

The Laboratory of Transcranial Brain Stimulation in Munich was one of the two psychiatric research centers in Germany where 1999 the »Working group on TMS in Psychiatry« (»Arbeitsgemeinschaft TMS in der Psychiatrie«) was founded. Currently, about 20 rTMS laboratories in Germany participate in this informal group meeting biannually and providing an active research structure for the recent multicenter trial mentioned above and a novel current multicenter project on the safety of rTMS. The Laboratory of Transcranial Brain Stimulation currently holds international collaborations with Dr. A. Zangen (Weizmann-Institut, Israel) and Dr. Y. Levkovitz (Tel Aviv University, Israel), Dr. U. Herwig (Psychiatrische Universitätsklinik Zürich, Switzerland), Dr. J. Rothwell (Sobell Department, Institute of Neurology, Queen Square, London) and Dr. F. Fregni (Department of Neurology, Beth

Israel Deaconess Medical Center, Harvard Medical School, Boston, MA, USA).

15.13   Research groups on bipolar affective disorders

Research and specialised treatment of bipolar affective disorders is represented twice in the hospital:
- First, by a group led by Waldemar Greil dedicated to the continuing analysis of a large multicenter study, the so-called MAP-Study,
- And secondly, by the Bipolar outpatient clinic, the continuation of the former Stanley Foundation Bipolar Outpatient Clinic (Heinz Grunze).

Research group MAP study

Head: Waldemar Greil

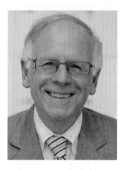

Current scientific members: Dorothee Giersch, Nicki Seitz, Emanuel Severus

Former scientific member: Niko Kleindienst

The research group continues to conduct more secondary analyses of the MAP Study, comparing the prophylactic efficacy of lithium and carbamazepine. As a primary result of the study, it has been demonstrated that lithium is especially helpful in classical forms of affective disorders, whereas carbamazepine seems to be advantageous in lithium non-responders and affective disorders with comorbidities of different kinds. Further analyses have demonstrated that higher lithium levels are especially helpful in preventing manic/mixed episodes whereas lower levels are at least equally effective in preventing depressive episodes. In addition, meta-analyses of studies of lithium in affective disorders yielded several predictors of response to lithium. At present, the creation of a »Lithium Response Scale« is under way. Finally, this large database is being analysed for the impact of personality characteristics and other potential prognostic markers on relapse prevention in the long-term treatment of bipolar disorders.

The group is further involved in »Continued Medical Education«, certified by the »Bavarian Board of Doctors«, providing a blended-learning based curriculum for bipolar disorder for board-examined psychiatrists in all parts of Germany. It implies a combination of conventional learning techniques (oral presentations, work shops) with e-learning based chats and case reports. This highly acclaimed curriculum is now in its 3rd year and will be continued at least throughout 2007/2008. It is accompanied by an extensive ongoing scientific evaluation regarding the different components of this learning program.

In November 2006, an integrated textbook on bipolar disorders has been published by Waldemar Greil and Dorothee Giersch. In contrast to conventional textbooks, the target audience for this book consists of professionals, patients as well as their relatives.

Research group Bipolar Outpatient Research clinic

Head: Heinz Grunze

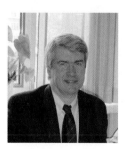

Current scientific member: Christoph Born

Former scientific members: Sandra Dittmann, Emanuel Severus, Sascha Dargel, Anna Forsthoff, Benedikt Amann, Florian Seemüller, Britta Bernhard, Nicole Matzner, Inge Schweiss

Part of the long-lasting tradition of the hospital in the research of bipolar disorders is the specialised Bipolar outpatient research clinic led by H. Grunze which was originally funded by the Stanley Foundation (from 1999 to 2004). This specialised outpatient clinic constituted the German centre of an international research group together with the Bipolar outpatient clinics of the University of Freiburg and the Charité in Berlin. Other centres were 5 centres in the US as well as a Dutch center (Utrecht). Between 1999 and 2004, prospective longitudinal data were collected from more than 300 bipolar patients which allow – together with the data of the other centres – sophisticated analyses about characteristics of morbidity over the time course of the illness, the impact of co-morbidities and, finally, the responsiveness to a multitude of innovative treatments tested within the network.

15.14   Research group on Addiction

Head: Michael Soyka

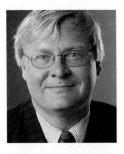

Current scientific members:
Brigitta Bondy, Peter Zill , Ulrich Preuss (genetics), Tobias Rüther (neuroimaging), Gabriele Koller, , Peggy Schmidt, Martin Lieb (therapeutic studies)

Former scientific member:
Miriam Bottlender (genetics, clinical research)

Starting in the mid-1980s a special ward for treatment of substance use disorders, mainly alcohol dependence, was established, followed by an outpatient clinic for patients with opioid dependence (methadone ambulance). Consequently, a broad spectrum of research efforts emerged from this basis. Research in substance use disorders has been very active over the past two decades with several hundred publications in this field. The focus has been both on basic mechanisms and treatment of substance use disorders

Basic mechanisms

The understanding of the neurobiological basis of substance use disorders, especially alcoholism, has dramatically increased over the past decades. Some 50% of the liability of becoming alcohol dependent is related to genetic vulnerability factors. Consequently, the genetics of alcoholism has been one of the key approaches in substance use research. Inspired by the US COGA group and other international groups, a well-defined gene bank for alcohol dependence was established with has been some 450 individuals included. Using this sample different aspects of alcoholism studied including the role of personality and temperament factors or medical disorders related to alcoholism. Special emphasis has been put on candidate genes for alcohol dependence and numerous studies have been performed and published focusing on very different genes encoding for GABA and glutamate receptors, among others. Especially, variations in GABA-A receptors have been identified as possible vulnerability markers for alcoholism.

Neuroimaging techniques offer unique opportunities to study basic mechanisms in substance use disorders. Unlike other psychiatric disorders, there are excellent animal models for substance use, and basic mechanisms of substance use such as craving or withdrawal, can directly be studied using neuroimaging techniques. A number of PET studies have been performed in this respect using both glucose or defined neurotransmitter tracers as ligands. Recent findings indicate that moderate alcohol consumption results in a dramatic decline of glucose utilization in all brain regions. In addition, using a special paradigm (dextrometorphan-challenge), the role of glutamate receptors in the development of alcohol-like effects and the mediation of craving was further elucidated.

Therapy research

Both psychotherapeutic and pharmacotherapeutic approaches have been studied intensively, often in close collaboration with other treatment centres.

With respect to psychotherapy of alcoholism, effects of setting were of special relevance. Several follow-up studies focused on the efficacy of novel outpatient services and treatment approaches indicating a positive outcome in many patients. In addition, the widely neglected topic »outpatient detoxification« was addressed in a model project funded by major health care providers. A treatment protocol was developed and tested in a consecutive number of studies. Meanwhile this model has entered clinical practice and has been adopted by other clinics.

From 2000-2006 a number of projects were funded within one of the four large national research networks for substance use research funded by the German Ministry of Science (BMBF, www.ASAT.de).

Pharmacologically based relapse prevention is a new field in the treatment of alcohol dependence. Starting with the putative NMDA modulator acamprosate, a broad range of substances has been tested including opioid antagonists, other glutamatergic drugs or most recently cannabis antagonists. This work has also inspired studies concerning basic mechanisms of addiction.

For opioid dependence, a number of full and mixed agonists have also been studied. In addition, the interaction of substitution treatment and setting effects as well as manual based psychotherapy have been studied in a number of projects within a research network funded by the German Ministry of Science (www.ASAT.de). Studies indicate that both methadone and buprenorphine are effective drugs in reducing mortality and morbidity in opioid dependence. The neurocognitive effects of different substitution drugs were studied in a number of experimental studies indicating cognitive deficits in some but not the majority of drug dependent patients, with some improvement during treatment.

Integrating addiction research into clinical practice

Many of the studies conducted so far have improved our understanding of treatment substance use disorders. Consequently, the Psychiatric Hospital of the University of Munich took part in various expert committees working on guidelines for sub-stance use treatment. This was the case for several national committees (AWMF-guidelines for substance use treatment). In addition, as part of a scientific project, guidelines for the inpatient rehabiltation of alcohol dependent patients funded by the German pension funds were developed.

15.15   Outpatient clinic/ Specialised clinics/Day clinic

Head: Michael Riedel

Current scientific members:
Emanuel Severus (outpatient clinic),
Florian Seemüller (day clinic)

Former scientific member: Ronald Bottlender

In the outpatient clinic, a range of therapies are being offered by a team of professionals from various specialities. This means that patients can be treated during both the acute and long-term stages of their illness with a therapy regime suited to their individual needs. The Psychiatric University Hospital has been cooperating with the district hospital in Haar since mid-2003 to offer complete psychiatric care to the 400,000 inhabitants of the southern area of Munich. As part of this project, specialised psychiatric clinics were founded at the Hospital for Psychiatry and Psychotherapy of the University of Munich.

Up to 2002, between 6,000 and 10,000 patients a year have made use of the outpatient clinic. Subsequent reorganisation enabled more kinds of therapy to be offered and also allowed a low-threshold access to the clinic helpingpatients with very difficult and complicated courses of illness. This has resulted in an almost threefold increase in the number of patient contacts, to 29,500 in 2005.

The research activities in the outpatient clinic and specialised clinics are mainly focussed on schizophrenia and affective psychoses. Studies are also performed in the field of compulsive disorders, Gilles de la Tourette syndrome, and acute and posttraumatic stress disorder.

In cooperation with the Munich public transportation services, employees (e.g. underground train drivers and tram drivers) are being treated who have been involved in job-related accidents where people have come to harm. The frequency of subsequent development of a posttraumatic stress disorder, with its negative consequences for the quality of life, is being evaluated.

Double-blind, randomised studies are being conducted to evaluate innovative psychopharmacological treatment approaches who been shown in routine clinical care to be better than the usual treatment strategies.

Studies of affective psychoses have recently been completed investigating the association between functional outcome and cognitive impairment in euthymic bipolar patients, as well as between homocystein levels and cognitive impairment. The efficacy of group interventions of cognitive psychoeducation is being evaluated in an ongoing case-control study.

Another project is being conducted to investigate the efficacy of light therapy in depressive syndromes occurring as a feature of various psychiatric disorders, i.e. the modulating effects of light therapy are being evaluated, for example when it is administered in addition to drug treatment.

The risk/benefit ratio must be critically considered when administering antidepressants to pregnant patients, especially if they are in this first trimester. A double-blind, randomised, placebo-controlled study is currently being performed to investigate this topic. This study is investigating the efficacy of eicosapentaenoic acid in the prevention of postnatal depression in patients who have had suffered from this depression in the past and who are pregnant again. The studies in the field of schizophrenia can be roughly summarised as investigating treatment optimisation, particularly in relation to long-term treatment.

Several double-blind, randomised, parallel-group studies have been performed to investigate the extent to which the different receptor profiles of atypical antipsychotics are responsible for differential effects in the treatment of cognitive impairments. A further focus of research has been the degree to which the impairment predicts the further course of this disorder. The occurrence of side effects has been investigated in a series of pharmacokinetic and pharmacogenetic studies, and cyto-

genetic studies have been performed with the aim to identify genetic risk factors in schizophrenia and the Gilles de la Tourette syndrome.

15.16 Research group documentation and disease course

Head: Michael Riedel, Hans-Jürgen Möller

Current scientific member: Anton Strauß

Former scientific members: Markus Jäger, Ronald Bottlender

Knowledge about the course of the different psychiatric disorders is highly relevant for acute and long-term treatment and for the initiation of rehabilitative procedures. The study of the course of psychiatric disorders is also of great importance since only a few psychiatric diseases could be characterised by consistent biological findings to date. The lack of such findings is the reason why Emil Kraepelin, who held the chair for psychiatry in Munich at the beginning of the 20th century, suggested using the long-term course to classify and diagnose psychiatric disorders.

Several large follow-up studies of the course of psychiatric disorders were performed in the 20th century. In the Department of Psychiatry and Psychotherapy of the LMU Munich, this research approach was followed more closely from 1994 onwards, with the commencement of ‚the Munich follow-up study'. At this time, the traditional psychiatric diagnosis and classification had been revised through the introduction of the so-called operationalised diagnosis systems, ICD-10 and DSM-IV. This has led to questions about the validity of these diagnosis systems.

The Munich 15-year follow-up study, which was performed under the leadership of Professor H.-J. Möller together with Dr. R. Bottlender and Dr. A. Strauß, included all patients diagnosed with a ‚functional psychosis' (schizophrenia and affective disorders) and who were first treated as inpatients in the Munich psychiatric hospital in the years 1980 to 1982 and who lived in Munich or the surrounding areas. The 323 patients were selected and their baseline data collected from the hospital's medical records retrospectively. A detailed follow-up evaluation of the patients was performed in the years 1995 to 1997. Standard evaluation instruments were used to measure the patients' psychopathological state, global and social level of functioning and quality of life.

The results of these studies showed that the operationalised diagnosis systems ICD-10 and DSM-IV have a high predictive validity since the diagnostic classification at the start of the illness is highly relevant for the prediction of the outcome. However, a large variability was found in those patients who were initially diagnosed with schizophrenia.

In 1998 a prospective study was initiated. This study also included first-episode patients with a 'functional psychosis' (ICD-10: F2, F30, F31, F32, F33), who were evaluated with standardised instruments during their inpatient treatment. The patients were then invited to a follow-up evaluation after one, two and five years. A total of 1271 patients (853 patients with F30-F33; 418 patients with F20) were included in the study.

In the year 2000 the competency networks on schizophrenia and depression were initiated, sponsored by the Federal Ministry for Education and Research. The ongoing, prospective, 5-year study of disease course was continued by Dr. M. Jäger, Dr. A. Strauß and Priv.-Doz. Dr. R. Bottlender within the framework of the two competency networks, whereby additional evaluation instruments were introduced. In contrast to the earlier investigations, not only first episode but also multiple episode patients were included. In addition, the competency network studies were performed as multi-centre studies in which university and other hospitals in the whole of Germany participated. This resulted in the recruitment of 400 patients with schizophrenic disorders, of which 129 had a first episode of schizophrenia and 279 multiple episodes (ICD-10: F2), as well as 1073 patients with affective disorders (ICD-10: F30, F31, F32, F33). Publications from these studies deal with the difference between first- and multiple-episode patients with a schizophrenic psychosis, the relevance of depressive symptoms occurring as part of a schizophrenic disorder, and with the possibility to predict the success of treatment of schizophrenic psychoses.

15.17   Research group Drug Surveillance in Psychiatry

Heads: Renate Grohmann, Rolf R. Engel

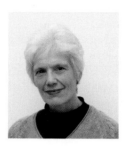

Current scientific members:
Susanne Stübner, Sylvia Brettschneider, Bettina Holtschmid-Täschner

Former scientific members:
Florian Müller-Siecheneder, Gabriele Neundörfer-Kohl, Susanne Steinwachs, Günter Wagner

This group of the hospital has a long tradition. The first drug surveillance program was established in 1978 as a collaboration between the psychiatric university hospitals in Berlin and Munich (»Drug Surveillance in Psychiatry« [»Arzneimittelüberwachung in der Psychiatrie«], AMÜP). Based on the knowledge gained in this 10-year project, a new drug safety program was established in 1990 called »Drug Safety in Psychiatry« (»Arzneimittelsicherheit in der Psychiatrie«, AMSP). It was founded by Hanns Hippius and Eckart Rüther. Renate Grohmann has organized the clinical and scientific work since the beginning. Currently, 55 psychiatric hospitals in Germany, Switzerland, Austria, Belgium and Hungary are working together this program. The aim of AMSP is (a) the documentation of severe adverse drug reactions (ADR) under routine, naturalistic therapy with psychotropic drugs in psychiatric inpatients, (b) the scientific analysis of possible antecedents and causes, and (c) the search for effective ways to reduce ADRs.

Clinically severe adverse drug reactions are systematically documented. The project has established guidelines for the classification of an event as 'severe'. The probability of a causal relationship between the application of a drug and the observed adverse event is rated according to usual international criteria. Imputations are not only given to single drugs but also to drug combinations. In addition, pharmacokinetic interactions are documented and considered as a further mechanism for the induction of an ADR.

Publications from the project include (a) descriptive overviews of the adverse effects of antipsychotic and antidepressant drugs, done as cross-section studies as well as comparative evaluations across time, (b) systematic studies on specific classes of adverse events (examples are: severe movement disorders, blood dyscrasias, cardiac ADRs, galactorrhea, and hyperglycemia) and (c) case studies of individual adverse effects. Current projects analyze dermatological side effects and rhabdomyolysis. The project is financed by grants from the drug industry and organized by independent societies in the three countries.

15.18   Research Group Epidemiology and Evaluation Research

Head: Manfred Fichter

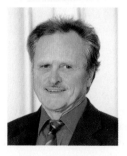

Current scientific members: Norbert Quadflieg, Gabriele Kohlböck, Marian Cebulla, Nadine Bachetzky, Kerstin Nisslmüller

Former scientific members: Markus Ladineo, Ingeborg Meller (senior researcher)

The main focus of this division is to conduct scientific epidemiological studies concerning prevalence, incidence, risk factors and course of mental illness in community populations. Another focus is the scientific evaluation of treatment, diagnosis and course of illness in patients with a mental or psychosomatic disorder.

Current major projects are as follows:

A. Psychiatric epidemiology
- Long-term longitudinal epidemiological study on the course of mental illness and predictors of outcome (Upper Bavarian Study). This series of projects was financed by the »Deutsche Forschungsgemeinschaft DFG (publication of data in preparation).
- Prevalence and course of mental illness in the very old – a longitudinal community study (all relevant data published).
- Prevalence of mental disorders and need for treatment of a representative sample of homeless people in the city of Munich (most data published).

B. Evaluation research
- Course of eating disorders and identification of risk factors for outcome.
- Treatment effects of a behavioral program on the long-term course of obesity.
- Long-term course of chronic tinnitus associated with anxiety and/or depression(C).
- Self-destructive behavior in eating disorders and candidate genes of serotonergic transmission (5-HTTLPR) / Promoter region of the 5-HT2A-receptor / Promoter region of the MAO-A gene.
- Mortality in eating disorders; based on data of 10,000 treated patients.
- Relapse prevention in anorexia nervosa based on in 9-month internet program with 18-month follow-up.
- NIH international collaborative study on phenotype and molecular genetics of anorexia nervosa.

15.19   Research group Suicide prevention and mental health research

Head: Ulrich Hegerl

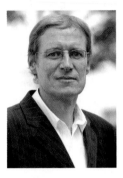

Current scientific members:
David Althaus, Rita Schäfer, Jörg Kunz,
Antje-Kathrin Allgaier

Former scientific members: Tim Pfeiffer-Gerschel,
Verena Henkel, Anja Ziervogel,

Several large projects have been implemented and conducted within the German Research Net on Depression and Suicidality (funded by the German Federal Ministry of Education and Research from 1999 up to 2008).

The »Nuremberg Alliance Against Depression« was a 2-year, 4-level, community based action programme in Nuremberg (500,000 inhabitants) with the aim to improve the care of depressed patients and to prevent suicidality. It has been evaluated both with respect to a 1-year baseline and a control region (city of Würzburg). The intervention took place on four different levels: *Co-operation with GPs* (Interactive workshops, screening instruments, videos, CD-ROM), a *Public relations campaign* (posters at public places, leaflets, information brochures, public events, cinema spot), *Community facilitators* (Educational workshops for teachers, counsellors, priests, geriatric nurses, policemen, pharmacists, local media) and *High risk groups* (»emergency card« for patients after suicide attempt, videos, CD-ROM, support of self-help activities). A significant and highly relevant reduction of suicidal acts (completed + attempted suicides: – 24%) was found during the

intervention years (2001, 2002) compared to these baseline (2000).

A further decline of the number of suicidal acts was found in the follow-up year 2003.

Many regions in Germany expressed interest in using the concept and materials developed within the Nuremberg Alliance Against Depression for starting own regional alliances. Up to October 2006 already 35 regions had started their own 4-level interventions under the common roof of the »German Alliance against Depression« (www.buendnis-depression.de).

Based on the work of the »German Alliance Against Depression«, 18 international partners representing 16 different countries started the »European Alliance Against Depression« (EAAD) in 2004. With support of the European Commission an international network has been built up. The successful basic principle of the action-oriented 4-level programme conducted in Nuremberg, is combinend with knowledge and expertise from international partners (www.EAAD.net). Starting first with local interventions, extension to other regions in different countries is the next step. In some of the European countries the concept has already been adopted by national authorities with the aim to promote an extension on a national level. EAAD has been included in the Green Paper of the European Commission as »best practice model« for improving the care of depressed patients and for preventing suicidality.

A study on minor forms of depression (MinD-study) was also run within the German Research Network on Depression and Suicidality in Nuremberg. The objective was to assess the efficacy of SSRI (sertraline) and cognitive-behavioral group therapy (CBT) for the treatment of a large group of primary care patients with minor and milder forms of depression and to evaluate if receiving treatment (pharmaco- or psychotherapy) according to randomization or free choice influences outcome. This randomized, controlled, single-center, 10-week, clinical trial with five arms was conducted between May 2000 and January 2006 in cooperation with a net of primary care providers in Nuremberg and a study center in Nuremberg. The SSRI sertraline showed superiority to placebo only in secondary analyses. The outcome of the CBT group was better than that of the unspecific support control group, but not better than that of the pill-placebo group. This superiority of CBT compared to unspecific support explained by negative unspecific effects (nocebo) of the latter. The outcome of the unspecific support group was also worse than that of the pill-placebo group. Patients who could freely chose their treatment (SSRI or CBT) did not differ in outcome from those who were randomized to their treatment.

15.20 Research group on Social Science in Psychiatry

Head: Anne-Maria Möller-Leimkühler

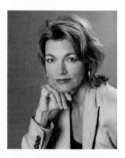

The Department of Psychiatry of the LMU is one of the few university hospitals in Germany where research on social science is performed, even though the research group is very small. The spectrum of the mainly biomedical dominated research domains is thereby specifically broadened and corresponds to modern concepts of mental health and illness.

Social science in psychiatry is related to Medical Sociology dealing with multiple social determinants of illnesses on different levels. Research was started in 1998. Main research fields are family burden and gender studies. In addition, patient satisfaction has also been a topic for research.

Patient satisfaction

In the context of quality assurance, patients´ satisfaction with treatment has gained much attention. However, when it is defined as consumer satisfaction, its validity as an indicator of quality of care has to be questioned because of numerous conceptual and methodological issues. In order to respond to these issues, the Munich Patient Satisfaction Scale (MPSS-24) was developed for psychiatric inpatients. The scale was validated on the basis of three independent samples, and the effects of moderating variables were controlled. In several steps of item selection, the initial pool of 133 items was reduced to 24. Psychometric properties were satisfactory. The MPSS-24 demonstrates one major principal component which indicates that doctor-patient communication is the essential source for satisfaction and dissatisfaction. The instrument is highly practicable for routine use, and has been adopted in several surveys on patient satisfaction (data not yet published).

In continuation of this work, another questionnaire has been developed for treatment evaluation of psychosomatic inpatients. It is currently under evaluation.

Family burden

Facing the increased responsibilities of the relatives of psychiatric patients due to deinstitutionalization, there is a growing need to better understand relatives´ burden within the course of illness; firstly because of their own health risk, and secondly because of their influence on the patients´ course of illness. While in past decades, the family of psychiatric patients had been perceived as a major cause of illness, it is now valued as the patients´ major source of social support. However, the burden experienced by the family has been neglected for a long time and only has been more systematically recently.

In order to identify family burden and its determinants a prospective 5-year follow-up study has been started with caregivers of first time hospitalized patients with schizophrenia and depression. Quantivative and qualitative methods were used for gaining comprehensive access to the relatives´ psychosocial context. The study was based on a transactional stress model including different dimensions of stress outcome, which were assumed to be the interactional product of the patients´ characteristics on one hand, and dispositions and resources of the relatives on the other, such as expressed emotion, coping strategies, perceived control, personality factors and life stressors not related to the illness. This design was also used in a cross-sectional survey of caregivers from a family support organization who had been predominantly caring for chronically ill family members.

Overall, findings show that relatives experience considerable objective and subjective burden including significantly elevated self-rated symptoms compared to norm values. Within the 2-year follow up period of the prospective study, objective and subjective burden decreased, but well-being did not improve. As expected, the burden was more strongly effected by the relatives´ own resources (in particular expressed emotion, neuroticism, negative coping strategies and life stressors) than by the patients´ psychopathology.

Findings support the transactional character of the stress process in caring for a patient with a severe mental disease. This will be documented more specifically by the qualitative analysis within the prospective study. The multidimensional methodology of this approach allows to identify the most important predictors of family burden in order to improve present family intervention strategies.

Gender studies

Gender studies are of emerging importance in medicine and psychiatry. Consistent gender differences are being observed in a broad range of somatic and psychiatric disorders, and it can be assumed that these differences are due to methodological, biological, psychological and social factors acting and interacting differently in men and women. In particular, evidence suggests that stress generated from gender-related social roles and gender-related stress response may play a dominant role in disease development, e.g. depression and alcohol dependence. Some reviews have been published by Möller-Leimkühler concerning socioeconomic status and gender, gender-related help-seeking behaviour, the gender-gap in suicide and premature death, gender role and mental disorders, and gender differences in cardiovascular disease and comorbid depression.

In several empirical studies, one aspect of the gender role has been studied in more detail: gender role orientation which is defined as the self-concept of being male or female with respect to instrumentality/masculinity and expressiveness/femininity.

▬ The dramatic change of the traditional female role, including gender role orientation, has been associated with changes in illness rates, e.g. increasing rates of alcohol dependence in women. In two studies with inpatients suffering from alcohol dependence (one of them with a 6-months follow-up), the question was analyzed whether alcohol dependence was related to higher levels of instrumentality/ masculinity in women. Findings of both studies did not support this hypothesis, but indicate that significantly lower levels of instrumentality/masculinity could be observed in female compared to male patients and norm values. Additionally, low instrumentality was associated with low scores in personal resources. Results give evidence to femininity being a risk factor for alcohol dependence and poor psychosocial resources in women under the condition of extended gender role options, and are in line with earlier findings on femininity. As gender role orientation is modifiable, further prospective studies will be needed to clarify the causal relationship between gender role orientation and alcohol dependence.

▬ A couple of studies have been conducted focussing on depression in men. These studies aim to contribute to further validating the concept of 'male depression' from a gender role perspective. It is assumed that men may mask depressive symptoms with typical male stress response patterns (e.g. risk taking behaviour) to protect their feelings of masculinity. As externalizing male coping strategies are not included in common depression inventories, the concept of 'male depression' may possibly explain lower diagnostic and treatment rates for depression in men, as well as their higher suicide rates.

In a community sample of male adolescents, well-being, depressive and distress symptoms, gender role orientation and help-seeking were assessed. The young men's general well-being was rather reduced, and 22% of them were seen to be at risk for male depression when typical male distress symptoms (e.g. irritability, aggressiveness, overconsumption of alcohol) were detected. There was no evidence that male adolescents are marking their depressive symptoms with typical male distress symptoms, however, a subgroup of 38% of those at risk for depression could be identified who reported significantly elevated male distress symptoms.

With respect to gender role orientation, the risk of 'male depression' was especially pronounced in males with low scores on instrumentality/masculinity, but high scores on 'negative' masculinity (e.g. arrogance, cynism, hostility). Nearly half of those at risk denied their emotional problems.

Further populations investigated with similar methods, include a large sample of male and female students, and a sample of outpatients with minor depression.

Future research activities will be aimed at deepening the previously attained findings in the two central research fields by focussing more on integrative biopsychosocial models on stress response.

15.21 Research group on the history of psychiatry

Heads: Hanns Hippius, Norbert Müller

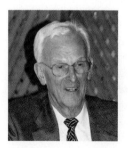

Former scientific member: Gabriele Neundörfer-Kohl

Documentation exists on all patients admitted to the clinic as of its opening in 1904. Barring this extensive archive of material, until K. Kolle joined the clinic in 1952 it remained more or less a matter of chance which material was kept at the clinic. Kolle instructed his secretary, Alma Kreuter

(1906–2005), who had been working at the clinic since 1924, to file and order the records, correspondence, certificates, photographs and other articles. This constituted the ground work for the publication of Kolle's three volumes of biographies on 61 »Great Psychiatrists and Neurologists« (Vol. I–III, 1956–1963). Following Kolle's retirement in 1966, Alma Kreuter processed the documents at her disposal and continued the task even after her retirement in 1970. The result of this work is the comprehensive, three-volume »Biographical, Bibliographical Lexicon of German-Speaking Neurologists and Psychiatrists«, published in 1996.

Among the documents stored in the clinic, was the unedited, typewritten manuscript by Emil Kraepelin, »Memoirs«. Originally, Kraepelin had intended the manuscript only for his family. However, it was possible to persuade Kraepelin's last living daughter (Eva Duerr, née Kraepelin) to give her permission for publication shortly before her death in 1983 (German version from 1983; English translation in 1987; Japanese translation in 2007).

Kolle's collection of biographies was continued by H. Hippius (together with H. Schliack and B. Holdorff) in »Nervenärzte«; Vol. 1: 1998, Vol. 2: 2006. Also, in 2007 a monography on Bernhard von Gudden was published.

In 1997 a psychiatry-historical study group was formed (H. Hippius, N. Müller, G. Neundörfer-Kohl) to process the historical clinic documents. On the occasion of the celebratory opening of the restored, old part of the clinic (the Emil Kraepelin building) in 1998, a museum on the history of psychiatry was opened in Alois Alzheimer's former microscopy hall. Documents, letters, certificates, photographs, historical microscopes and other collectable items are exhibited in eleven glass cabinets. G. Neundörfer-Kohl prepared a catalogue of the exhibition in the museum.

One special exhibit in the Alzheimer cabinet of the museum are the historical documents and materials on the case of Johann F (► Chapter 7). This case was the center of attention, in particular with respect to the theoretical aspects, in Alzheimer's publication in 1911 about Alzheimer's disease. On discovery of Johann F's case history, the Neuropathological Institute of the LMU (Professor Dr. P. Mehraein, PD Dr. M. Graeber) was able to connect history with modern neurobiological research and confirmed Alzheimer's findings, using molecular biological analysis methods on still existing histological brain sections.

Another important topic of the study group was the change from the diagnosis »dementia praecox« to »schizophrenia« only a few months after the retirement of Emil Kraepelin. Moreover, the role of O. Bumke, important members of his medical team and hospital staff in general during the Third Reich and especially during the action T4, is also a subject of the study group's work.

15.22   Teaching

Head: Heinz Grunze

Since 1999 major changes have occurred in the teaching of psychiatry. Until the end of the 1990s, 450 medical students per year were trained, mostly by the senior faculty of the department. The traditional psychiatry curriculum stretched across several semesters and was divided into an introductory course, plenary lectures, hand-on seminars and special lectures for advanced students. With the amendment of the regulations for medical licensure, the previous discipline-specific education was discontinued; a consequence was the integration of psychiatry into a longitudinal course spanning across the whole medical study curriculum as well as into an interdisciplinary course running over one semester. In addition, the new medical licensing regulations gave much more weight to interactive small groups and bedside teaching limiting the amount of plenary lectures.

Since the mid-1990s in preparation of this amendment, the medical faculty of the LMU introduced the so-called »Harvard-Courses«, developed in close cooperation with the Harvard Medical School. In these courses, teachers and students became familiar with the 'new pathway' of teaching with a 4-week intensive course integrated in the traditional study curriculum. Between the winter semester 1999 until the winter semester 2004/2005, the so-called »NerV-Kursus« (»Nervensystem und Verhalten«, Nervous system and behaviour) combined selected topics of psychiatry, neurology, child- and adolescent psychiatry, medical psychology, developmental neurology, pharmacology, and ophthalmology in common tutorials, labs and bedsides. The overall concept was to introduce problem-oriented and evidence-based learning instead of comprehensive accumulation of facts. This »NerV-Kursus« was the germ cell from which – starting in the summer of 2005 – psychiatry became involved in the new study curriculum, the so-called »MECUM« (»Medical Curriculum of the University of Munich«, »Medizinisches Curriculum der Universität München«). The main part of teaching in psychiatry is now taking place in the 5th clinical semester, integrated into a course lasting for one semester, the so-called »Module 4«. This interdisciplinary »Module 4« unites psychiatry, neurology, psychosomatics, ophthalmology, dermatology, pharmacology, and otorinolaryngology. Elements of this course are – besides a daily plenary lecture – seminars, tutorials and bedside teaching in small groups. Because nowadays more than 500 students per year are taught in staff-intensive small groups, a more intensive recruitment of all resources of the department is needed nowadays compared to previous times. This means that teaching is not only a responsibility of senior faculty members now but a daily task for the whole medical staff of the department.

Psychiatry as a discipline has also been integrated into another track of the MECUM. As part of the longitudinal course accompanying the students throughout their whole studies, students receive a crash course on the basics of a psychiatric interview, including taking history and psychopathological examination at an early stage. Students with a special interest in psychiatry also have the opportunity to deepen their knowledge in a one-week intensive course as part of the so-called »Module 5« towards the end of their studies. In addition, and in the same way it was at the time of the traditional medical study curriculum, a multitude of special lectures and seminars of different specialist groups within the department are still offered on a voluntary basis.

In summary, during the last 10 years not only the way of teaching psychiatry changed considerably but also, as a consequence, the capacity utilisation of the department with all its doctors now intensively involved in teaching.

Scientific publications since 2000

Only papers with an impact factor > 2 are listed, apart from a few exceptions

2000

Akiskal HS, Bourgeois M, Angst J, Post R, Möller HJ, Hirschfeld RM (2000) Re-evaluating the prevalence of and diagnistic composition within the broad clinical sprectrum of bipolar disorders. J Aff Disord 59 (Suppl 1):5-30

Akiyama H, Barger S, Barnum S, Bradt B, Bauer J, Cole GM, Cooper NR, Eikelenboom P, Emmerling M, Fiebich BL, Finch CE, Frautschy S, Griffin WST, Hampel H, Hull M, Landreth G, Lue L-F, Mrak R, Mackenzie IR, O'Banion MK, Pachter J, Pasinetti G, Plata-Salaman C, Rogers J, Rydel R, Shen Y, Streit W, Strohmeyer R, Tooyoma I, Van Muiswinkel FL, Veerhuis R, Walker D, Webster S, Wegrzyniak B, Wenk G, Wyss-Coray A (2000) Proceedings of the Neuroinflammation Working Group. Inflammation and Alzheimer's disease. Neurobiol Aging 21:383-421

Amann B, Hummel B, Rall-Autenrieth H, Walden J, Grunze H (2000) Bupropion-induced isolated impairement of sensory trigeminal nerve function. Int Clin psychopharmacol 15:115-116

Averback P, Kahle P, Teipel SJ, Hampel H, Murphy GM Jr (2000) Combined assessment of tau and neuronal thread protein in Alzheimer's disease CSF. Neurology 55:1068-1069

Bondy B, Erfurth A, de Jong S, Krüger M, Meyer H (2000) Possible association of the short allele of the serotonin transporter promoter gene polymorphism (5-HTTLPR) with violent suicide. Mol Psychiatry 5:193-195

Bondy B, Kuznik J, Baghai T, Schüle C, Zwanzger P, Minov C, de Jonge S, Rupprecht R, Meyer H, Eisenmenger W, Ackenheil M (2000) Lack of association of serotonin 2A receptor (5HT2A) gene polymorphism with suicidal ideation and suicide. Am J Med Genet 96:831-835

Bottlender R, Rudolf D, Strauss A, Möller HJ (2000) Are low basal serum levels of the thyroid stimulating hormone (b-TSH) a risk factor for switches into states of expansive syndromes (known in German as »maniform syndromes«) in bipolar I depression? Pharmacopsychiatry 33:75-77

Bottlender R, Strauss A, Möller HJ (2000) Impact of duration of symptoms prior to first hospitalization on acute outcome in 998 schizophrenic patients. Schizophr Res 44:145-150

Bowden CL, Lecrubier Y, Bauer M, Goodwin G, Greil W, Sachs G, von Knorring L (2000) Maintenance therapies for classic and other forms of bipolar disorder. J Affect Disord 59 (Suppl 1): S57-S67

Gallinat J, Boetsch T, Padberg F, Hampel H, Herrmann WM, Hegerl U (2000) Is the EEG helpful in diagnosing and monitoring lithium intoxication? A case report and review of the literature. Pharmacopsychiatry 33:169-173

Gallinat J, Bottlender R, Juckel G, Munke-Puchner A, Stotz G, Kuss HJ, Mavrogiorgou P, Hegerl U (2000) The loudness depemdemcy of the acute SSRI response in depression. Psychopharmacology 148:404-411

Göbels N, Soyka M (2000) Dementia associated with vitamin B12 deficiency: presentation of two cases and review of the literature. J Neuropsychiatry Clin Neurosci 12:389-394

Greene R, Bergeron R, McCarley R, Coyie JT, Grunze H (2000) Short-term and long-term effects of N- methyl-D-aspartate receptor hypofunction. Arch Gen Psychiatry 57:1180-1181

Grunze H, Schlosser S, Walden J (2000) New perspectives in the acute treatment of bipolar depression. World J Biol Psychiatry. 1:129-13

Halmi K, Sunday S, Strober M, Kaplan A, Woodside B, Fichter MM, Treasure J, Berrettini W, Kaye W (2000) Perfectionism in anorexia nervosa: variation by clinical subtype, obsessionality, and pathological behavior. Am J Psychiatry 157:1799-1805

Herrmann B, Landgraf R, Keck ME, Wigger A, Morrow AL, Strohle A, Holsboer F, Rupprecht R (2000) Pharmacological characterisation of cortical gamma-aminobutyric acid type A (GABAA) receptors in two Wistar rat lines selectively bred for high and low anxiety-related behaviour. World J Biol Psychaitry 1:137-143

Juckel G, Hegerl U, Mavrogiorgou P, Gallinat J, Mager T, Tigges P, Dresel S, Schroter A, Stotz G, Meller I, Greil W, Möller HJ (2000) Clinical and biological findings in a case with 48-hour bipolar ultrarapid cycling before and during valproate treatment. J Clin psychiatry 61:585-593

Kahle PJ, Jakowec M, Teipel SJ, Hampel H, Petzinger GM, di Monte DA, Silverberg GD, Möller HJ, Yesavage JA, Tinklenberg JR, Shooter EM, Murphy GM (2000) Combined assessment of tau and neuronal threas protein in Alzheimer's disease CSF. Neurology 54:1498-1503

Kaye WH, Lilenfeld LR, Berrettini WH, Strober M, Devlin B, Klump KL, Goldman D, Bulik CM, Halmi KA, Fichter MM, Kaplan A, Woodside DB, Treasure J, Plotnicov KH, Pollice C, Rao R, McConaha CW (2000) A Search for Susceptibility Loci in Anorexia Nervosa: Methods and Sample Description. Biol Psychiatry 47:794-803

Keck ME, Engelmann M, Müller MB, Henniger MS, Hermann B, Rupprecht R, Neumann ID, Toschi N, Landgraf R, Post A (2000) Repititive transcranial magnetic stimulation induced active coping strategies and atttenuates the neuroendocrine stress response in rats. J Psychiatr Res 34:265-276

Kleindienst N, Greil W (2000) Differential efficacy of lithium and carbamazepine in the prophylaxis of bipolar disorder: results of the MAP study. Neuropsychobiology 42 (Suppl 1):2-10

Kohnken R, Buerger K, Zinkowski R, Miller C, Kerkman D, de Bernadis J, Shen J, Möller HJ, Davies P, Hampel H (2000) Detection of tau phosphorylated at threonine 231 in cerebrospinal fluid of Alzheimer's disease patients. Neurosci Lett 287:187-190

Laakmann G, Schüle C, Baghai T, Waldvogel E, Bidlingmaier M, Strasburger C (2000) Mirtazapine: An inhibitor of cortisol secretion that does not influence growth hormone and prolactin secretion. J Clin Psychopharmacol 20:101-103

Langosch JM, Zhou XY, Frick A, Grunze H, Weiden J (2000) Effects of lamotrigine on field potentials and long-term potentiation in guinea pig hippocampal slices. Epilepsie 41:1102-1106

Maurer I, Zierz S, Möller HJ (2000) A selective defect of cytochrome c oxidase is present in brain of Alzheimer disease patients. Neurobiol Aging 21:455-462

Meisenzahl EM, Dresel S, Frodl T, Schmitt GJE, Preuss UW, Rossmüller B, Tatsch K, Mager T, Hahn K, Möller HJ (2000) D2 receptor occupancy under recommended and high doses of olanzapine: an iodine-123-iodobenzamide SPECT study. J Psychopharmacol 14:364-370

Meisenzahl EM, Frodl T, Zetzsche T, Leinsinger G, Heiss D, Maag K, Hegerl U, Hahn K, Möller HJ (2000) Adhesio interthalamica in male patients with schizophrenia. Am J Psychiatry 157:823-825

Möller HJ (2000) Are all antidepressants the same? J Clin Psychiatry 61 (Suppl 6):24-28

Möller HJ (2000) Rating depressed patients: observer- vs self-assessment. Eur Psychiatry 15:160-172

Möller HJ (2000) State of the art of drug treatment of schizophrenia and the future position of the novel/atypical antipsychotics. World J Biol Psychiatry 1:204-214

Möller HJ, Glaser K, Leverkus F, Göbel C (2000) Double-blind, multicenter comparative study of sertraline versus amitriptyline in outpatients with major depression. Pharmacopsychiatry 33:206-212

Möller HJ, Grunze H (2000) Have some guidelines for the treatment of acute bipolar depression gone too far in the restriction of antidepressants? Eur Arch Psychiatry Clin Neurosci 250:57-68

Preuss UW, Koller G, Bahlmann M, soyka M, Bondy B (2000) No association between suicidal behavior and 5-HT2A-T102C polymorphism in alcohol dependents. Am J Med Genet 96:877-878

Rothenhäusler HB, Haberl C, Ehrentraut S, Kapfhammer HP, Weber MM (2000) Suicide attempt by pure citalopram overdose causing long-lasting severe sinus bradycardia, hypotension and syncopes: succesful therapy with a temporary pacemaker. Pharmacopsychiatry 33:150-152

Pukrop R, Möller HJ, Steinmeyer EM (2000) Quality of life in psychiatry: a systematic contribution to construct validation and the development of the integrative assessment tool »modular system for quality of life«. Eur Arch Psychiatry Clin Neurosci 250 (3):120-132

Rief W, Trenkamp S, Auer C, Fichter MM (2000) Cognitive Behavior Therapy in Panic Disorder and Comorbid Major Depression: A Naturalistic Study. Psychother Psychosom 69:70-78

Romeo E, Pompili E. di Michele F, Face M, Rupprecht R, Bernardi G, Pasinib A (2000) Effects of fluoxetine, indomethacine and placebo on 3 alpha, 5 alpha tetrahydroprogesterone (THP) plasma levels in uncomplicated alcohol withdrawal. Worl J Biol Psychaitry 1:101-104

Soyka M (2000) Alcoholism and schizophrenia. Addiction 95:1613-1618

Soyka M (2000) Substance misuse, psychiatric disorder and violent and disturbed behaviour. Br J Psychiatry 176:345-350

Soyka M, Bottlender R, Möller HJ (2000) Epidemiological evidence for a low abuse potential of zolpidem. Pharmacopsychiatry 33:138-141

Soyka M, de Vry J (2000) Flupenthixol as a potential pharmacotreatment of alcohol and cocaine abuse/dependence. Eur Neuropsychopharmacol 10:325-332

Soyka M, Zetzsche T, Dresel S, Tatsch K (2000) FDG-PET and IBMZ-SPECT suggest reduced thalamic activity but no dopaminergic dysfunction in chronic alcohol hallucinosis. J Neuropsychiatry Clin Neurosci 12:287-288

Schäfer M, Boetsch T, Laakmann G (2000) Psychosis in a methadone-substituted patient during interferon-alpha treatment of hepatitis C. Addiction 95:1101-1104

Schelling G, Stoll C, Vogelmeier C, Hummel T, Behr J, Kapfhammer HP, Rothenhäusler HB, Haller M, Durst K, Krausneck T, Briegel J (2000) Pulmonary function and health-related quality of life in a sample of long-term survivors of the acute respiratory distress syndrome. Intensive Care Med 26:1304-1311

Schütz C, Soyka M (2000) Dextromethorphan challenge in alcohol-dependent patients and controls. Arch Gen Psychiatry 57:291-292

Stoll S, Schelling G, Goetz AE, Kilger E, bayer A, Kapfhammer HP, Rothenhäusler HB, Kreuzer E, Reichart B, Peter K (2000) Health-related quality of life and post-traumatic stress disorder in patients after cardiac surgery and intensive care treatment. J Thorac Cardiovasc Surg 120:505-512

Ströhle A, Holboer F, Rupprecht R (2000) Increased ACTH concentrations associated with cholecystokinin tetrapeptide-induced panic attacks in patients with panic disorder. Neuropsychopharmacology 22:251-256

Ströhle A, Pasini A, Romeo E, Hermann B, Spalletta G, di Michele F, Holsboer F, Rupprecht R (2000) Fluoxetine decreases concentrations of 3α, 5α- terahydrodeoxycorticosterone (THDOC) in major depression. J Psychiatric Res 34:183-186

Stübner S, Padberg F, Grohmann R, Hampel H, Hollweg m, Hippius H, Möller HJ, Rüther E (2000) Pisa syndrome (pleurothotonus): report of a multicenter drug safety surveillance project. J Clin Psychiatry 61:569-574

Tigges P, Mergl R, Frodl T; Meisenzahl EM, Galliant, Schröter A, Riedel M, Müller N, Möller HJ, Hegerl U (2000) Digitized analysis of abnormal hand-motor performance in schizophrenic patients. Schizophr Res 45:133-143

Volz HP, Möller HJ, Reimann I, Stoll KD (2000) Opipramol for the treatment of somatoform disorders results from a placebo-controlled trial. Eur Neuropsychopharmacol 10:211-217

Walden J, Schaerer L, Schloesser S, Grunze H (2000) An open longitudinal study of patients with bipolar rapid cycling treated with lithium or lamotrigine for mood stabilization. Bipolar Disord 2:336-339

Zill P, Baghai TC, Zwanzger P, Schüle C, Minov C, Riedel M, Neumeier K, Rupprecht R, Bondy B (2000) Evidence for an association between a G-protein beta3-gene variant with depression and response to antidepressant treatment. Neuroreport 11:1892-1897

Zill P, Bürger K, Behrens S, Hampel H, Padberg F, Boetsch T, Möller HJ, Ackenheil M, Bondy B (2000) Polymorphisms in the α-2 macroglobulin gene in psychogeriatric patients. Neurosci Lett 294:69-72

Zill P, Padberg F, de Jong S, Hampel H, Bürger K, Stübner S, Boetsch T, Möller HJ, Ackenheil M, Bondy B (2000) Serotonin transporter (5-HTT) gene polymorphism in psychogeriatric patients. Neurosci Lett 284:113-115

2001

Baghai TC, Schüle C, Zwanzger P, Minow C, Schwarz MJ, de Jong S, Rupprecht R, Bondy B (2001) Possible influence of the insertation/deletion polymorphism in the angiotensin I-converting enzyme gene on therapeutic outcome in affective disorders. Mol Psychiatry 6:258-259

Biberthaler P, Mussack T, Wiedemann E, Gilg T, Soyka M, Koller G, Pfeifer KJ, Linsenmaier U, Mutschler W, Gippner-Steppert C, Jochum M (2001) Elevated serum levels of S-100B reflect the extent of brain injury in alcohol intoxicated patients after mild head trauma. Shock 16:97-101

Blennow K, Vanmechelen E, Hampel H (2001) CSF total tau, $A\beta_{42}$ and phosphorylated tau protein as biomarkers for Alzheimer's disease. Mol Neurobiol 24:87-97

Cuntz U, Leibbrand R, Ehrig C, Shaw R, Fichter MM (2001) Predictors of post-treatment weight reduction after in-patient behavioural therapy. Int J Obes 25 (Suppl 1):99-101

Dahmen N, Müller MJ, Germeyer S, Rujescu D, Anghelescu I, Hiemke C, Wetzel H (2001) genetic polymorphisms of the dopamine D2 and D3 receptor and neuroleptic drug effects in schizophrenic patients. Schizophr Res 49:223-229

Damianisch K, Rupprecht R, Lancel M (2001) The influence of subchronic administration of the neurosteroid allopregnanolone on sleep in the rat. Neuropsychopharmacology 25:576-584

Du Y, Dodel R, Hampel H, Buerger K, Lin S, Eastwood B, Bales K, Gao F, Möller HJ, Oertel W, Farlow M, Paul S (2001) Reduced levels of amyloid ß-peptide antibody in Alzheimer disease. Neurology 57:801-805

Fichter M, Quadflieg N (2001) The structured interview for anorexic and bulimic disorders for DSMIV and ICD-10 (SIAB-EX): reliability and validity. Eur Psychiatry 16:38-48

Fichter MM, Quadflieg N (2001) Prevalence of mental illness in homeless men in Munich, Germany: Results from a representative sample. Acta Psychiatr Scand 103:94-104

Friess E, Kuempfel T, Winkelmann J, Schmid D, Uhr M, Rupprecht R, Holsboer F, Trenkwalder C (2001) Increased growth hormone response to apomorphine in Parkinson disease compared with multiple system atrophy. Arch Neurol 58:241-246

Frodl T, Meisenzahl EM, Müller D, Greiner J, Juckel G, Leinsinger G, Hahn H, Möller HJ, Hegerls U. (2001) Corpus callosum and P300 in schizophrenia. Schizophr Res 49:107-120

Frodl T, Meisenzahl EM, Müller D, Leinsinger G, Juckel G, Hahn K, Möller HJ, Hegerl U (2001) The effect of the skull on event-related P300. Clin Neurophysiol 112:1773-1776

Galliant J, Riedel M, Juckel G, Sokullu S, Frodl T, Moukhtieva R, Mavrogiorgou P, Nissle S, Müller N, Danker-Hopfe H, Hegerl U (2001) P300 and symptom improvement in schizophrenia. Psychopharmacology 158:55-65

Greil W, Horvath A, Sassim N, Erazo N, Grohmann R (2001) Disinhibition of libido: an adverse affect of SSRI? J Affect Disord 62:225-228

Grunze H, Normann C, Langosch J, Schaefer M, Amann B, Sterr A, Schloesser S, Kleindienst N, Weiden J (2001) Antimanic efficacy of topiramate in 11 patients in an open trial with an on-off-on design. Clin Psychiatry 62:464-468

Hampel H, Bürger K, Kohnken R, Teipel SJ, Zinkowski R, Möller HJ, Rapoport SI, Davies P (2001) Tracking of Alzheimer's disease progression with cerebrospinal fluid tau protein phosphorylated at threonine 231. Ann Neurol 49:545-546

Hampel H, Kötter HU, Padberg F, Berger C (2001) Severe Hirsutism associated with psychopharmacological treatment in major depression. World J Biol Psychiatry 2:48-49

Hartmann A, Rujescu D, Giannakouros T, Nikolakaki E, Gödert M, Mandelkow EM, Gao QS, Andreadis A, Stamm S (2001) Regulation of alternative splicing of human tau exon 10 by phosphorylation of splicing factors. Mol Cell Neurosci 18:80-90

Henkel V, Mergl R, Juckel G, Rujescu P, Mavrogiorgou P, Giegling I, Möller HJ, Hegerl U (2001) Assessment of handedness using a digitalizing tablet: a new method. Neuropsychologia 39:1158-1166

Hermann B, Vollmer I, Holsboer F, Rupprecht R (2001) Antidepressants do not modulate estrogen receptor alpha-mediated gene expression. J Neural Transm 108:1197-1202

Herwig U, Padberg F, Unger J, Spitzer M, Schönfeldt-Lecuona C (2001) Transcranial magnetic stimulation in therapy studies: examination of the reliability of »standard« coil positioning by neuronavigation. Biol Psychiatry 42:58-62

Hiller W, Cuntz U, Rief W, Fichter M (2001) Searching for a gastrointestinal subgroup within the somatoform disorders. Original Research Reports. Psychosomatics 42:14-20

Itoh N, Arai H, Urakami K, Ishiguro K, Ohno H, Hampel H, Bürger K, Wiltfang J, Otto M, Kretzschmar H, Möller HJ, Imagawa M, Kohno H, Nakashima K, Kuzuhara S, Sasaki H, Imahori K (2001) A large-scale, multi-centre study of cerebrospinal fluid tau protein phosphorylated at serine 199 for the antemortem diagnosis of Alzheimer's disease. Ann Neurol 50:150-156

Kojima T, Matsushima E, Ohta K, Toru M, Han YH, Shen YC, Moussaoui D, David I, Sato K, Yamashita I, Kathmann N, Hippius H, Thavundayil JX, Lal S, Nair V, Potkin SG, Prilipko L (2001) Stability of exploratory eye movements as a marker of schizophrenia – a WHO multi-centre study. Schizophr Res 52:203-213

Lilenfeld R, Devlin B, Kaye W H, Bulik C, Strober M, Berrettini W, Fichter MM, Goldman D, Halmi K, Kaplan A, Woodside DB, Treasure J (2001) Deriving behavioural phenotypes in an international, multi-centre study of eating disorders. Psychol Med 31:635-645

Lue LF, Rydel R, Brigham EF, Yang lB, Hampel H, Murphy GM, Brachova L, Yan SD, Walker DG, Shen Y, Rogers J (2001) Inflammatory repertoire of Alzheimer's disease and nondemented elderly microglia in vitro. GLIA 35:72-79

Maurer I, Zierz S, Möller HJ (2001) Evidence for am mitochondrial oxidative phosphorylation defect in brains from patients with schizophrenia. Schizophr Res 48:125-136

Meisenzahl EM, Rujescu D, Kirner A, Giegling I, Kathmann N, Leinsinger G, Maag K, Hegerl U, Hahn K, Möller HJ (2001) Association of an interleukin 1ß genetic polymorphism with altered brain structure in patients with schizophrenia. Am J Psychiatry 158:1316-1318

Minov C, Baghai TC, Schüle C, Zwanzger P, Schwarz MJ, Zill P, Rupprecht R, Bondy B (2001) Serotonin-2A-receptor and –transporter polymorphisms: lack of association in patients with major depression. Neurosci Lett 303:119-122

Möller HJ (2001) Amisulpride: efficacy in the management of chronic patients with predominant negative symptoms of schizophrenia . Eur Arch Psychiatry Clin Neurosci 251:217-224

Möller HJ (2001) Are atypicals better than antipsychotics in long-term schizophrenia? Eur Neuropsychopharmacol 11 (Suppl 3):S119-S120

Möller HJ (2001) Methodological issues in psychiatry: psychiatry as an empirical science. World J Biol Psychiatry 2:38-47

Möller HJ (2001) Past, present and future of biological psychiatry. World J Biol Psychiatry 2:156-158

Möller HJ, Bottlender R, Grunze H, Strauss A, Wittmann J (2001) Are antidepressants less effective in the acute treatment of bipolar 1 compared to unipolar depression? J Affect Disord 67:141-146

Möller HJ, Volz HP, Reimann IW, Stoll KD (2001) Opipramol for the treatment of generalized anxiety disorder: a placebo-controlled trial including an alprazolam-treated group. J Clin Psychiatry 21:59-65

Mulert C, Galliant J, Pascual-Marqui R, Dorn H, Frick K, Schlattmann P, Mientus S, Herrmann WM, Winterer G (2001) Neuroimage 13:589-600

Niesler B, Weiss B, Fischer C, Nöthen MM, Propping P, Bondy B, Rietschel M, Maier W, Albus M, Franzek E, Rappold GA (2001) Serotonin receptor gene HTR3A variants in schizophrenic and bipolar affective patients. Pharmacogenetics 11:21-27

Otto B, Cuntz U, Frühauf E, Wawarta R, Folwaczny C, Riepl RL, Heiman ML, Lehnert P, Fichter M, Tschöp M (2001) Weight gain decrease elevated plasma ghrelin concentrations of patients with anorexia nervosa. Eur J Endocrinol 145: 669-673

Padberg F, Haase CG, Feneberg W, Schwarz MJ, Hampel H (2001) No association between anti-myelin oligodendocyte glycoprotein antibodies and serum/cerebrospinal fluid levels of the soluble interleukin-6 receptor complex in multiple sclerosis. Neurosci Lett 305:13-16

Parnetti L, Lunari A, Amici S, Gallai V, Vanmechelen E, Hulstaert F (2001) CSF phosphorylated tau is a possible marker for discriminating Alzheimer's disease from dementia with Lewy bodies. Neuroschience 22:77-78

Pedrosa F, Grohmann R, Rüther E.(2001) Asymptomatic bradycardia associated with amisulpride. Pharmacopsychiatry 34:259-261

Pitschel-Walz G, Leucht S, Bäuml J, Kissling W, Engel RR (2001) The effect of family interventions on relapse and rehospitalisation in schizophrenia. Schizophr Bull 27:73-92

Post RM, Nolen WA, Kupka RW, Denicoff KD, Leverich GS, Keck PE, McElroy SL, Rush AJ, Suppes T, Altshuler LL, Frye MA, Grunze H, Weiden J (2001) The Stanley Foundation Bipolar Network I. Rationale and methods. Br J Psychiatry 41:169-176

Preuss UW, Koller G, Soyka M, Bondy B (2001) Association between suicide attempts and 5-HT-TLPR-S-Allele in alcohol dependent and control subjects: further evidence from a German alcohol dependent inpatient sample. Biol Psychiatry 50:636-639

Rammes G, Rupprecht R, Ferrari U, Zieglgansberger W, Parsons CG (2001) The N.methyl-D-aspartate receptor channel blockers memantine, MRZ 2/579 and other amino-alkyl-cyclohexanes antagonise 5-HT(3) receptor currents in cultured HEK-293 and N1E-115 cell systems in a non-competitive manner. Neurosci Lett 306:81-84

Rothenhäusler HB, Ehrentraut S, Kapfhammer HP (2001) Changes in patterns of psychiatric referral in a german general hospital: results of a comparison of two 1-year surveys 8 years apart. Gen Hosp Psychiatry 23:205-214

Rothenhäusler HB, Ehrentraut S, Stoll C, Schelling G, Kapfhammer HP (2001) The relationship between cognitive performance and employment and health status in long-term survivors of the acute respiratory distress syndrome: results of an exploratory study. Gen Hosp Psychiatry 23:90-96

Rupprecht R, Holsboer F (2001) Neuroactive steroids in neuropsychopharmacology. Int Rev Neurobiol 46:461-477

Rupprecht R, di Michele F, Hermann B, Ströhle A, Lancel M Romeo E, Holsboer F (2001) Neuroactive steroids: molecular mechanisms of action and implications for neuropsychopharmacology. Brain Res Brain Res Rev 37:59-67

Soyka M (2001) Antipsychotic treatment of schizophrenics at risk for violence. Pharmacopsychiatry 34:43-44

Schäfer M, Rujescu D, Giegling I, Guntermen A, Erfurth A, Bondy B, Möller HJ (2001) Association of short-term response to haloperidol treatment with polymorphism in the dopamine D2 receptor gene. Am J Psychiatry 158:802-804

Schelling G, Briegel J, Roozendaal B, Stoll C, Rothenhäusler HB, Kapfhammer HP (2001) The effect of stress doses of hydrocortisone during septic shock on posttraumatic stress disorder. Biol Psychiatry 50:978-985

Schüle C, Baghai T, Zwanzger P, Minow C, Padberg F, Rupprecht R (2001) Sleep deprivation and hypothalamic-pituitary-adrenal (HPA) axis activity in depressed patients. J Psychiatry Res 35:239-247

Schüle C, Baghai T, Zwanzger P, Rupprecht R (2001) Attenuation of HPA axis hyperactivity and simultaneous clinical deterioration in a depressed patient treated with mirtazapine. World J Biol Psychiatry 2:103-105

Zwanzger P, Baghai T, Boerner RJ, Möller HJ, Rupprecht R (2001) Anxiolytic effects of vigabatrin in panic disorder. J Clin Psychopharmacol 21:539-540

Zwanzger P, Baghai T, Schüle C, Minov C, Padberg F, Möller HJ, Rupprecht R (2001) Tiagabine improves panic and agoraphobia in panic disorder patients. J Clin Psychiatry 62:656-657

Zwanzger P, Baghai T, Schuele C, Ströhle A, Padberg F, Kathmann N, Schwarz M, Möller HJ, Rupprecht R (2001) Vigabatrin decreases cholecystokinin-tetrapeptide (CCK-4) induced panic in health volunteers. Neuropsychopharmacology 25:699-703

2002

Baghai TC, Schüle C, Zwanzger P , Minov C, Holme C, Padberg F, Bidlingmaier M, Strasburger CJ, Rupprecht R (2002) Evaluation of a salivary based combined dexamethasone/CRH test in patients with major depression. Psychoneuroendocrinology 27:385-399

Baghai TC, Schüle C, Zwanzger P , Minov C, Zill P, Ella R, Eser D, Oezer S, Bondy B, Rupprecht R (2002) Hypothalamic-pituitary-adrenocortical axis dysregulation in patients with major depression is influenced by the insertion/deletion polymorphism in the angiotensin I-converting enzyme gene. Neurosci Lett 328:299-303

Bauer M, Whybrow PC, Angst J, Versiani M, Möller HJ, WFSBP Task Force on Treatment Guidelines for Unipolar Depressive Disorders (2002) World Federation of Societies of Biological Psychiatry (WFSBP) guidelines for biological treatment of unipolar depressive disorders, Part 2; Maintenance treatment of major depressive disorder and treatment of chronic depressive disorders and subthreshold depressions. World J Biol Psychiatry 3:69-86

Bauer M, Whybrow PC, Angst J, Versiani M, Möller HJ, WFSBP Task Force on Treatment Guidelines for Unipolar Depressive Disorders (2002) World Federation of Societies of Biological Psychiatry (WFSBP) guidelines for biological treatment of unipolar depressive disorders, Part 1: Acute and continuation treatment of major depressive disorder. World J Biol Psychiatry 3:5-43

Bondy B, Baghai TC, Zill P, Bottlender R, Jäger M, Minov C, Schüle C, Zwanzger P, Rupprecht R, Engel RR (2002) Combined action of the ACE D- and G-protein beta3 T-allel in major depression: a possible link to cardiovascular disease? Mol Psychiatry 7:1120-1126

Bokde ALW, Teipel SJ, Zebuhr Y, Leinsinger G, Gootjes L, Schwarz R, Buerger K, Scheltens P, Möller HJ, Hampel H (2002) A new rapid landmark-based regional MRI segmentation method of the brain. J Neuroll Sci 194:35-40

Bottlender R, Rudolf D, Jäger M, Strauss A, Möller HJ (2002) The impact of duration of untreated psychosis and premorbid functioning on outcome of first inpatient treatment in schizophrenic and schizoaffective patients. Eur Arch Psychiatry Clin Neurosci 252:226-231

Buerger K, Teipel SJ, Zinkowski R, Blennow K, Arai H, Engel R, Hofmann-Kiefer K, McCulloch C, Ptok U, Heun R, Andreasen N, DeBernardis J, Kerkman D, Möller HJ, Davies P, Hampel H (2002) CSF tau protein phosphorylated at threonine 231 correlates with cognitive decline in MCI subjects. Neurology 59:627-629

Buerger K, Zinkowski R, Teipel SJ, Tapiola T, Arai H, Blennow K, Andreasen N, Hofmann-Kiefer K, DeBernardis J, Kerkman D, McCulloch C, Kohnken R, Padberg F, Pirttila T, Schapiro MB, Rapoport SI, Möller HJ, Davies P, Hampel H (2002) Differential diagnosis of Alzheimer's disease with cerebrospinal fluid levels of tau protein phosphorylated at threonine 231. Arch Neurology 59:1267-1272

Carta MG, Hardoy MC, Grunze H, Carpiniello B (2002) The use of tiagabine in affective disorders. Pharmacopsychiatry 35:33-34

Chiang SS, Schütz CG, Soyka M (2002) Effects of irritability on carving before and after cue exposure in abstinent alcoholic inpatients: experimental data subjective response and heart rate. Neuropsychobiology 46:150-160

Devlin B, Bacanu SA, Klump KL, Bulik CM, Fichter MM, Halmi KA, Kaplan AS, Strober M, Treasure J, Woodside DB, Berrettini WH, Kaye WH (2002) Linkage analysis of anorexia nervosa incorporating behavioural covariates. Hum Mol Genet 11:689-696

Dittmann S, Biedermann NC, Grunze H, Hummel B, Scharer LO, Kleindienst N, Forsthoff A, Matzner N, Walser S, Walden J (2002) The Stanley Foundation Bipolar Network: results of the naturalistic follow-up study after 2.5 years of follow-up in German centres. Neuropsychobiology 46 (Suppl1):2-9

Dodel R, Hampel H, Depboylu C, Lin S, Gao F, Schock S, Jäckel S, Wei X, Buerger K, Höft C, Hemmer B, Möller HJ, Farlow M, Oertel WH, Sommer N, Du Y (2002) Human antibodies against amyloid β-peptide: a potential treatment for Alzheimer's disease. Ann Neurol 52:25325-6

Ella R, Zwanzger P, Stampfer R, Preuss UW, Müller-Sicheneder F, Möller HJ, Padberg F (2002) Switch to mania after slow rTMS of the right prefrontal cortex. J Clin Psychiatry 63:249

Frodl T, Hampel H, Juckel G, Bürger K, Padberg F, Engel RR, Möller HJ, Hegerl U (2002) Value of event related P300 subcomponents in the clinical diagnosis of mild cognitive impairment and Alzheimer's disease. Psychophysiology 39:175-181

Frodl T, Meisenzahl EM, Müller D, Holder J, Juckel G, Möller HJ, Hegerl U (2002) P300 subcomponents and clinical symptoms in schizophrenia. Int J Psychophysiol 43:237-246

Frodl T, Meisenzahl EM, Zetzsche T, Born C, Groll C, Jäger M, Leinsinger G, Bottlender R, Hahn K, Möller HJ (2002) Hippocampal changes in patients with first episode of major depression. Am J Psychiatry 159:1112-1118

Frodl T, Meisenzahl EM, Zetzsche T, Bottlender R, Born C, Groll C, Jäger M, Leinsinger G, Hahn K, Möller HJ (2002) Enlargement of the amygdala in patients with first episode of major depression. Biol Psychiatry 51:708-714

Gao F, Bales K, Dodel R, Chen XM, Liu JY, Hampel H, Farlow M, Paul SM, Du Y (2002) NF-kappa-b mediates IL-1beta-induced synthesis/release of alpha-2-macroglobulin in human glial cell line. Brain Res Mol Brain Res 105:108-114

Gastpar M, Bonnet U, Boning J, Mann K, Schmidt LG, Soyka M, Wetterling T, Kielstein V, Labriola D, Croop R (2002) Lack of efficacy of naltrexone in the prevention of alcohol relapse: results from a German multicenter study. J Clin Psychopharmacol 22:592-598

Grice DE, Halmi KA, Fichter MM, Strober M, Woodside DB, Treasure JT, Kaplan AS, Magistretti PJ, Goldman D, Bulik CM, Kaye WH, Berrettini WH (2002) Evidence for a susceptibility gene for anorexia nervosa on chromosome 1. Am J Hum Genet 70:787-792

Grunze H, Amann B, Dittmann S, Walden J (2002) Clinical relevance and treatment possibilities of bipolar rapid cycling. Neuropsychobiology 45 (Suppl 1):20-26

Grunze H, Marcuse A, Scharer LO, Born C, Walden J (2002) Nefazodone in psychotic unipolar and bipolar depression: a retrospective chart analysis and open prospective study on its efficacy and safety versus combined treatment with amitriptyline and haloperidol. Neuropsychobiology 46 (Suppl 1):31-35

Grunze H, Kasper S, Goodwin G, Bowden C, Baldwin D, Licht R, Vieta E,. Möller HJ (2002) World Federation of Societies of Biological Psychiatry (WFSBP) Guidelines for biological treatment of bipolar disorders. Part 1: Treatment of bipolar depression. World J Biol Psychiatry 3 :115-124

Grunze H, Walden J (2002) Relevance of new and newly rediscovered anticonvulsants for atypical forms of bipolar disorder. J Affect Disord 72 (Suppl 1):S15-S21

Hampel H, Teipel SJ, Alexander GE, Pogarell O, Rapoport SI, Möller HJ (2002) In vivo image of region and cell type specific neocortical neurodegeneration in Alzheimer's disease. Perspectives of MRI derived corpus callosum measurement for mapping disease progression and effects of therapy. Evidence from studies with MRI, EEG and PET. J Neural Transm 109:837-855

Hampel H, Teipel SJ, Bayer W, Alexander GE, Schwarz R, Schapiro MB, Rapoport SI, Möller HJ (2002) Age-transformation of combined hippocampus amygdala volume improves diagnostic accuracy in Alzheimer's disease. J Neuroll Sci 194:15-19

Hapfelmeier G, Haseneder R, Lampadius K, Rammes G, Rupprecht R, Zieglgansberger W (2002) Cloned human and murine serotonin(3A) receptors expressed in human embryonic kidney 293 cells display different single-channel kinetics. Neurosci Lett 335:44-48

Henkel V., Bussfeld P., Möller H.J., Hegerl U. (2002) Cognitive-behavioural theories of helplessness: valid models of depression? Eur Arch Psychiatry Clin Neurosci 252:240-249

Hebebrand J, Fichter M, Gerber G, Görg T, Hermann H, Geller F, Schäfer H, Remschmidt H, Hinney A (2002) Molecular Genetic Evidence for an Association Between Bulimia Nervosa and Obesity: A Mutation Screen of the Melanocortin-4 Receptor Gene in Females with Bulimia Nervosa. Mol Psychiatry 7:647-651

Henkel V, Mergl R, Kohnen R, Maier W, Möller HJ, Hegerl U (2002) Identifying depression in primary care: a comparison of different methods in a prospective cohort study. BMJ 326:200-201

Hiller W, Leibbrand R, Rief W, Fichter MM (2002) Predictors of course and outcome in hypochondriasis after cognitive-behavioural treatment. Psychother Psychosom 71:318-325

Hiller W, Rief W, Fichter MM (2002) Dimensional and categorical approaches to hypochondriasis. Psychol Med 32:707-718

Hirano S, Sato T, Narita T, Kusunoki K, Ozaki N, Rimura S, Takahashi T, Sakado K, Uehara T (2002) Evaluating the state dependency of the temperament and character inventory dimensions in patients with major depression: a methodological contribution. J Affect Disord 69:31-38

Hirschfeld RM, Montgomery SA, Aguglia E, Amore M, Delgado PL, Gastpar M, Hamley C, Kasper S, Linden M, Massana J, Mendlewicz J, Möller HJ, Nemeroff CB, Saiz J, Such P, Torta R, Versiani M (2002) Partial response and non-response to antidepressant therapy: current approaches and treatment options. J Clin Psychiatry 63:826-837

Hummel B, Walden J, Stampfer R, Dittmann S, Amann B, Sterr A, Schaefer M, Frye MA, Grunze H (2002) Acute antimanic efficacy and safety of oxcarbazepine in an open trial with an on-off-on design. Bipolar Disord 4:412-417

Kathmann N, Frodl-Bauch T, Hegerl U (2002) Stability of the mismatch negativity different stimulus and attention conditions. Clin Neurophysiol 110:317-323

Kleindienst N, Greil W (2002) Inter-episodic morbidity and drop-out under carbamazepine and lithium in the maintenance treatment of bipolar disorder. Psychol Med 32:493-501

Koller G, Preuss UW, Bottlender M, Wenzel K, Soyka M (2002) Impulsivity and aggression as predictors of suicide attempts in alcoholics? Eur Arch Psychiatry Clin Neurosci 252:155-160

Leibbrand R, Fichter MM (2002) Maintenance of weight loss after obesity treatment: Is continuous support necessary? Behaviour Research and Therapy 40: 1275-1289

Leucht S, Pitschel-Walz G, Engel RR, Kissling W. (2002) Amisulpride, an unusual »atypical« antipsychotic: a meta-analysis of randomized controlled trials. Am J Psychiatry 159:180-190

Mavrogiorgou P, Juckel G, Frodl T, Galliant J, Hauke W, Zaudig M, Dammann G, Möller HJ, Hegerl U (2002) P300 subcomponents in obsessive-compulsive disorder. J Psychiatr Res 36:399-406

McElroy SL, Frye MA, Suppes T, Dhavale D, Keck PE, Leverich GS, Altshuler L, Denicoff KD, Nolen WA, Kupka R, Grunze H, Walden J, Post RM (2002) Correlates of overweight and obesity in 644 patients with bipolar disorder. J Clin Psychiatry 63:207-213

Meisenzahl EM, Frodl T, Zetzsche T, Leinsinger G, Maag K, Hegerl U, Hahn K, Möller HJ (2002) Investigation of a possible diencephalic pathology in schizophrenia. Psychiatr Res Neuroimaging 115:127-135

Meisenzahl EM, Zetzsche T, Preuss U, Frodl T, Leinsinger G, Möller HJ (2002) Does the definition of borders of the planum temporale influence the results in schizophrenia? Am J Psychiatry 159:1198-200

Möller HJ (2002) Anxiety associated with comorbid depression. J Clin Psychiatry 63 (Suppl 14):22-26

Möller HJ (2002) Appearance of the first WFSBP treatment guidelines. World J Biol Psychiatry 3:2-3

Möller HJ, Bottlender R, Groß A, Hoff P, Wittmann J, Wegner U, Strauss A (2002) The Kraepelinian dichotomy: preliminary results of a 15-year follow-up study on functional psychoses: focus on negative symptoms. Schizophr Res 56:87-94

Möller HJ, Bottlender M, Strauss A, Grunze H (2002) The switch-real threat or overestimated danger? Antidepressant-associated maniform states in acute treatment of patients with bipolar-I depression in the Munich study. Bipolar Disord 4:115

Möller-Leimkühler AM (2002) Barriers to help-seeking by men: a review of sociocultural and clinical literature with particular reference to depression. J Affect Disord 71:1-9

Möller-Leimkühler AM, Dunkel R, Müller P, Pukies G, de Fazio S, Lehmann E (2002) Is patient satisfaction a undimensional construct? Factor analysis of the Munich patient satisfaction scale (MPSS-24). Eur Arch Psychiatry Clin Neurosci 252:19-23

Montgomery SA, Bech P, Blier P, Möller HJ, Nierenberg AA, Pinder RM, Quitkin FM, Reimitz PE, Rosenbaum JF, Rush AJ, Stassen HH, Thase ME (2002) Selecting methodologies fort he evaluation of differences in time to response between antidepressants. J Clin Psychiatry 63:694-699

Müller N (2002) Neuroimmunology of schizophrenia. Biol Psychiatry 17:613-623

Müller N, Riedel M, Scheppach C, Brandstatter B, Sokullu S, Krampe K, Ulmschneider M, Engel RR, Möller HJ, Schwarz MJ (2002) Beneficial antipsychotic effects of celecoxib add-on therapy compared to risperidone alone in schizophrenia. Am J Psychiatry 159:1029-1034

Müller-Preuss P, Rupprecht R, lancel M (2002) The effects of the neuroactive steroid 3α, 5α-THDOC on sleep in the rat. Neuroreport 13:487-490

Mulert C, Juckel G, Augustin H, Hegerl U (2002) Comparison between the analysis of the loudness dependency of the auditory N1/P2 component with LORETA and dipole source analysis in the prediction of treatment response to the selective serotonin reuptake inhibitor citalopram in major depression. Clin Neurophysiol 113:1566-1572

Neumeister A, Konstantinidis A, Stastny J, Schwarz MJ, Vitouch O, Willeit M, Praschak-Rie-derer N, Zach J, de Zwaan M, Bondy B, Ackenheil M, Kasper S (2002) Association between serotonin transporter gene promoter polymorphism (5HT-TLPR) and behavioural responses to tryptophan depletion in healthy woman with and without family history of depression. Arch Gen Psychiatry 59:613-620

Normann C, Hummel B, Scharer LO, Horn M, Grunze H, Walden J (2002) Lamotrigine as adjunct to paroxetine in acute depression: a placebo-controlled, double-blind study. J Clin Psychiatry 63:337-344

Padberg F, Möller HJ (2003) Repetitive transcranial magnetic stimulation : does it have potential in the treatment of depression? CNS Drugs 17:383-403

Padberg F, Michele F, Zwanzger P, Romeo E, bernardi G, Schüle C, baghai TC, Ella R, Pasini A, Rupprecht R (2002) Plasma concentrations of neuroactive steroids before and after repetitive transcranial magnetic stimulation (RTMS) in major depression. Neuropsychopharmacology 27:874-878

Padberg F, Schüle C, Zwanzger P, Baghai T, Ella R, Mikhaiel P, Hampel H, Möller HJ, Rupprecht R (2002) Relation between response to repetitive transcranial magnetic stimulation and partial sleep deprevation in major depression J Psychiatr Res 36:131-135

Padberg F, Zwanzger P, Keck ME, Kathmann N, Mikhaiel P, Ella R, Rupprecht P, Thoma H, Hampel H, Toschi N, Möller HJ (2002) Repetitive transcranial magnetic stimulation (rTMS) in major depression: relation between efficacy and stimulation intensity. Neuropsychopharmacology 27:636-645

Peuskens J, Möller HJ, Puech A (2002) Amisulpride improves depressive symptoms in acute exacerbations of schizophrenia: comparison with haloperidol and risperidone. Eur Neuropsychopharmacol12:305-310

Pogarell O, Gasser T, van Hilten JJ, Spieker S, Pollentier S, Meier D, Oertel WH (2002) Pramipexole in tremordominant Parkinson's disease. Results of a double-blind placebo-controlled study. J Neurol Neurosurg Psychiat 72:713-720

Praschkak-Rieder N, Willeit M, Winkler D, Neumeister A, Hilger E, Zill P, Hornik K, Stastny J, Thierry N, Ackenheil M, Bondy B, Kasper S (2002) Role of family history and 5-HTTLPR) polymorphism in female seasonal affective disorder patients with and without premenstrual dysphoric disorder. Eur Neuropsychopharmacol12:129-134

Riedel M, Kronig H, Schwarz MJ, Engel RR, Kuhn KU, Sikorski C, Sokullu S, Ackenheil M, Möller HJ, Müller N (2002) No association between the G308A polymorphism ot the tumor necrosis factor-alpha gene and schizophrenia. Eur Arch Psychiatry Clin Neurosci 252:232-234

Rothenhäusler HB, Ehrentraut S, Kapfhammer HP, Lang C, Zachoval R, Bilzer M, Schelling G, Gerbes AL (2002) Psychiatric and psychosocial outcome of orthotopic liver transplantation. Psychother Psychosom 71:285-297

Rujescu D, Giegling I, Bondy B, Gietl A, Zill P, Möller HJ (2002) Association of anger-related traits with SNPs in the TPH gene. Mol Psychiatry 7:1023-1029

Rujescu D, Meisenzahl EM, Giegling I, Kirner A, Leisinger G, Hegerl U, Hahn K, Möller HJ (2002) Methionine homozygosity at codon 129 in the prion protein is associated with white matter reduction and enlargement of CSF compartments in healthy volunteers and schizophrenic patients. Neuroimage 15:200-206

Sato T, Bottlender R, Kleindienst N, Möller HJ (2002) Syndromes and phenomenological subtypes underlying acute mania: a factor analytic study of 576 manic patients. Am J Psychiatry 159:968-974

Sato T, Bottlender R, Kleindienst N, Tanaba A, Möller HJ (2002) The boundary between mixed and manic episodes in the ICD-10 classification. Acta Psychiatr Scand 106:109-116

Schaefer M, Engelbrecht MA, Gut O, Fiebich BL, Bauer J, Schmidt F, Grunze H, Lieb K (2002) Interferon alpha (IFNalpha) and psychiatric syndromes: a review. Prog Neuropsychopharmacol Biol Psychiatry 26:731-746

Schaefer M, Schmidt F, Neumer R, Scholler G, Schwarz M (2002) Interferon-alpha, cytokines and possible implications for mood disorders. Bipolar Disord 4 (Suppl 1):111-113

Scharer LO, Hartweg V, Valerius G, Graf M, Hoern M, Biedermann C, Walser S, Boensch A, Dittmann S, Forsthoff A, Hummel B, Grunze H, Walden J (2002) Life charts on a palmtop computer: first results of a feasibility study with an electronic diary for bipolar patients. Bipolar Disord 4 (Suppl 1):107-108

Schmitt GJ, Meisenzahl EM, Dresel S, Tatsch K, Rossmüller B, Frodl T, Preuss UW, Hahn K, Möller HJ (2002) Striatal dopamine D2 receptor binding of risperidone in schizophrenic patients as assessed by 123I.iodobenzamide SPECT: a comparative study with olanzapine. J Psychopharmacol 16:200-206

Schüle C, Baghai T, Goy J, Bidlingmaier M, Srasburger C, Laakmann G (2002) The influence of mirtazapine on anterior pituitary hormone secretion in healthy male subjects. Psychopharmacology 163:95-101

Soyka M, Morhart-Klute V, Horak M (2002) A combination of carbamazepine/tiapride in outpatient alcohol detoxification. Results from an open clinical study. ? Eur Arch Psychiatry Clin Neurosci 252:197-200

Soyka M, Preuss U, Schütz C (2002) Dopamine D4 receptor gene polymorphism and extraversion revisted:results from the Munich gene bank project for alcoholism. J Psychiatry Res 36:429-435

Strohle A, Romeo E, di Michele F, Pasini A, Yassouridis A, Holsboer F, Rupprecht R (2002) GABA(A) receptor-modulating neuroactive steroid composition in patients with panic disorder before and during paroxetine treatment. Am J Psychiatry 159:145-147

Teipel SJ, Bayer W, Alexander GE, Zebuhr Y, Teichberg D, Kulic L, Schapiro MB, Möller HJ, Rapoport SI, Hampel H (2002) Progression of corpus callosum atrophy in Alzheimer's disease. Arch Neurology 59:243-248

Tiemeier H, Pelzer E, Jonck L, Möller HJ, Rao ML (2002) Plasma catecholamines and selective slow wave sleep deprivation. Neuropsychobiology 45:81-85

Volz HP, Möller HJ, Gerebtzoff A, Bischoff S (2002) Savoxepine versus haloperidol. Reasons for a failed controlled clinical trial in patients with an acute episode of schizophrenia. Eur Arch Psychiatry Clin Neurosci 252:76-80

Volz HP, Murck H, Kasper S, Möller HJ (2002) St John's wort extract (LI 160) in somatoform disorders: results of a placebo-controlled trial. Psychopharmacology 164:294-300

Walden J, Langosch J, Born C, Schaub A, Grunze H (2002) Levetiracetam and ethosuximide in the treatment of acute mania in an open study with an on-off-on design. Bipolar Disord 4:114

Winkler D, Willeit M, Praschak-Rieder N., Lucht MJ, Hilger E, Konstantinidis A, Stastny J, Thierry N, Pjrek E, Neumeister A, Möller HJ, Kasper S (2002) Changes of clinical pattern in seasonal affective disorder (SAD) over time in a German-speaking sample. Eur Arch Psychiatry Clin Neurosci 252:54-62

Woodside BD., Bulik CM, Halmi KA, Fichter MM, Kaplan A, Berrettini Wade H, Strober M, Treasure J, Lilenfeld L, Klump K ,Kaye WH (2002) Personality, Perfectionism, and Attitudes Toward Eating in Parents of Individuals with Eating Disorders. Int J Eat Disord 31:290-299

Zill P, Baghai TC, Zwanzger P, Schüle C, Minov C, Behrens S, Rupprecht R, Möller HJ, Engel R, Bondy B (2002) Association analysis of a polymorphism in the G.protein stimulatory alpha subunit in patients with major depression. Am J Med Genet 114:530-532

Zill P, Engel R, Baghai TC, Juckel G, Frodl T, Müller-Sicheneder F, Zwanzger P, Schüle C, Minov C, Behrens S, Rupprecht R, Hegerl U, Möller HJ, Bondy B (2002) Identification of a naturally occurring polymorphism in the promoter region of the norepinephirne transporter and analysis in major depression. Neuropsychopharmacology 26:489-493

Zwanzger P, Ella R, Keck ME, Rupprecht R, Padberg F (2002) Occurrence of delusions during repetitive transcranial magnetic stimulation (rTMS) in major depression. Biol Psychiatry 52:602-603

Zwanzger P, Minov C, Ella R, Schüle C, Baghai TC, Möller HJ, Rupprecht R (2002) Transcranial magnetic stimulation for panic. Am J Psychiatry 159:315-316

2003

Adli M, Rush J, Möller HJ, Bauer M (2003) Algorithms for optimizing the treatment of depression: making the right decision at the right time. Pharmacopsychiatry 36 (Suppl 3):S222-S229

Altshuler L, Suppes T, Black D, Nolen WA, Keck PE, Frye MA, McElroy S, Kupka R, Grunze H, Walden J, Leverich G, Denicoff K, Luckenbaugh D, Post R (2003) Impact of antidepressant discontinuation after acute bipolar depression remission on rates of depressive relapse at 1-year follow-up. Am J Psychiatry 160:1252-1262

Baghai TC, Schüle C, Zwanzger P, Zill P, Ella R, Eser D, Deiml T, Minov C, Rupprecht R, Bondy B (2003) No influence of a functional polymorphism within the serotonin transporter gene on partial sleep deprevation in major depression. World J Biol Psychiatry 4:111-114

Baghai TC, Schüle C, Zwanzger P, Zill P, Ella R, Eser D, Deiml T, Minov C, Rupprecht R, Bondy B (2003) Influence of a functional polymorphism within the angiotensin I-converting enzxme gene on partial sleep deprevation in patients with major depression. Neurosci Lett 339:223-226

Bagli M, Papassotiropoulos A, Hampel H, Becker K, Jessen F, Bürger K, Ptok U, Rao ML, Möller HJ, Maier W, Heun R (2003) Polymorphisms of the gene encoding the inflammatory cytokine interleukin-6 determine the magnitude of the increase in soluble interleukin-6 receptor levels in Alzheimer's disease. Results of a pilot study. Eur Arch Psychiatry Clin Neurosci 253:44-48

Baldwin D, Broich K, Fritze J, Kasper S, Westenberg H, Möller HJ (2003) Placebo-controlled studies in depression: necessary, ethical and feasible. Eur Arch Psychiatry Clin Neurosci 253:22-28

Bandelow B, Zohar J, Hollander E, Kasper S, Möller HJ, WFSBP Task Force on Treatment Guidelines for Anxiety O-CaPSD (2003) World Federation of Societies of Biological Psychiatry (WFSBP) guidelines for the pharmacological treatment of anxiety, obsessive-compulsive and post-traumatic stress disorders. World J Biol Psychiatry 3:171-199

Benamer HT, Oertel WH, Patterson J, Hadley DM, Pogarell O, Hoffken H, Gerstner A, Grosset DG (2003) Prospective study of presynaptic dopaminergic imaging in patients with mild parkinsonism and tremor disorders: Part1. Baseline and 3-month observations. Mov Disord 18:977-984

Bergen AW, van den Bree M B M, Yeager M, Welch R, Ganjei JK, Haque K, Bacanu S, Berrettini WH, Grice DE, Goldman D, Bulik CM, Klump K, Fichter M, Halmi K, Kaplan A, Strober M, Treasure J, Woodside B, Kaye WH (2003) Candidate genes for anorexia nervosa in the 1p33-36 linkage region: serotonin 1D and delta opioid receptor loci exhibit significant association to anorexia nervosa. Mol Psychiatry 8:397-406

Blennow K, Hampel H (2003) CSF markers for incipient Alzheimer's disease. Lancet Neurol 2:605-613

Bondy B, Baghai TC, Minov C, Schüle C, Schwarz MJ, Zwanzger P, Rupprecht R, Möller HJ (2003) Substance P serum levels are increased in major depression: preliminary results. Biol Psychiatry 53:538-542

Bottlender R, Sato T, Groll C, Jäger M, Kunze I, Möller HJ (2003) Negative symptoms in depressed and schizophrenic patients: how do they differ? J Clin Psychiatry 64:954-958

Bottlender R, Sato T, Jäger M, Kunze I, Groll C, Borski I, Möller HJ (2003) Does considering duration of negative symptoms increase their specificity for schizophrenia? Schizophr Res 60:321-322

Bottlender R, Sato T, Jäger M, Wegener U, Wittmann J, Strauß A, Möller HJ (2003) The impact of the duration of untreated psychosis prior to first psychiatric admission on the 15-year outcome in schizophrenia. Schizophr Res 62:37-44

Bottlender R, Sato T, Möller HJ (2003) Summer birth and deficit schizophrenia. Am J Psychiatry 160:594-595

Bulik CM, Devlin B, Bacanu SA, Thornton L, Klump K, Fichter MM, Halmi KA, Kaplan AS, Strober M, Woodside B, Bergen AW, Ganjei JK, Crow S, Mitchell J, Rotondo A, Mauri M, Cassano G, Keel P, Berrettini WH, Kaye WH, (2003) Significant linkage on chromosome 10p in families with bulimia nervosa. Am J Hum Genet 72:200-207

Bürger K, Zinkowski R, Teipel ST, Arai H, DeBernardis J, Kerkman D, McCulloch C, Padberg F, Faltraco F, Goernitz A, Tapiola T, Rapoport SI, Pirttilä T, Möller HJ, Hampel H (2003) Differentiation of geriatric major depression from Alzheimer's disease with CSF tau protein phosphorylated at threonine 231. Am J Psychiatry 160:376-379

Carta MG, Hardoy MC, Hardoy MJ, Grunze H, Carpiniello B (2003) The clinical use of gabapentin in bipolar spectrum disorders. J Affect Disord 75:83-91

Dodel RC, Hampel H, Yansheng D (2003) Immunotherapy for Alzheimer's disease. Lancet Neurol 2:215-220

Du Y, Wei X, Dodel R, Sommer N, Hampel H, Gao F, Ma Z, Zhao L, Oertel WH, Farlow M (2003) Human anti-abeta-amyloid antibodies block abeta-amyloid fibril formation and prevent abeta-amyloid-induced neurotoxicity. Brain 126:1935-1939

Eisensamer B, Rammes G, Gimpl G, Shapa M, Ferrari U, Hapfelmeier G, Bondy B, Parsons C, Gilling K, Zieglgänsberger W, Holsboer F, Rupprecht R (2003) Antidepressants are functional antagonists at the serotonin type 3 (5-HT3) receptor. Mol Psychiatry 8:994-1007

Empl M, Sostak P, Riedel M, Schwarz M, Müller N, Förderreuther S, Straube A (2003) Decreased sTNF-RI in migraine patients? Cephalalgia 23:55-58

Eser D, Zwanzger P, Rupprecht R (2003) Carbamazepine treatment of adverse psychiatric effects after treatment with the nonsteroidal anti-inflammatory drug piroxicam. J Clin Psychiatry 64:852-854

Faltraco F, Bürger K, Zill P, Teipel SJ, Möller HJ, Hampel H, Bondy B, Ackenheil M (2003) Interleukin-6-174 G/C promoter gene polymorphism C allele reduces Alzheimer's disease risk.
J Am Geriatr Soc 51:578-579

Frank RA, Galasko D, Hampel H, Hardy J, deLeon MJ, Mehta PD, Rogers J, Siemers E, Trojanowski JQ (2003) Biological markers for therapeutic trials in Alzheimer's disease. Proceedings of the biological markers working group; NIA initiative on neuroimaging in Alzheimer's disease. Neurobiol Aging 24:521-536

Frye MA, Altshuler LL, McElroy SL, Suppes T, Keck PE, Denicoff K, Nolen WA, Kupka R, Leverich GS, Pollio C, Grunze H, Walden J, Post RM (2003) Gender differences in prevalence, risk, and clinical correlates of alcoholism comorbidity in bipolar disorder. Am J Psychiatry 160:883-889

Frodl T, Meisenzahl EM, Zetzsche T, Born C, Jäger M, Groll C, Bottlender R, Leinsinger G, Möller HJ (2003) Larger amygdala volumes in first depressive episode as compared to recurrent major depression and healthy control subjects. Biol Psychiatry 53:338-344

Greil W, Kleindienst N (2003) Concepts in the treatment of bipolar disorder. Acta Psychiatr Scand 108 (Suppl 418):41-46

Grunze H (2003) Lithium in the acute treatment of bipolar disorders - a stocktaking. Eur Arch Psychiatry Clin Neurosci 253:115-119

Grunze H, Kasper S, Goodwin G, Bowden C, Baldwin D, Ucht RW, Vieta E, Möller HJ (2003) The World Federation of Societies of Biological Psychiatry (WFSBP) Guidelines for the Biological Treatrnent of Bipolar Disorders, Part II: Treatmentof Mania. World J Biol Psychiatry. 4:5-13

Grunze H, Langosch J, Born C, Schaub G, Walden J (2003) Levetiracetam in the treatment of acute mania: an open add-on study with an on-off-on design. J Clin Psychiatry 64:781-784

Gupta RK, Möller HJ (2003) St. John's Wort. An option for the primary care treatment of depressive patients? Eur Arch Psychiatry Clin Neurosci 253:140-148

Hampel H, Goernitz A, Bürger K (2003) Advances in the development of biomarkers for Alzheimer's disease: from CSF total tau and Abeta(1-42) proteins to phosphorylated tau protein. Brain Res Bull 61:243-253

Hapfelmeier G, Tredt C, Haseneder R, Zieglgansberger W, Eisensamer B, Rupprecht R, Rammes G (2003) Co-expression of the 5-HT3B serotonin receptor subunit alters the biophysics of the 5-HT3 receptor. Biophys J 84:1720-1733

Hegerl U, Mergl R, Henkel V, Gallinat J, Kotter G, Müller-Siecheneder F, Pogarell O, Juckel G, Schröter A, Bahra R, Emir B, Laux G, Möller HJ (2003) Kinematic analysis of the effects of donepezil hydrochloride on hand motor function in patients with Alzheimer dementia. J Clin Psychopharmacol 23:214-216

Henkel V, Mergl R, Kohnen R, Maier W, Möller HJ, Hegerl U (2003) Identifying depression in primary care: a comparison of different methods in a prospective cohort study. BMJ 326:200-201

Hiller W, Fichter MM, Rief W (2003) A controlled treatment study of somatoform disorders including analysis of healthcare utilization and cost-effectiveness. J Psychosom Res 54:369-380

Holtkamp K, Herpertz-Dahlmann B, Mika C, Heer M, Heussen N, Fichter MM, Herpertz S, Senf W, Blum W, Schweiger U, Warnke A, Ballauff A, Remschmidt H, Hebebrand J (2003) Elevated Physical Activity and Low Leptin Levels Co-occur in Patients with Anorexia Nervosa. J Clin Endocrinol Metab 88:5169-5174

Jäger M, Hintermayr M, Bottlender R, Strauß A, Möller HJ (2003) Course and outcome of first-admitted patients with acute and transient psychotic disorders (ICD-10:F23) Focus on relapses and social adjustment. Eur Arch Psychiatry Clin Neurosci 253:209-215

Johansson C, Willeit M, Levitan R, Partonen T, Smedh C, del Favero J, Bel Kacem S, Praschak-Rieder N, Neumeister A, Masellis M, Basile V, Zill P, Bondy B, Paunio T, Kasper S, van Broeckhoven C, Nilsson LG, Lam R, Schalling M, Adolfsson R (2003) The serotonin transporter promoter repeat length polymorphism, seasonal affective disorder and seasonality. Psychol Med 33:785-792

Juckel G, Schüle C, Pogarell O, Rupp D, Laakmann G, Hegerl U (2003) Epileptiform EEG patterns induced by mirtazapine in both psychiatric patients and healthy volunteers. J Clin Psychopharmacol 23:421-422

Kathmann N, Hochrein A, Uwer R, Bondy B (2003) Deficits in gain of smooth pursuit eye movements in schizophrenia and affective disorder patients and their unaffected relatives. Am J Psychiatry 160:696-702

Kleindienst N, Greil W (2003) Lithium in the long-term treatment of bipolar disorders. Eur Arch Psychiatry Clin Neurosci 253:120-125

Laumbacher B, Müller N, Bondy B, Schlesinger B, Gu S, Fellerhoff B, Wank R (2003) Significant frequency deviation of the class I polymorphism HLA-A10 in schizophrenic patients. J Med Genet 40:217-219

Leverich GS, Altshuler LL, Frye MA, Suppes T, Keck PE, McElroy SL, Denicoff KD, Obrocea G, Nolen WA, Kupka R, Walden J, Grunze H, Perez S, Luckenbaugh DA, Post RM (2003) Factors associated with suicide attempts in 648 patients with bipolar disorder in the Stanley Foundation Bipolar Network. J Clin Psychiatry. 64:506-515

Mergl R, Vogel M, Mavrogiorgou P, Göbel C, Zaudig M, Hegerl U, Juckel G (2003) Kinematical analysis of emotionally induced facial expressions in patients with obsessive-compulsive disorder. Psychol Med 33:1453-1462

Möller HJ (2003) Bipolar disorder and schizophrenia: distinct illnesses or a continuum? J Clin Psychiatry 64 (Suppl 6):23-27

Möller HJ (2003) Is lithium still the gold standard in the treatment of bipolar disorders? Eur Arch Psychiatry Clin Neurosci 253:113-114

Möller HJ (2003) Management of the negative symptoms of schizophrenia. New treatment options. CNS Drugs 17:793-823

Möller HJ (2003) Suicide, suicidality and suicide prevention in affective disorders. Acta Psychiatr Scand 108 (Suppl 418):73-80

Möller HJ, Demyttenaere K, Sacchetti E, Rush AJ, Montgomery SA (2003) Improving the chance of recovery from the short- and long-term consequences of depression. Int Clin Psychopharmacol 18:219-225

Möller HJ, Nasrallah HA (2003) Treatment of bipolar disorder. J Clin Psychiatry 64 (Suppl 6):9-17

Möller-Leimkühler AM (2003) The gender gap in suicide and premature death or: why are men so vulnerable? European Eur Arch Psychiatry Clin Neurosci 253:1-8

Olsson A, Höglund K, Sjögren M, Andreasen N, Minthon L, Lannfelt L, Bürger K, Möller HJ, Hampel H, Davidsson P, Blennow K (2003) Measurement of alpha- and beta-secretase cleaved amyloid precursor protein in cerebrospinal fluid from Alzheimer patients. Exp Neurol 183:74-80

Padberg F, Möller HJ (2003) Repetitive transcranial magnetic stimulation: does it have potential in the treatment of depression? CNS Drugs 17:383-403

Pogarell O, hamann C, Pöpperl G, Juckel G, Choukèr M, Zaudig M, Riedel M, Möller HJ, hegerl U, Tatsch K (2003) Elevated brain serotonin transporter availability in patients with obsessive-compulsive disorder. Boil Psychiatry 54:1406-1413

Post RM, Leverich GS, Altshuler LL, Frye MA, Suppes TM, Keck PE, McElroy SL, Kupka R, Nolen WA, Grunze H, Walden J (2003) An overview of recent findings of the Stanley Foundation Bipolar Network (Part 1). Bipobar Disord 5:310-319

Post RM, Leverich GS, Nolen WA, Kupka RW, Altshuler LL, Frye MA, Suppes T, McElroy S, Keck

P, Grunze H, Walden J (2003) A re-evaluation of the role of antidepressants in the treatment of bipolar depression: data from the Stanley Foundation Bipolar Network. Bipolar Disord 5:396-406

Preuss UW, Koller G, Zill P, Bondy B, Soyka M (2003) Alcoholism-related phenotypes and genetic variants of the CB1 receptor. European Archives of Psychiatry and Clinical Neuroscience 253:275-280

Riedel M, Krönig H, Schwarz MJ, Engel RR, Sikorski C, Kühn KU, Behrens S, Möller HJ, Ackenheil M, Müller N (2003) Investigation of the ICAM-1 G241A and A469G gene polymorphisms in schizophrenia. Mol Psychiatry 8:257-258

Rujescu D, Giegling I, Gietl A, Gonnermann C, Kirner A, Möller HJ (2003) Association study of a SNP coding for a M129V substitution in the prion protein in schizophrenia.Schizophr Res 62:289-291

Rujescu D, Giegling I, Gietl A, Hartmann AM, Möller HJ (2003) A functional single nucleotide polymorphism (V158M) in the COMT gene is associated with aggressive personality traits. Biol Psychiatry 54:34-39

Rujescu D, Giegling I, Sato T, Hartmann AM, Möller HJ (2003) Genetic variations in tryptophan hydroxylase in suicidal behavior: analysis and meta-analysis. Biol Psychiatry 54:465-473

Rupprecht R (2003) Neuroactive steroids: mechanisms of action and neuropsycho-pharmacological properties. Psychoneuroendocrinology 28:139-168

Rupprecht R (2003) Editorial: The World Journal of Biological Psychiatry -Past, present and future. World J Biol Psychiatry 4:46-47

Sato T, Bottlender R, Schröter A, Möller HJ (2003) Frequency of manic symptoms during a depressive episode and unipolar 'depressive mixed state' as bipolar spectrum. Acta Psychiatr Scand 107:268-274

Sato T, Bottlender R, Sievas M, Schröter A, Hecht S, Möller HJ (2003) Long-term inter-episode stability of syndromes underlying mania. Acta Psychiatr Scand 108:310-313

Schaefer M, Schmidt F, Folwaczny C, Lorenz R, Martin G, Schindlbeck N, Heldwein W, Soyka M, Grunze H, Koenig A, Loeschke K (2003) Adherence and mental side effects during hepatitis C treatment with interferon alfa and ribavirin in psychiatric risk groups. Hepatology 37:443-451

Schröter A, Mergl R, Bürger K, Hampel H, Möller HJ, Hegerl U (2003) Kinematic analysis of handwriting movements in patients with Alzheimer's disease, mild cognitive impairment, depression and healthy subjects. Dement Geriatr Cogn Disord 15:132-142

Schüle C, Baghai T, Zwanzger P, Ella R, Eser D, Padberg F, Möller HJ, Rupprecht R (2003) Attenuation of hypothalamic-pituitary-adrenocortical hyperactivity in depressed patients by mirtazapine. Psychopharmacology 166:271-275

Schüle C, di Michele F, Baghai T, Romeo E, Bernardi G, Zwanzger P, Padberg F, Pasini A, Rupprecht R (2003) Influence of sleep deprivation on neuroactive steroids in major depression. Neuropsychopharmacology 28:577-581

Schüle C, Zwanzger P, Baghai T, Mikhaiel P, Thoma H, Möller HJ, Rupprecht R, Padberg F (2003) Effects of antidepressant pharmacotherapy after repetitive transcranial magnetic stimulation in major depression: an open follow-up study. J Psychiatr Res 37:145-153

Schumann G, Rujescu D, Kissling C, Soyka M, Dahmen N, Preuss UW, Wieman S, Depner M, Wellek S, Lascorz J, Bondy B, Giegling I, Anghelescu I, Cowen MS, Poustka A, Spanagel R, Mann K, Henn FA, Szegedi A (2003) Analysis of genetic variations of protein tyrosine kinase fyn and their association with alcohol dependence in two independent cohorts. Biol Psychiatry 54:1422-1426

Ströhle A, Romeo E, di Michele F, Pasini A, Hermann B, Gajewsky G, Holsboer F, Rupprecht R (2003) Induced panic attecks shift gamma-aminobutyric acid type A receptor modulatory neuroactive steroid composition in patients with panic disorder: preliminary results. Arch Gen Psychiatry 60:161-168

Tadic A, Rujescu D, Szegedi A, Giegling I, Singer P, Möller HJ, Dahmen N (2003) Association of a MAOA gene variant with generalized anxiety disorder, but not with panic disorder or major depression. Am J Med Genet 117B:1-6

Teipel SJ, Bayer W, Alexander GE, Bokde ALW, Zebuhr Y, Teichberg D, Müller-Spahn F, Schapiro F, Möller HJ, Rapoport SI, Hampel H (2003) Regional pattern of hippocampus and corpus callosum atrophy in Alzheimer's disease in relation to dementia severity – evidence for early neocortical degeneration. Neurobiol Aging 24:85-94

Teipel SJ, Schapiro MB, Alexander GE, Krasuski JS, Horwitz B, Hoehne C, Möller HJ, Rapoport SI, Hampel H (2003) Relation of corpus callosum and hippocampal size to age in nondemented adults with Down's syndrome. Am J Psychiatry 160:1-9

Willeit M, Praschak-Rieder N, Zill P, Neumeister A, Ackenheil M, Kasper S, Bondy B (2003) C825T polymorphism in the G protein beta3-subunit gene is associated with seasonal affective disorder. Biol Psychiatry 54:682-686

Wiltfang J, Esselmann H, Smirnov A, Bibl M, Cepek L, Steinacker P, Mollenhauer B, Buerger K, Hampel H, Paul S, Neumann M, Maler M, Zerr I, Kornhuber J, Kretzschmar HA, Poser S, Otto M (2003) Pattern of beta-amyloid peptides in cerebrospinal fluid of patients with Creutzfeldt-Jakob disease. Ann Neurol 54:263-267

Zill P, Malitas PN, Bondy B, Engel R, Boufidou F, Behrens S, Alevizos BE, Nikolaou CK, Christodoulou GN (2003) Analysis of polymorphisms in the alpha-subunit of the olfactory G-protein Golf in lithium-treated bipolar patients. Psychiatr Genet 13:65-69

Zwanzger P, Baghai TC, Padberg F, Ella R, Minov C, Mikhaiel P, Schüle C, Thoma H, Rupprecht R (2003) The combined dexamethasone-CRH test before and after repetitive transcranial magnetic stimulation (rTMS) in major depression. Psychoneuroendocrinology 28:376-385

Zwanzger P, Eser D, Aicher S, Schüle C, Baghai TC, Padberg F, Ella R, Möller HJ, Rupprecht R (2003) Effects of alprazolam on cholecystokinin-tetrapeptide-induced panic and hypothalamic-pituitary-adrenal-axis activity: a placebo-controlled study. Neuropsychopharmacology 28:979-984

Zwanzger P, Eser D, Padberg F, Baghai TC, Schüle C, Rotzer F, Ella R, Möller HJ, Rupprecht R (2003) Effects of tiagabine on cholecystokinin-tetrapeptide (CCK-4)-induced anxiety in healthy volunteers. Depress Anxiety 18:140-143

Zwanzger P, Jarry H, Eser D, Padberg F, Baghai T, Schüle C, Ella R, Möller HJ, Rupprecht R (2003) Plasma gamma-amino-butyric acid (GABA) levels in cholecystokinine-tetrapeptide (CCK-4) induced anxiety. J Neural Transm 110:313-316

2004

Baghai TC, Schule C, Zill P, Deiml T, Eser D, Zwanzger P, Ella R, Rupprecht R, Bondy B (2004) The angiotensin I converting enzyme insertion/deletion polymorphism influences therapeutic outcome in major depressed women, but not in men. Neurosci Lett 363:38-42

Baumann P, Hiemke C, Ulrich S, Eckermann G, Gaertner I, Gerlach M, Kuss HJ, Laux G, Müller-Oerlinghausen B, Rao ML, Riederer P, Zernig G (2004) The AGNP-TDM expert group consensus guidelines: therapeutic drug monitoring in psychiatry. Pharmacopsychiatry 37:243-265

Baumann P, Hiemke C, Ulrich S, Gaertner I, Rao ML, Eckermann G, Gerlach M, Kuss HJ, Laux G, Müller-Oerlinghausen B, Riederer P, Zernig G (2004) Therapeutic monitoring of psychotropic drugs: an outline of the AGNP-TDM expert group consensus guideline. Ther Drug Monit 26:167-170

Bender S, Grohmann R, Engel RR, Degner D, Dittmann-Balcar A, Rüther E (2004) Severe adverse drug reactions in psychiatric inpatients treated with neuroleptics. Pharmacopsychiatry 37 (Suppl 1):S46-S53

Binder EB, Salyakina D, Lichtner P, Wochnik GM, Ising M, Pütz B, Papiol S, Seaman S, Lucae S, Kohli MA, Nickel T, Künzel HE, Fuchs B, Majer M, Pfennig A, Kern N, Brunner J, Modell S, Baghai T, Deiml T, Zill P, Bondy B, Rupprecht R, Messer T, Köhnlein O, Dabitz H, Brückl T, Müller N, Pfister H, Lieb R, Mueller JC, Lohmussaar E, Strom TM, Bettecken T, Meitinger T, Uhr M, Rein T, Holsboer F, Muller-Myhsok B (2004) Polymorphisms in FKBP5 are associated with increased recurrence of depressive episodes and rapid response to antidepressant treatment. Nat Genet 36:1319-1325

Bondy B, Zill P (2004) Pharmacogenetics and psychopharmacology. Curr Opin Pharmacol 4:72-78

Bottlender R, Sato T, Kleindienst N, Strauß A, Möller HJ (2004)Mixed depressive features predict maniform switch during treatment of depression in bipolar I disorder. J Affect Disord 78:149-152

Brunnauer A, Laux G, Geiger E, Möller HJ (2004) The impact of antipsychotics on psychomotor performance with regards to car driving skills. J Clin Psychopharmacol 24:155-160

Bulik C, Klump K, Thornton L, Kaplan A, Devlin B, Fichter MM, Halmi K, Strober M, Woodside B, Crow S, Mitchell J, Rotondo A, Mauri M, Cassano G, Keel P, Berrettini W, Kaye W (2004) Alcohol use disorder comorbidity in eating disorders: A multicenter study. J Clin Psychiatry 65:1000-1006

Degner D, Grohmann R, Kropp S, Rüther E, Bender S, Engel RR, Schmidt LG (2004) Severe adverse drug reactions of antidepressants: results of the German multicenter drug surveillance program AMSP. Pharmacopsychiatry 37 (Suppl 1): S39-S45

Deiml T, Haseneder R, Zieglgansberger W, Rammes G, Eisensamer B, Rupprecht R, Hapflemeier G (2004) Alpha-thujone reduces 5-HT3 receptor activity by an effect on the agonist-reduced desensitization. Neuropharmacology 46:192-201

Dodel RC, Du Y, Depboylu C, Hampel H, Frölich L, Haag A, Hemmeter U, Paulsen S, Teipel SJ, Brettschneider S, Spottke A, Nölker C, Möller HJ, Wei X, Farlow M, Sommer N, Oertel WH (2004) Intravenous immunoglobulins containing antibodies against beta-amyloid for the treatment of Alzheimer's disease. Journal Neurol Neurosurg Psychiatry 75:1472-1474

Fichter MM, Quadflieg N (2004) Twelve-year course and outcome of bulimia nervosa. Psychol Med 34:1395-1406

Fichter MM, Xepapadakos F, Quadflieg N, Georgopoulou E, Fthenakis WE (2004) A comparative study of psychopathology in Greek adolescents in Germany and in Greece in 1980 and 1998 - 18 years apart. Eur Arch Psychiatry Clin Neurosci 254:27-35

Frick E, Borasio GD, Zehentner H, Fischer N, Bumeder I (2004) Individual quality of life of patients undergoing autologous peripheral blood stem cell transplantation. Psychooncology 13:116-124

Frodl T, Meisenzahl EM, Zetzsche T, Höhne T, Banca S, Schorr C, Jäger M, Leinsinger G, Bottlender R, Reiser M, Möller HJ (2004) Hippocampal and amygdale changes in patients with major depressive disorders and healthy controls during a 1-year follow-up. J Clin Psychiatry

Frodl T, Meisenzahl EM, Zill P, Baghai T, Rujescu D, Leinsinger G, Bottlender R, Schüle C, Zwanzger P, Engel RR, Rupprecht R, Bondy B, Reiser M, Möller HJ (2004) Reduced hippocampal volumes associated with the long variant of the serotonin transporter polymorphism in major depression. Arch Gen Psychiatry 61:177-183

Frölich L, Fox J, Padberg F, Maurer K, Möller HJ, Hampel H (2004) Targets of antidementive therapy: drugs with a specific pharmacological mechanism of action. Curr Pharml Des 10:223-229

Goodwin GM, Bowden CL, Calabrese JR, Grunze H, Kasper S, White R, Greene P, Leadbetter R (2004) A pooled analysis of 2 placebo-controlled 18-month trials of lamotrigine and lithium maintenance in bipolar I disorder. J Clin Psychiatry 65:432-441

Gootjes L, Teipel SJ, Zebuhr Y, Schwarz R, Leinsinger G, Scheltens P, Möller HJ, Hampel H Regional distribution of white matter hyperintensities in vascular dementia, Alzheimer's disease and healthy aging. Dement Geriatr Cogn Disord 18:180-188

Grohmann R, Engel RR, Geissler KH, Rüther E (2004) Psychotropic drug use in psychiatric inpatients: recent trends and changes over time-data from the AMSP study. Pharmacopsychiatry 37 (Suppl 1):S27-S38

Grohmann R, Engel RR, Rüther E, Hippius H (2004) The AMSP drug safety program: methods and global results. Pharmacopsychiatry 37 (Suppl 1):S4-S11

Grohmann R, Hippius H, Helmchen H, Rüther E, Schmidt LG (2004) The AMÜP study for drug surveillance in psychiatry - a summary of inpatient data. Pharmacopsychiatry 37 (Suppl 1):S16-S26

Grunze H, Kasper S, Goodwin G, Bowden C, Möller HJ (2004) The World Federation of Societies of Biological Psychiatry (WFSBP) guidelines tor the biological treatment of bipolar disorders, part III: maintenance treatment. World J Biol Psiatry 5:120-135

Hampel H, Buerger K, Zinkowski R, Teipel SJ, Goernitz A, Andreasen N, Sjoegren M, deBernardis J, Kerkman D, Ishiguro K, Ohno H, Vanmechelen E, Vanderstichele H, McCulloch C, Möller HJ, Davies P, Blennow K (2004) Measurement of phosphorylated tau epitopes in the differential diagnosis of Alzheimer disease: a comparative cerebrospinal fluid study. Arch Gen Psychiatry 61:95-102

Hampel H, Mitchell A, Blennow K, Frank RA, Brettschneider S, Weller L, Möller HJ (2004) Core biological marker candidates of Alzheimer's disease - perspectives for diagnosis, prediction of outcome and reflection of biological activity. J Neural Transm 111:247-272

Hampel H, Teipel SJ (2004) Total and phosphorylated tau proteins: evaluation as core biomarker candidates in frontotemporal dementia. Dement Geriatr Cogn Disord 17 350-354

Hampel H, Teipel SJ, Fuchsberger T, Andreasen N, Wiltfang J, Otto M, Shen Y, Dodel R, Du Y, Farlow M, Möller HJ, Blennow K, Buerger K (2004) Value of CSF beta-amyloid1-42 and tau as predictors of Alzheimer's disease in patients with mild cognitive impairment. Mol Psychiatry 9:705-710

Henkel V, Baghai TC, Eser D, Zill P, Mergl R, Zwanzger P, Schüle C, Bottlender R, Jäger M, Rupprecht R, Hegerl U, Möller HJ, Bondy B (2004) The gamma amino butyric acid (GABA) receptor alpha-3 subunit gene polymorphism in unipolar depressive disorder: a genetic association study. Am J Med Genet B Neuropsychiatr Genet 126B:82-87

Henkel V, Mergl R, Coyne JC, Kohnen R, Allgaier AK, Rühl E, Möller HJ, Hegerl U (2004) Depression with atypical features in a sample of primary care outpatients: prevalence, specific characteristics and consequences. J Affect Disord 83:237-242

Henkel V, Mergl R, Schäfer M, Rujescu D, Möller HJ, Hegerl U (2004) Kinematical analysis of motor function in schizophrenic patients: a possibility to separate negative symptoms from extrapyramidal dysfunction induced by neuroleptics? Pharmacopsychiatry 37:110-118

Hiller W, Fichter MM (2004) High utilizers of medical care: A crucial subgroup among somatizing patients. J Psychosom Res 56:437-443

Jäger M, Bottlender R, Strauss A, Möller HJ (2004) Fifteen-year follow-up of ICD-10 schizoaffective disorders compared with schizophrenia and affective disorders. Acta Psychiatr Scand 109:30-37

Jeck N, Waldegger S, Lampert A, Boehmer C, Waldegger P, Lang PA, Wissinger B, Friedrich B, Risler T, Moehle R, Lang UE, Zill P, Bondy B, Schaeffeler E, Asante-Poku S, Seyberth H, Schwab M, Lang F (2004) Activating mutation of the renal epithelial chloride channel ClC-Kb predisposing to hypertension. Hypertension 43:1175-1181

Kapfhammer HP, Rothenhäusler HB, Krauseneck T, Stoll C, Schelling G (2004) Posttraumatic stress disorder and health-related quality of life in long-term survivors of acute respiratory distress syndrome. Am J Psychiatry 161:45-52

Kaye WH, Bulik C, Thornton L, Barbarich N, Masters K, Fichter MM, Plotnicov K, Pollice C, Devlin B, Quadflieg N, Halmi KA, Kaplan AS, Woodside DB, Strober M, Bergen AW, Crow S, Mitchell J, Rotondo A, Mauri M, Keel P, Klump KL, Lilenfeld LR, Berrettini WH (2004) Comorbidity of Anxiety Disorders with Anorexia and Bulimia Nervosa. Am J Psychiatry 161:2215-2221

Kaye WH, Devlin B, Barbarich N, Bulik C, Thornton L, Bacanu S, Fichter MM, Halmi KA, Kaplan AS, Strober M, Woodside B, Bergen A, Crow S, Mitchell J, Rotondo A, Mauri M, Cassano G, Keel P, Plotnicov K, Pollice C, Klump KL, Lilenfeld LR, Ganjei JK, Quadflieg N, Berrettini WH (2004) Genetic analysis of bulimia nervosa: Methods and sample description. Int J Eat Disord 35:556-570

Keel PK, Fichter MM, Quadflieg N, Bulik CM, Baxter MG, Thornton L, Halmi KA, Kaplan AS, Strober M, Woodside DB, Crow SJ, Mitchell JE, Rotondo, A, Mauri M, Cassano G, Treasure J, Goldman D, Berrettini W, Kaye WH (2004) Application of a latent class analysis to empirically define eating disorder phenotypes. Arch Gen Psychiatry 61:192-200

Kleindienst N, Greil W (2004) Are illness concepts a powerful predictor of adherence to prophylactic treatment of bipolar disorder? J Clin Psychiatry 65:966-974

Klump K, Strober M, Johnson C, Thornton L, Bulik C, Devlin B, Fichter MM, Halmi K, Kaplan A, Woodside B, Crow S, Mitchell J, Rotondo A, Keel P, Berrettini W, Ploticov K, Pollice C, Lilenfeld L, Kaye W (2004) Personality characteristics of women before and after recovery from an eating disorder. Psychol Med 34:1407-1418

Kropp S, Grohmann R, Hauser U, Rüther E, Degner D (2004) Hyperglycemia associated with antipsychotic treatment in a multicenter drug safety project. Pharmacopsychiatry 37 (Suppl 1): S79-S83

Kropp S, Ziegenbein M, Grohmann R, Engel RR, Degner D (2004) Galactorrhea due to psychotropic drugs. Pharmacopsychiatry 37 (Suppl 1): S84-S88

Li R, Yang L, Lindholm K, Konishi Y, Yue X, Hampel H, Zhang D, Shen Y (2004) Tumor necrosis factor death receptor signaling cascade is required for amyloid-ß protein-induced neuron death. J Neurosci 24:1760-1771

Lieb K, Walden J, Grunze H, Fiebich BL, Berger M, Normann C (2004) Serum levels of substance P and response to antidepressant pharmacotherapy. Pharmacopsychiatry 37:238-239

Meisenzahl EM, Frodl T, Müller D, Schmitt G, Gallinat J, Zetzsche T, Marcuse A, Juckel G, Leinsinger G, Hahn K, Möller HJ, Hegerl U (2004) Superior temporal gyrus and P300 in schizophrenia: a combined ERP/structural magnetic resonance imaging investigation. J Psychiatr Res 38:153-162

Mergl R, Juckel G, Rihl J, Henkel V, Karner M, Tigges P, Schröter A, Hegerl U (2004) Kinematical analysis of handwriting movements in depressed patients. Acta Psychiatr Scand 109: 383-391

Möhrenschlager M, Henkel V, Ring J (2004) Fabry disease: more than angiokeratomas. Arch Dermatol140:1526-1528

Möhrenschlager M, Henkel HV, Ring J (2004) Fabry outcome survey: need for documentation of dermatological, ophthalmological and psychiatric affections. Eur J Clin Invest 34:515-516

Möller HJ (2004) Course and long-term treatment of schizophrenic psychoses. Pharmacopsychiatry 37 (Suppl 2):S126-S135

Möller HJ (2004) Novel antipsychotics in the long-term treatment of schizophrenia. World J Biol Psychiatry 5:9-19

Möller HJ (2004) SSRIs: Are the Accusations Justified? World J Biol Psychiatry 5:174-175

Möller HJ, Riedel M, Müller N, Fischer W, Kohnen R (2004) Zotepine versus placebo in the treatment of schizophrenic patients with stable primary negative symptoms: a randomized double-blind multicenter trial. Pharmacopsychiatry 37:270-278

Möller-Leimkühler AM, Bottlender R, Strauß A, Rutz W (2004) Is there evidence for a male depressive syndrome in inpatients with major depression? J Affect Disord 80:87-93

Müller N, Riedel M, Schwarz MJ (2004) Psychotropic effects of COX-2 inhibitors - a possible new approach for the treatment of psychiatric disorders. Pharmacopsychiatry 37:266-269

Müller N, Strassnig M, Schwarz MJ, Ulmschneider M, Riedel M (2004) COX-2 inhibitors as adjunctive therapy in schizophrenia. Expert Opin Investig Drugs 13:1033-1044

Mulert C, Jäger L, Schmitt R, Bussfeld P, Pogarell O, Möller HJ, Juckel G, Hegerl U (2004) Integration of fMRI and simultaneous EEG: Toward a comprehensive understanding of localisation and time-course of brain activity in target detection. NeuroImage 22:83-94

Neumeister A, Nugent AC, Waldeck T, Geraci M, Schwarz M, Bonne O, Bain EE, Luckenbaugh DA, Herscovitch P, Charney DS, Drevets WC (2004) Neural and behavioral responses to tryptophan depletion in unmedicated patients with remitted major depressive disorder and controls. Arch Gen Psychiatry 61:765-773

Normann C, Hörn M, Hummel B, Grunze H, Walden J (2004) Paroxetine in major depression: correlating plasma concentrations and clinical response. Pharmacopsychiatry 37:123-126

Pogarell O, Juckel G, Mulert C, Amann B, Möller HJ, Hegerl U (2004) EEG Abnormalities under treatment with atypical antipsychotics: Effects of Olanzapine and Amisulpride as compared to Haloperidol. Pharmacopsychiatry 37:304-305

Pogarell O, Tatsch K, Juckel G, Hamann C, Mulert C, Pöpperl G, Folkerts M, Chouker M, Riedel M, Zaudig M, Möller HJ, Hegerl U (2004) Serotonin and dopamine transporter availabilities correlate with the loudness dependence of auditory evoked potentials in patients with obsessive-compulsive disorder. Neuropsychopharmacology 29:1910-1917

Rujescu D, Giegling I, Sato T, Möller HJ (2003) Lack of association between serotonin 5-HT1B receptor gene polymorphism and suicidal behaviour. Am J Med Genet 116:69-71

Rujescu D, Hartmann AM, Gonnermann C, Möller HJ, Giegling (2003) A M129V variation in the prion protein which influences white matter volume also influences cognitive performance. Mol Psychiatry 8:937-941

Sato T, Bottlender R, Schröter A, Möller HJ (2004) Psychopathology of early-onset versus late-onset schizophrenia revisited: an observation of 473 neuroleptic-naive patients before and after first-admission treatments. Schizophr Res 67:175-183

Sato T, Bottlender R, Sievers M, Schröter A, Kleindienst N, Möller HJ (2004) Evaluating the inter-episode stability of depressive mixed states. J Affect Disord 81:103-113

Schelling G, Kilger E, Roozendaal B, de Quervain D, Briegel J, Dagge A, Rothenhäusler HB, Krauseneck T, Nollert G, Kapfhammer HP (2004) Stress doses of hydrocortisone, traumatic memories, and symptoms of posttraumatic stress disorder in patients after cardiac surgery: a randomized study. Biol Psychiatry 55:627-633

Schmid C, Grohmann R, Engel RR, Rüther E, Kropp S (2004) Cardiac adverse effects associated with psychotropic drugs. Pharmacopsychiatry 37 (Suppl 1):S65-S69

Schuhmann G, Rujescu D, Szegedi A, Singer P, Wiemann S, Wellek S, Giegling I, Klawe C, Anghelescu I, Heinz A, Spanagel R, Mann K, Henn FA, Dahmen N (2003) No association of alcohol dependence with a NMDA-receptor 2B gene variant. Mol Psychiatry 8:11-12

Soyka M, Preuss UW, Koller G, Zill P, Bondy B (2004) Association of 5-HT1B receptor gene and antisocial behavior in alcoholism. J Neural Transm 111:101-109

Stefulj J, Büttner A, Skavic J, Zill P, Balija M, Eisenmenger W, Bondy B, Jernej B (2004) Serotonin 1B (5HT-1B) receptor polymorphism (G861C) in suicide victims: association studies in German and Slavic population. Am J Med Genet B Neuropsychiatr Genet 127B:48-50

Stübner S, Grohmann R, Engel R, Bandelow B, Ludwig W-D, Wagner G, Müller-Oerlinghausen B, Möller HJ, Hippius H, Rüther E (2004) Blood dyscrasias induced by psychotropic drugs. Pharmacopsychiatry 37 (Suppl 1):S70-S78

Stübner S, Rustenbeck E, Grohmann R, Wagner G, Engel R, Neundörfer G, Möller HJ, Hippius H, Rüther E (2004) Severe and uncommon involuntary movement disorders due to psychotropic drugs. Pharmacopsychiatry 37 (Suppl 1):S54-S64

Tadic A, Rujescu D, Szegedi A, Giegling I, Singer P, Möller HJ, Dahmen N (2003) Association of a MAO-A gene variant with generalized anxiety disorder bur not with panic disorder or major depression. Am J Med Genet 117B:1-6

Teipel SJ, Alexander GE, Schapiro MB, Möller HJ, Rapoport SI, Hampel H (2004) Age-related cortical grey matter reductions in non-demented Down's syndrome adults determined by MRI with voxel-based morphometry. Brain 127:811-824

Thierry N, Willeit M, Praschak-Rieder N, Zill P, Hornik K, Neumeister A, Lenzinger E, Stastny J, Hilger E, Konstantinidis A, Aschauer H, Ackenheil M, Bondy B, Kasper S (2004) Serotonin transporter promoter gene polymorphic region (5-HTTLPR) and personality in female patients with seasonal affective disorder and in healthy controls. Eur Neuropsychopharmacol 14: 53-58

Thompson R, Henkel V, Coyne JC (2004) Suicidal ideation in primary care: ask a vague question, get a confusing answer. Psychosom Med 66:455-457

Wei X, Zhao L, Ma Z, Holtzman DM, Yan C, Dodel R, Hampel H, Oertel W, Farlow MR, Du Y (2004) Caffeic acid phenethyl ester prevents neonatal hypoxic-ischaemic brain injury. Brain 127:2629-2635

Willeit M, Praschak-Rieder N, Neumeister A, Zill P, Leisch F, Stastny J, Hilger E, Thierry N, Konstantinids A, Winkler D, Fuchs K, Sieghart W, Aschauer H, Ackenheil M, Bondy B, Kasper S (2003) A polymorphism (5-HTTLPR) in the serotonin transporter promoter gene is associated with DSM-IV depression subtypes in seasonal affective disorder. Mol Psychiatry 8:942-946

Woodside DB, Bulik C, Thornton L, Klump K, Tozzi F, Fichter MM, Halmi K, Kaplan A, Strober M, Devlin B, Bacanu S, Ganjei K, Crow S, Mitchell J, Rotondo A, Mauri M, Cassano G, Keel P, Berrettini W, Kaye W (2004) Personality in men with eating disorders. J PsychosomRes 57:273-278

Zill P, Baghai TC, Engel R, Zwanzger P, Schüle C, Eser D, Behrens S, Rupprecht R, Möller HJ, Ackenheil M, Bondy B (2004) The dysbindin gene in major depression: an association study. Am J Med Genet B Neuropsychiatr Genet 129B:55-58

Zill P, Büttner A, Eisenmenger W, Bondy B, Ackenheil M (2004) Regional mRNA expression of a second tryptophan hydroxylase isoform in postmortem tissue samples of two human brains. Eur Neuropsychopharmacology 14:282-284

Zimmermann U, Spring K, Koller G, Holsboer F, Soyka M (2004) Hypothalamic-pituitary-arenal system regulation in recently detoxified alcoholics is not altered by one week of treatment with Acamprosate. Pharmacopsychiatry 37:98-102

Zwanzger P, Eser D, Padberg F, Baghai TC, Schüle C, Rupprecht R (2004) Neuroactive steroids are not affected by panic induction with 50 microg cholecystokinin-tetrapeptide (CCK-4) in healthy volunteers. J Psychiatric Res 38:215-217

Zwanzger P, Rupprecht R (2004) Vigabatrin and tiagabine might have antipanic properties. J Psychopharmacol 18:440

2005

Adam D, Kasper S, Möller HJ, Singer EA (2005) Placebo-controlled trials in major depression are necessary and ethically justifiable. How to improve the communication between researchers and ethical committees. Eur Arch Psychiatry Clin Neurosci 255:258-260

Amann B, Grunze H (2005) Neurochemical underpinnings in bipolar disorder and epilepsy. Epilepsia 46 (Suppl 4):26-30

Amann B, Sterr A, Mergl R, Dittmann S, Seemüller F, Dobmeier M, Orth M, Schaefer M,

Grunze H (2005) Zotepine loading in acute and severely manic patients: a pilot study. Bipolar Disord 7:471-476

Bacanu SA, Bulik CM, Klump KL, Fichter MM, Halmi KA, Keel P, Kaplan AS, Mitchell JE, Rotondo A, Strober M, Treasure J, Woodside DB, Sonpar VA, Xie W, Bergen AW, Berrettini WH, Kaye WH, Devlin B (2005) Linkage analysis of anorexia and bulimia nervosa cohorts using selected behavioral phenotypes as quantitative traits or covariates. Am J Med Genet B Neuropsychiatr Genet 139B:61-68

Baghai TC, di Michele F, Schüle C, Eser D, Zwanzger P, Pasini A, Romeo E, Rupprecht R (2005) Plasma concentrations of neuroactive steroids before and after electroconvulsive therapy in major depression. Neuropsychopharmacology 30:1181-1186

Bechdolf A, Ruhrmann S, Wagner M, Kühn KU, Janssen B, Bottlender R, Wieneke A, Schulze-Lutter F, Maier W, Klosterkötter J (2005)Interventions in the initial prodromal states of psychosis in Germany: concept and recruitment. Br J Psychiatry 187 (Suppl 48):s45-s48

Bergen AW, Yeager M, Welch RA, Haque K, Ganjei JK, van den Bree MBM, Mazzanti C, Nardi I, Fichter MM, Halmi KA, Kaplan AS, Strober M,

Treasure J, Woodside DB, Bulik CM, Bacanu SA, Devlin B, Berrettini WH, Goldman D, Kaye WH (2005) Association of multiple DRD2 polymorphisms with anorexia nervosa. Neuropsychopharmacology 30:1703-1710

Bokde ALW, Dong W, Born C, Leinsinger G, Meindl T, Teipel SJ, Reiser M, Hampel H (2005) Task difficulty in a simultaneous face matching task modulates activity in face fusiform area. Brain Res Cogn Brain Res 25:701-710

Bokde ALW, Teipel SJ, Drzezga A, Thissen J, Bartenstein P, Dong W, Leinsinger G, Born C, Schwaiger M, Moeller HJ, Hampel H (2005) Association between cognitive performance and cortical glucose metabolism in patients with mild Alzheimer's disease. Dement Geriatr Cogn Disord 20:352-357

Bokde AL, Teipel SJ, Schwarz R, Leinsinger G, Buerger K, Moeller T, Möller HJ, Hampel H (2005) Reliable manual segmentation of the frontal, parietal, temporal, and occipital lobes on magnetic resonance images of healthy subjects. Brain Res Brain Res Protoc 14:135-145

Biringer E, Lundervold A, Stordal K, Mykletun A, Egeland J, Bottlender R, Lund A (2005) Exekutive function improvement upon remission of recurrent unipolar depression. Eur Arch Psychiatry Clin Neurosci 255:373-380

Bondy B, Baghai TC, Zill P, Schüle C, Eser D, Deiml T, Zwanzger P, Ella R, Rupprecht R (2005) Genetic variants in the angiotensin I-converting-enzyme (ACE) and angiotensin II receptor (AT1) gene and clinical outcome in depression. Prog Neuro-Psychopharmacol Biol Psychiatry 29:1094-1099

Bowden CL, Grunze H, Mullen J, Brecher M, Paulsson B, Jones M, Vagerö M, Svensson K (2005) A randomized, double-blind, placebo-controlled efficacy and safety study of quetiapine or lithium as monotherapy for mania in bipolar disorder. J C Psychiatry 66:111-121

Braam AW, Prince MJ, Beekman ATF, Delespaul P, Dewey ME, Geerlings SW, Kivelä SL, Lawlor BA, Magnusson H, Meller I, Pérès K, Reischies FM, Roelands M, Schoevers RA, Saz P, Skoog I, Turrina C, Versporten A, Copeland JRM (2005) Physical health and depressive symptoms in older Europeans. Results from EURODEP. Br J Psychiatry 187:35-42

Brettschneider S, Morgenthaler NG, Teipel SJ, Fischer-Schulz C, Bürger K, Dodel R, Du Y, Möller HJ, Bergmann A, Hampel H (2005) Decreased serum amyloid β1–42 autoantibody levels in Alzheimer's disease, determined by a newly developed immuno-precipitation assay with radiolabeled amyloid β1–42 peptide. Biol Psychiatry 57:813-816

Buerger K, Ewers M, Andreasen N, Zinkowski R, Ishiguro K, Vanmechelen E, Teipel SJ, Graz C, Blennow K, Hampel H (2005) Phosphorylated tau predicts rate of cognitive decline in MCI subjects: a comparative CSF study. Neurology 65:1502-1503

Buerger K, Teipel S, Zinkowski R, Sunderland T, Andreasen N, Blennow K, Ewers M, DeBernardis J, Shen Y, Kerkman D, Du Y, Hampel H (2005) Increased levels of CSF phosphorylated tau in apolipoprotein E ε4 carriers with mild cognitive impairment. Neurosci Lett 391:48-50

Bulik CM, Bacanu SA, Klump KL, Fichter MM, Halmi KA, Keel P, Kaplan AS, Mitchell JE, Rotondo A, Strober M, Treasure J, Woodside DB, Sonpar VA, Xie W, Bergen AW, Berrettini WH, Kaye WH, Devlin B (2005) Selection of eating-disorder phenotypes for linkage analysis. Am J Med Genet B Neuropsychiatr Genet 139B:81-87

Chiang SSW, Schütz C, Soyka M (2005) Effects of cue exposure on the subjective perception of alcohol dependents with different types of cue reactivity. J Neural Transm 112: 1275-1278

Degner D, Kropp S, Porzig J, Grohmann R, Rüther E (2005) Pseudohallucinations associated with moclobemide: a case report. Pharmacopsychiatry 38:179-181

Dehning S, Riedel M, Müller N (2005) Aripiprazole in a patient vulnerable to side effects. Am J Psychiatry 162:625

Eisensamer B, Uhr M, Meyr S, Gimpl G, Deiml T, Rammes G, Lambert JJ, Zieglgänsberger W, Holsboer F, Rupprecht R (2005)Antidepressants and antipsychotic drugs colocalize with 5-HT3 receptors in raft-like domains. J Neurosci 25:10198-10206

Eser D, di Michele F, Zwanzger P, Pasini A, Baghai TC, Schüle C, Rupprecht R, Romeo E (2005) Panic induction with cholecystokinin-tetrapeptide (CCK-4) increases plasma concentrations of the neuroactive steroid 3α, 5α tetrahydrodeoxycorticosterone (3α, 5α-THDOC) in healthy volunteers. Neuropsychopharmacology 30:192-195

Falkai P, Wobrock T, Lieberman J, Glenthoj B, Gattaz WF, Möller HJ (2005) WFSBP Task Force on Treatment Guidelines for Schizophrenia World Federation of Societies of Biological Psychiatry (WFSBP) guidelines for biological treatment of schizophrenia, Part 1: acute treatment of schizophrenia. World J Biol Psychiatry 6:132-191

Fichter MM, Quadflieg N (2005) Three year course and outcome of mental illness in homeless men. A prospective longitudinal study based on a representative sample. Eur Arch Psychiatry Clin Neurosci 255:111-120

Fichter MM, Quadflieg N, Georgopoulou E, Xepapadakos F, Fthenakis WE (2005) Time Trends in Eating Disturbances in Young Greek Migrants. Int J Eating Disord 38:310-322

la Fougère C, Meisenzahl E, Schmitt G, Stauss J, Frodl T, Tatsch K, Hahn K, Möller HJ, Dresel S (2005) D2 receptor occupancy during high- and low-dose therapy with the atypical antipsychotic amisulpride: A 123I-iodobenzamide SPECT study. J Nucl Med 46:1028-1033

Frick E, Motzke C, Fischer N, Busch R, Bumeder I (2005) Is perceived social support a predictor of survival for patients undergoing autologous peripheral blood stem cell transplantation? Psychooncology 14:759-770

Gajwani P, Forsthoff A, Muzina D, Amann B, Gao K, Elhaj O, Calabrese JR, Grunze H (2005) Antiepileptic drugs in mood-disordered patients. Epilepsia 46 (Suppl 4):38-44

Genius D, Dong-Si T, Grau AP, Lichy C (2005) Postacute C-reactive protein levels are elevated in cervical artery dissection. Stroke 36:e42-e44

Grünblatt E, Schlößer R, Fischer P, Fischer MO, Li J, Koutsilieri E, Wichart I, Sterba N, Rujescu D, Möller HJ, Adamcyk W, Dittrich B, Müller F, Oberegger K, Gatterer G, Jellinger KJ, Mostafaie N, Jungwirth S, Huber K, Tragl KH, Danielczyk W, Riederer P (2005) Oxidative stress related markers in the »VITA« and the centenarian projects. Neurobiol Aging 26:429-438

Grunze H (2005) Reevaluating Therapies for Bipolar Depression. J Clin Psychiatry 66 (Suppl 5):17-25

Halmi KA, Tozzi F, Thornton LM, Crow S, Fichter MM, Kaplan AS, Keel P, Klump KL, Lilenfeld LR, Mitchell JE, Plotnicov KH, Pollice C, Rotondo A, Strober M, Woodside DB, Berrettini WH, Kaye WH, Bulik CM (2005) The Relation among Perfectionism, Obsessive-Compulsive Personality Disorder and Obsessive-Compulsive disorder in Individuals with Eating Disorders. Int J Eat Disord 38:371-374

Hampel H, Bürger K, Pruessner JC, Zinkowski R, DeBernardis J, Kerkman D, Leinsinger G, Evans AC, Davies P, Möller HJ, Teipel SJ (2005) Correlation of cerebrospinal fluid levels of tau protein phosphorylated at threonine 231 with rates of hippocampal atrophy in Alzheimer disease. Arch Neurol 62:770-773

Hampel H, Haslinger A, Scheloske M, Padberg F, Fischer P, Unger J, Teipel SJ, Neumann M, Rosenberg C, Oshida R, Hulette C, Pongratz D, Ewers M, Kretzschmar HA, Möller HJ (2005) Pattern of interleukin-6 receptor complex immunoreactivity between cortical regions of rapid autopsy normal and Alzheimer's disease brain. Eur Arch Psychiatry Clin Neurosci 255:269-278

Hegerl U, Mergl R, Henkel V, Pogarell O, Müller-Siecheneder F, Frodl T, Juckel G (2005) Differential effects of reboxetine and citalopram on hand-motor function in patients suffering from major depression. Psychopharmacology 178:58-66

Heinze M, Andreae D, Grohmann R (2005) Pharmacotherapy of personality disorders in German speaking countries: state and changes in the last decade. Pharmacopsychiatry 38:201-205

Hesselbrock V, Higuchi S, Soyka M (2005) Recent Developments in the Genetics of Alcohol-Related Phenotypes. Alcohol Clin Exp Res 29:1321-1324

Hiller W, Leibbrand R, Rief W, Fichter MM (2005) Differentiating hypochondrias from panic disorder. J Anxiety Disord 19:29-49

Hock B, Schwarz M, Domke I, Grunert VP, Wuertemberger M, Schiemann U, Horster S, Limmer C, Stecker G, Soyka M (2005) Validity of carbohydrate-deficient transferrin (%CDT), γ-glutamyltransferase (γ-GT) and mean corpuscular erythrocyte volume (MCV) as biomarkers for chronic alcohol abuse: a study in patients with alcohol dependence and liver disorders of non-alcoholic and alcoholic origin. Addiction 100:1477-1486

Johansson A, Zetterberg H, Hampel H, Buerger K, Prince JA, Minthon L, Wahlund LO, Blennow K (2005) Genetic Association of CDC2 with Cerebrospinal Fluid Tau in Alzheimer's Disease. Dement Geriatr Cogn Disord 20:367-374

Kleindienst N, Engel RR, Greil W (2005) Which clinical factors predict response to prophylactic lithium? A systematic review for bipolar disorders .Bipolar Disord 7:404-417

Kleindienst N, Severus WE, Möller HJ, Greil W (2005) Is polarity of recurrence related to serum lithium level in patients with bipolar disorder? Eur Arch Psychiatry Clin Neurosci 255:72-74

Kleindienst N, Engel RR, Greil W (2005) Psychosocial and demographic factors associated with response to prophylactic lithium: a systematic review for bipolar disorders. Psychol Med 35:1-10

Krause J, la Fougere C, Krause KH, Ackenheil M, Dresel SH (2005) Influence of striatal dopamine transporter availability on the response to methylphenidate in adult patients with ADHD. Eur Arch Psychiatry Clin Neurosci 255:428-431

Kupka RW, Luckenbaugh DA, Post RM, Suppes T, Altshuler LL, Keck PE, Frye MA, Denicoff KD, Grunze H, Leverich GS, McElroy SL, Walden J, Nolen WA (2005) Comparison of rapid-cycling and non-rapid-cycling bipolar disorder based on prospective mood ratings in 539 outpatients. Am J Psychiatry 162:1273-1280

Lerch JP, Pruessner JC, Zijdenbos A, Hampel H, Teipel SJ, Evans AC (2005) Focal decline of cortical thickness in Alzheimer's disease identified by computational neuroanatomy. Cerebral Cortex 15:995-1001

Leucht S, Kane JM, Kissling W, Hamann J, Etschel E, Engel R (2005)Clinical implications of Brief Psychiatric Rating Scale scores. Br J Psychiatry 187:366-371

Leucht S, Kane JM, Kissling W, Hamann J, Etschel E, Engel RR (2005) What does the PANSS mean? Schizophr Res 79:231-238

Maier W, Möller HJ (2005) Metaanalyses – highest level of empirical evidence? Eur Arch Psychiatry Clin Neurosci 255:369-370

Mann JJ, Apter A, Bertolote J, Beautrais A, Currier D, Haas A, Hegerl U, Lonnqvist J, Malone K, Marusic A, Mehlum L, Patton G, Philips M, Rutz W, Rihmer Z, Schmidtke A, Shaffer D, Silverman

M, Takahashi Y, Varnik A, Wassermann D, Yin P, Hendin H (2005) Suicide prevention strategies: a systematic review. JAMA 294:2064-2074

McElroy SL, Suppes T, Keck PE, Black D, Frye MA, Altshuler LL, Nolen WA, Kupka RW, Leverich GS, Walden J, Grunze H, Post RM (2005) Open-Label Adjunctive Zonisamide in the Treatment of Bipolar Disorders: A Prospective Trial. J Clin Psychiatry 66:617-624

Mergl R, Mavrogiorgou P, Hegerl U, Juckel G (2005) Kinematical analysis of emotionally induced facial expressions: a novel tool to investigate hypomimia in patients suffering from depression. J Neurol Neurosurg Psychiatry 76:138-140

Mergl R, Mavrogiorgou P, Juckel G, Zaudig M, Hegerl U (2005) Can a subgroup of OCD patients with motor abnormalities and poor therapeutic response be identified? Psychopharmacology 179: 826-837

Möhrenschlager M, Henkel V, Ring J (2005) Angiokeratomas, Fabry disease and enzyme replacement therapy: still a challenge. Br J Dermatol 152:177-178

Möller HJ (2005) Antidepressive effects of traditional and second generation antipsychotics: a review of the clinical data. Eur Arch Psychiatry Clin Neurosci 255:83-93

Möller HJ (2005) Antipsychotic and antidepressive effects of second generation antipsychotics. Two different pharmacological mechanisms? Eur Arch Psychiatry Clin Neurosci 255:190-201

Möller HJ (2005) Are placebo-controlled studies required in order to prove efficacy of antidepressants? World J Biol Psychiatry 6:130-131

Möller HJ (2005) Are the new antipsychotics no better than the classical neuroleptics? The problematic answer from the CATIE study. Eur Arch Psychiatry Clin Neurosci 255:371-372

Möller HJ (2005) Problems associated with the classification and diagnosis of psychiatric disorders. World J Biol Psychiatry 6:45-56

Möller HJ (2005) Occurrence and treatment of depressive comorbidity/cosyndromality in schizophrenic psychoses: conceptual and treatment issues. World J Biol Psychiatry 6:247-263

Möller HJ, Llorca PM, Sacchetti E, Martin SD, Medori R, Parellada E, for the StoRMi Study Group (2005) Efficacy and safety of direct transition to risperidone long-acting injectable in patients treated with various antipsychotic therapies. Int Clin Psychopharm 20:121-130

Möller-Leimkühler AM (2005) Burden of relatives and predictors of burden. Baseline results from the Munich 5-year-follow-up study on relatives of first hospitalized patients with schizophrenia or depression. Eur Arch Psychiatry Clin Neurosci 255:223-231

Mourao-Miranda J, Bokde ALW, Born C, Hampel H, Stetter M (2005) Classifying brain states and determining the discriminating activation patterns: Support Vector Machine on functional MRI data. NeuroImage 28:980-995

Müller N, Riedel M, Schwarz MJ, Engel RR (2005) Clinical effects of COX-2 inhibitors on cognition in schizophrenia. Eur Arch Psychiatry Clin Neurosci 255:149-151

Mulert C, Jäger L, Propp S, Karch S, Störmann S, Pogarell O, Möller HJ, Juckel G, Hegerl U (2005) Sound level dependence of the primary auditory cortex: Simultaneous measurement with 61-channel EEG and fMRI. NeuroImage 28:49-58

Mulert C, Menzinger E, Leicht G, Pogarell O, Hegerl U (2005)Evidence for a close relationship between conscious effort and anterior cingulate cortex activity. Int J Psychophysiol 56:65-80

Naber D, Riedel M, Klimke A, Vorbach EU, Lambert M, Kühn KU, Bender S, Bandelow B, Lemmer W, Moritz S, Dittmann RW (2005) Randomized double blind comparison of olanzapine vs. clozapine on subjective well-being and clinical outcome in patients with schizophrenia. Acta Psychiatr Scand 111:106-115

Offenbaecher M, Ackenheil M (2005) Current trends in neuropathic pain treatments with special reference to fibromyalgia. CNS Spectr 10:285-297

Otto BH, Tschop M, Frühauf E, Heldwein W, Fichter M, Otto C, Cuntz U (2005) Postprandial ghrelin release in anorectic patients before and after weight gain. Psychoneuroendocrinology 30:577-581

Pogarell O, Ehrentraut S, Rüther T, Mulert C, Hegerl U, Möller HJ, Henkel V (2005) Prolonged confusional state following electroconvulsive therapy - diagnostic clues from serial electroencephalography. Pharmacopsychiatry 38: 316-320

Pogarell O, Hegerl U, Boutrous N (2005) Clinical neurophysiology services in psychiatry departments. Psychiatric Serv 56:871

Pogarell O, Poepperl G, Mulert C, Hamann C, Sadowsky N, Riedel M, Möller HJ, Hegerl U, Tatsch K (2005) SERT and DAT availabilities under citalopram treatment in obsessive-compulsive disorder (OCD). Eur Neuropsychopharmacology 15:521-524

Pogarell O, Teipel SJ, Juckel G, Gootjes L, Möller T, Bürger K, Leinsinger G, Möller HJ, Hegerl U, Hampel H (2005) EEG coherence reflects regional corpus callosum area in Alzheimer's disease. J Neurol Neurosurg Psychiatry 76:109-111

Post RM, Altshuler LL, Frye MA, Suppes T, McElroy SL, Keck PE, Leverich GS, Kupka R, Nolen WA, Luckenbaugh DA, Walden J, Grunze H (2005) Preliminary observations on the effectiveness of levetiracetam in the open adjunctive treatment of refractory bipolar disorder. J Clin Psychiatry 66:370-374

Praschak-Rieder N, Willeit M, Zill P, Winkler D, Thierry N, Konstantinidis A, Masellis M, Basile VS, Bondy B, Ackenheil M, Neumeister A, Kaplan AS, Kennedy JL, Kasper S, Levitan R (2005) A Cys 23-Ser 23 substitution in the 5-HT(2C) receptor gene influences body weight regulation in females with seasonal affective disorder: an Austrian-Canadian collaborative study. J Psychiatric Res 39:561-567

Praschak-Rieder N, Wilson AA, Hussey D, Carella A, Wei C, Ginovart N, Schwarz MJ, Zach J, Houle S, Meyer JH (2005) Effects of tryptophan depletion on the serotonin transporter in healthy humans. Biol Psychiatry 58:825-830

Preuss UW, Zetzsche T, Jäger M, Groll C, Frodl T, Bottlender R, Leinsinger G, Hegerl U, Hahn K, Möller HJ, Meisenzahl EM (2005) Thalamic volume in first-episode and chronic schizophrenic subjects: volumetric MRI study.Schizophr Res 73:91-101

Rasgon NL, Altshuler LL, Fairbanks L, Elman S, Bitran J, Labarca R, Saad M, Kupka R, Nolen WA, Frye MA, Suppes T, McElroy SL, Keck PE Jr, Leverich G, Grunze H, Walden J, Post R, Mintz J (2005) Reproductive function and risk for PCOS in women treated for bipolar disorder. Bipolar Disord 7:246-259

Reba L, Thornton L, Tozzi F, Klump KL, Brandt H, Crawford S, Crow S, Fichter MM, Halmi KA, Johnson C, Kaplan AS, Keel P, LaVia M, Mitchell J, Strober M, Woodside DB, Rotondo A, Berrettini WH, Kaye WH, Bulik CM (2005) Relationships Between Features Associated with Vomiting in Purging-Type Eating Disorders. Int J Eat Disord 38:287-294

Riedel M, Müller N, Strassnig M, Spellmann I, Engel RR, Musil R, Dehning S, Douhet A, Schwarz MJ, Möller HJ (2005) Quetiapine has equivalent efficacy and superior tolerability to risperidone in the treatment of schizophrenia with predominantly negative symptoms. Eur Arch Psychiatry Clin Neurosci 255:432-437

Riedel M, Schwarz MJ, Strassnig M, Spellmann I, Müller-Arends A, Weber K, Zach J, Müller N, Möller HJ (2005) Risperidone plasma levels, clinical response and side-effects. Eur Arch Psychiatry Clin Neurosci 255:261-268

Riedel M, Strassnig M, Müller N, Zwack P, Möller HJ (2005) How representative of everyday clinical populations are schizophrenia patients enrolled in clinical trials? Eur Arch Psychiatry Clin Neurosci 255:143-148

Riedel M, Strassnig M, Schwarz MJ, Müller N (2005) COX-2 inhibitors as adjunctive therapy in schizophrenia: rationale for use and evidence to date. CNS Drugs 19:805-819

Rothenhäusler HB, Grieser B, Noller G, Reichart B, Schelling G, Kapfhammer HP (2005) Psychiatric and psychosocial outcome of cardiac surgery with cardiopulmonary bypass: a prospective 12-month follow-up study. Gen Hosp Psychiatry 27:18-28

Rujescu D, Soyka M, Dahmen N, Preuß U, Hartmann AM, Giegling I, Koller G, Bondy B, Möller HJ, Szegedi A (2005) GRIN1 locus may modify the susceptibility to seizures during alcohol withdrawal. Am J Med Genet B Neuropsychiatr Genet 133B:85-87

Sato T, Bottlender R, Kleindienst N, Möller HJ (2005) Irritable psychomotor elation in depressed inpatients: a factor validation of mixed depression. J Affect Disord 84:187-196

Sato T, Bottlender R, Sievers M, Möller HJ (2005) Evidence of depressive mixed states. Am J Psychiatry 162:193-194

Schmitt GJE, Meisenzahl EM, Frodl T, la Fougère C, Hahn K, Möller HJ, Dresel S (2005) The striatal dopamine transporter in first-episode, drug-naive schizophrenic patients: evaluation by the new SPECT-ligand[99mTc]TRODAT-1. J Psychopharmacology 19:488-493

Schüle C, Baghai TC, Alajbegovic L, Schwarz M, Zwanzger P, Eser D, Schaaf L, Möller HJ, Rupprecht R (2005) The influence of 4-week treatment with sertraline on the combined T3/TRH test in depressed patients. Eur Arch Psychiatry Clin Neurosci 255:334-340

Schüle C, Baghai TC, Tsikolata V, Zwanzger P, Eser D, Schaaf L, Rupprecht R (2005) The combined T3/TRH test in depressed patients and healthy controls. Psychoneuroendocrinology 30:341-356

Selle H, Lamerz J, Buerger K, Dessauer A, Hager K, Hampel H, Karl J, Kellmann M, Lannfelt L, Louhija J, Riepe M, Rollinger W, Tumani H, Schrader M, Zucht HD (2005) Identification of Novel Biomarker Candidates by Differential Peptidomics Analysis of Cerebrospinal Fluid in Alzheimer's Disease. Comb Chem High Throughput Screen 8:801-806

Severus WE, Grunze H, Kleindienst N, Frangou S, Möller HJ (2005) Is the prophylactic antidepressant efficacy of lithium in bipolar I disorder dependent on study design and lithium level? J Clin Psychopharmacology 25:457-462

Sievers M, Sato T, Möller HJ, Bottlender R (2005) Obsessive-compulsive disorder (OCD) with psychotic symptoms and response to treatment with SSRI. Pharmacopsychiatry 38:104-105

Soyka M, Hock B, Kagerer S, Lehnert R, Limmer C, Kuefner H (2005) Less impairment on one portion of a driving-relevant psychomotor battery in buprenorphine-maintained than in methadone-maintained patients: Results of a randomized clinical trial. J Clin Psychopharmacology 25:490-493

Soyka M, Koch W, Möller HJ, Rüther T, Tatsch K (2005) Hypermetabolic pattern in frontal cortex and other brain regions in unmedicated schizophrenia patients. Results from a FDG-PET study. Eur Arch Psychiatry Clin Neurosci 255:308-312

Soyka M, Winter C, Kagerer S, Brunnauer M, Laux G, Möller HJ (2005) Effects of haloperidol and risperidone on psychomotor performance relevant to driving ability in schizophrenic patients

compared to healthy controls. J Psychiatric Res 39:101-108

Spanagel R, Pendyala G, Abarca C, Zghoul T, Sanchis-Segura C, Magnone MC, Lascorz J, Depner M, Holzberg D, Soyka M, Schreiber S, Matsuda F, Lathrop M, Schumann G, Albrecht U (2005) The clock gene Per2 influences the glutamatergic system and modulates alcohol consumption. Nat Med 11:35-42

Suppes T, Mintz J, McElroy SL, Altshuler LL, Kupka RW Frye MA, Keck PE, Nolen WA, Leverich GS, Grunze H, Rush AJ, Post RM (2005) Mixed hypomania in 908 patients with bipolar disorder evaluated prospectively in the Stanley Foundation Bipolar Treatment Network: a sex-specific phenomenon. Arch Gen Psychiatry 62:1089-1096

Szegedi A, Rujescu D, Tadic A, Müller MJ, Kohnen R, Stassen HH, Dahmen N (2005) The catechol-O-methyltransferase Val108/158Met polymorphism affects short-term treatment response to mirtazapine, but not to paroxetine in major depression. Pharmacogenomics J 5:49-53

Tadic A, Dahmen N, Szegedi A, Rujescu D, Giegling I, Koller G, Anghelescu I, Fehr C, Klawe C, Preuss UW, Sander T, Toliat MR, Singer P, Bondy B, Soyka M (2005) Polymorphisms in the NMDA subunit 2B are not associated with alcohol dependence and alcohol withdrawal-induced seizures and delirium tremens. Eur Arch Psychiatry Clin Neurosci 255: 129-135

Teipel SJ, Flatz WH, Heinsen H, Bokde AL, Schoenberg SO, Stöckel S, Dietrich O, Reiser MF, Möller HJ, Hampel H (2005) Measurement of basal forebrain atrophy in Alzheimer's disease using MRI. Brain 128:2626-2644

Tohen M, Greil W, Calabrese JR, Sachs GS, Yatham LN, Müller-Oerlinghausen B, Koukopoulos A, Cassano GB, Grunze H, Licht RW, Dell'Osso L, Evans AR, Risser R, Baker RW, Crane H, Dossenbach MR, Bowden CL (2005) Olanzapine versus lithium in the maintenance treatment of bipolar disorder: a 12-month, randomized, double-blind, controlled clinical trial. Am J Psychiatry 162:1281-1290

Tozzi F, Thornton LM, Klump KL, Fichter MM, Halmi KA, Kaplan AS, Strober M, Woodside DB, Crow S, Mitchell J, Rotondo A, Mauri M, Cassano G, Keel P, Plotnicov KH, Pollice C, Lilenfeld

LR, Berrettini WH, Bulik CM, Kaye WH (2005) Symptom Fluctuation in Eating Disorders: Correlates of Diagnostic Crossover. Am J Psychiatry 162:732-740

Vieta E, Nolen WA, Grunze H, Licht RW, Goodwin G (2005) A European perspective on the Canadian guidelines for bipolar disorder. Bipolar Disord 7 (Suppl 3):73-76

Wiltfang J, Lewczuk P, Riederer P, Grünblatt E, Hock C, Scheltens P, Hampel H, Vanderstichele H, Iqbal K, Galasko D, Lannfelt L, Otto M, Esselmann H, Henkel AW, Kornhuber J, Blennow K (2005) Consensus paper of the WFSBP Task Force on Biological Markers of Dementia: the role of CSF and blood analysis in the early and differential diagnosis of dementia. World J Biol Psychiatry 6:69-84

Yatham LN, Goldstein JM, Vieta E, Bowden CL, Grunze H, Post RM, Suppes T, Calabrese JR (2005) Atypical antipsychotics in bipolar depression: potential mechanisms of action. J Clin Psychiatry 66 (Suppl 5):40-48

Zwanzger P, Rupprecht R (2005) Selective GABAergic treatment for panic? Investigations in experimental panic induction and panic disorder. J Psychiatry Neurosci 30: 167-175

2006

Alexander G, Chen K, Merkley TL, Reimann EM, Caselli RJ, Aschenbrenner M, Santerre-Lemmon L, Lewis D, Pietrini P, Teipel SJ, Hampel H, Rapoport SI, Moeller JR (2006) Regional network of MRI gray matter volume in healthy aging. Neuroreport 17:951-956

Altshuler LL, Suppes T, Black DO, Nolen WA, Leverich G, Keck PE, Frye MA, Kupka R, McElroy SL, Grunze H, Kitchen CM, Post R (2006) Lower switch rate in depressed patients with bipolar II than bipolar I disorder treated adjunctively with second-generation antidepressants. Am J Psychiatry 163:313-315

Baghai TC, Marcuse A, Brosch M, Schüle C, Eser D, Nothdurfter C, Steng Y, Noack I, Pietschmann K, Möller HJ, Rupprecht R (2006) The influence of concomitant antidepressant medication on safety, tolerability and clinical effectiveness of electroconvulsive therapy. World J Biol Psychiatry 7:82-90

Baghai TC, Volz HP, Möller HJ (2006) Drug treatment of depression in the 2000s: an overview of achievements in the last 10 years and future possibilities. World J Biol Psychiatry 7:198-222

Baghai TC, Binder EB, Schule C, Salyakina D, Eser D, Lucae S, Zwanzger P, Haberger C, Zill P, Ising M, Deiml T, Uhr M, Illig T, Wichmann HE, Modell S, Nothdurfter C, Holsboer F, Muller-Myhsok B, Möller HJ, Rupprecht R, Bondy B (2006) Polymorphisms in the angiotensin-converting enzyme gene are associated with unipolar depression, ACE activity and hypercortisolism. Mol Psychiatry 11:1003-1015

Baghai TC, Möller HJ, Rupprecht R (2006) Recent progress in pharmacological and non-pharmacological treatment options of major depression. Curr Pharm Des 12:503-515

Bender S, Dittmann-Balcar A, Schall U, Wolstein J, Klimke A, Riedel M, Vorbach EU, Kuhn KU, Lambert M, Dittmann RW, Naber D (2006) Influence of atypical neuroleptics on executive functioning in patients with schizophrenia: a randomized, double-blind comparison of olanzapine vs. clozapine. Int J Neuropsychopharmacol 9: 135-145

Bender W, Albus M, Möller HJ, Tretter F (2006) Towards systemic theories in Biological Psychiatry. Pharmacopsychiatry 39 (Suppl 1):S4-S9

Bokde ALW, Lopez-Bayo P, Meindl T, Pechler S, Born C, Faltraco F, Teipel SJ, Möller HJ, Hampel H (2006) Functional connectivity of the fusiform gyrus during a face-matching task in subjects with mild cognitive impairment. Brain 129:1113-1124

Bondy B, Buettner A, Zill P (2006) Genetics of suicide. Mol Psychiatry 11:336-351

Bottlender M, Preuss UW, Soyka M (2006) Association of personality disorders with Type A and Type B alcoholics. Eur Arch Psychiatry Clin Neurosci 256:55-61

Brunnauer A, Laux G, Geiger E, Soyka M, Möller HJ (2006) Antidepressants and Driving Ability: Results from a Clinical Study. J Clin Psychiatry 67:1776-1781

Buerger K, Otto M, Teipel SJ, Zinkowski R, Blennow K, DeBernardis J, Kerkman D, Schröder J, Schönknecht P, Cepek L, McCulloch C, Möller HJ, Wiltfang J, Kretzschmar H, Hampel H (2006) Dissociation between CSF total tau and tau protein phosphorylated at threonine 231 in Creutzfeldt-Ja-kob disease. Neurobiol Aging 27:10-15

Buerger K, Ewers M, Pirttila T, Zinkowski R, Alafuzoff I, Teipel SJ, DeBernardis J, Kerkman D, McCulloch C, Soininen H, Hampel H (2006) CSF phosphorylated tau protein correlates with neo-cortical neurofibrillary pathology in Alzheimer's disease. Brain 129:3035-3041

de la Fontaine L, Schwarz MJ, Riedel M, Dehning S, Douhet A, Spellmann I, Kleindienst N, Zill P, Plischke H, Gruber R, Muller N (2006) Investigating disease susceptibility and the nega-tive correlation of schizophrenia and rheumatoid arthritis focusing on MIF and CD14 gene poly-morphisms. Psychiatry 144:39-47

de Leon MJ, deSanti S, Zinkowski R, Mehta PD, Pratico D, Segal S, Rusinek H, Li J, Tsui W, Saint Louis LA, Clark CM, Tarshish C, Li Y, Lair L, Javier E, Rich K, Lesbre P, Mosconi L, Reisberg B, Sadowski M, deBernardis JF, Kerkman DJ, Hampel H, Wahlund LO, Davies P (2006) Longitudinal CSF and MRI biomarkers improve the diagnosis of mild cognitive impairment. Neurobiol Aging 27:394-401

Eser D, Romeo E, Baghai TC, di Michele F, Schule C, Pasini A, Zwanzger P, Padberg F, Rupprecht R (2006) Neuroactive steroids as modulators of depression and anxiety. Neuroscience 138:1041-1048

Eser D, Schule C, Baghai TC, Romeo E, Uzu-nov DP, Rupprecht R (2006) Neuroactive steroids and affective disorders. Pharmacol Biochem Behav 84:656-666

Eser D, Schule C, Romeo E, Baghai TC, di Mi-chele F, Pasini A, Zwanzger P, Padberg F, Rupprecht R (2006) Neuropsychopharmacological properties of neuroactive steroids in depression and anxiety disorders. Psychopharmacology 186:373-387

Ewers M, Teipel SJ, Dietrich O, Schonberg SO, Jessen F, Heun R, Scheltens P, Pol L, Freymann NR, Moeller HJ, Hampel H (2006) Multicenter assess-ment of reliability of cranial MRI. Neurobiol Aging 27:1051-1059

Falkai P, Wobrock T, Lieberman J, Glenthoj B, Gattaz WF, Möller HJ (2006) World Federation of Societies of Biological Psychiatry (WFSBP) guide-lines for biological treatment of schizophrenia, part 2: long-term treatment of schizophrenia. World J Biol Psychiatry 7:5-40

Fichter MM, Quadflieg N (2006) Intervention effects of supplying homeless individuals with per-manent housing: a 3-year prospective study. Acta Psychiatr Scand 113 (Suppl 429):36-40

Fichter MM, Quadflieg N, Hedlund S (2006) Twelve-year course and outcome predictors of an-orexia nervosa. Int J Eat Disord 39:87-100

Frodl T, Schaub A, Banac S, Charypar M, Jager M, Kummler P, Bottlender R, Zetzsche T, Born C, Leinsinger G, Reiser M, Möller HJ, Meisenzahl EM (2006) Reduced hippocampal volume correlates with executive dysfunctioning in major depression. J Psychiatry Neurosci 31:316-323

Gallinat J, Meisenzahl E, Jacobsen LK, Kalus P, Bierbrauer J, Kienast T, Witthaus H, Leopold K, Seifert F, Schubert F, Staedtgen M (2006) Smoking and structural brain deficits: a volumetric MR in-vestigation. Eur J Neurosci 24:1744-1750

Gauthier S, Reisberg B, Zaudig M, Petersen RC, Ritchie K, Broich K, Belleville S, Brodaty H, Bennett D, Chertkow H, Cummings JL, de Leon M, Feldman H, Ganguli M, Hampel H, Scheltens P, Tierney MC, Whitehouse P, Winblad B, on behalf of the participants (2006) Mild cognitive impair-ment. The Lancet 367:1262-1270

Giegling I, Hartmann AM, Möller HJ, Rujescu D (2006) Anger- and aggression-related traits are associated with polymorphisms in the 5-HT-2A gene.J Affect Disord 96:75-81

Glatz DC, Rujescu D, Tang Y, Berendt FJ, Hart-mann AM, Faltraco F, Rosenberg C, Hulette C, Jellinger K, Hampel H, Riederer P, Möller HJ, An-dreadis A, Hohagen F, Stamm S (2006) The alterna-tive splicing of tau exon 10 and its regulatory pro-teins CLK2 and TRA2-BETA1 changes in sporadic Alzheimer's disease. J Neurochem 96:635-644

Hegerl U (2006) Antidepressants and suicidali-ty. Eur Arch Psychiatry Clin Neurosci 256:199-200

Hegerl U, Althaus D, Schmidtke A, Niklewski G (2006) The alliance against depression: 2-year evaluation of a community-based intervention to reduce suicidality. Psychol Med 36:1225-1233

Heinsen H, Hampel H, Teipel SJ (2006) Com-puter-assisted 3D reconstruction of the Nucleus basalis complex in response to the suggestons of Boban et al. Brain 129:E43

Henkel V, Mergl R, Allgaier AK, Kohnen R, Möller HJ, Hegerl U (2006) Treatment of depression with atypical features: a meta-analytic approach. Psychiatry Res 141:89-101

Johannsen P, Salmon P, Hampel H, Xu Y, Richardson S, Qvitzau S, Schindler R, The AWARE Study Group (2006) Assessing therapeutic efficacy in a progressive disease : a study of donepezil in Alzheimer's disease. CNS Drugs 20:311-325

Krause J, Dresel SH, Krause KH, la Fougere C, Zill P, Ackenheil M (2006) Striatal dopamine transporter availability and DAT-1 gene in adults with ADHD: no higher DAT availability in patients with homozygosity for the 10-repeat allele. World J Biol Psychiatry 7:152-157

Lauterbach E, Brunner J, Hawellek B, Lewitzka U, Ising M, Bondy B, Rao ML, Frahnert C, Rujescu D, Muller-Oerlinghausen B, Schley J, Heuser I, Maier W, Hohagen F, Felber W, Bronisch T (2006) Platelet 5-HT2A receptor binding and tryptophan availability in depression are not associated with recent history of suicide attempts but with personality traits characteristic for suicidal behavior. J Affect Disord 91:57-62

Leverich GS, Altshuler LL, Frye MA, Suppes T, McElroy SL, Keck PE, Jr., Kupka RW, Denicoff KD, Nolen WA, Grunze H, Martinez MI, Post RM (2006) Risk of switch in mood polarity to hypomania or mania in patients with bipolar depression during acute and continuation trials of venlafaxine, sertraline, and bupropion as adjuncts to mood stabilizers. Am J Psychiatry 163:232-239

Lichy C, Dong-Si T, Reuner K, Genius J, Rickmann H, Hampe T, Dolan T, Stoll F, Grau A (2006) Risk of cerebral venous thrombosis and novel gene polymorphisms of the coagulation and fibrinolytic systems. J Neurol 253:316-320

Meisenzahl EM, Scheuerecker J, Zipse M, Ufer S, Wiesmann M, Frodl T, Koutsouleris N, Zetzsche T, Schmitt G, Riedel M, Spellmann I, Dehning S, Linn J, Bruckmann H, Möller HJ (2006) Effects of treatment with the atypical neuroleptic quetiapine on working memory function: a functional MRI follow-up investigation. Acta Psychiatr Scand 256:522-531

Möller HJ (2006) Long-acting risperidone: focus on safety. Clin Ther 28:633-651

Möller HJ (2006) Is there evidence for negative effects of antidepressants on suicidality in depressive patients? : A systematic review. Eur Arch Psychiatry Clin Neurosci 256:476-496

Möller HJ (2006) Ethical aspects of publishing. World J Biol Psychiatry 7:66-69

Möller HJ (2006) Long-Acting Risperidone: Focus on Safety. Clin Ther 28:633-651

Möller HJ (2006) Evidence for beneficial effects of antidepressants on suicidality in depressive patients : A systematic review. Eur Arch Psychiatry Clin Neurosci 256:329-343

Möller HJ, Bottlender R (2006) Severe mental illness in depression. Acta Psychiatr Scand Suppl 429:64-68

Möller HJ, Grunze H, Broich K (2006) Do recent efficacy data on the drug treatment of acute bipolar depression support the position that drugs other than antidepressants are the treatment of choice? A conceptual review. Eur Arch Psychiatry Clin Neurosci 256:1-16

Möller-Leimkühler AM (2006) Multivariate prediction of relatives' stress outcome one year after first hospitalization of schizophrenic and depressed patients. Eur Arch Psychiatry Clin Neurosci 256:122-130

Mulert C, Juckel G, Giegling I, Pogarell O, Leicht G, Karch S, Mavrogiorgou P, Möller HJ, Hegerl U, Rujescu D (2006) A Ser9Gly polymorphism in the dopamine D3 receptor gene (DRD3) and event-related P300 potentials. Neuropsychopharmacology 31:1335-1344

Müller N (2006) Obituary to Prof. Dr. med. Manfred Ackenheil (1939-2006). Eur Arch Psychiatry Clin Neurosci 256:541

Müller N, Schwarz MJ, Dehning S, Douhe A, Cerovecki A, Goldstein-Muller B, Spellmann I, Hetzel G, Maino K, Kleindienst N, Möller HJ, Arolt V, Riedel M (2006) The cyclooxygenase-2 inhibitor celecoxib has therapeutic effects in major depression: results of a double-blind, randomized, placebo controlled, add-on pilot study to reboxetine. Mol Psychiatry 11:680-684

Nothdurfter C, Eser D, Schüle C, Zwanzger P, Marcuse A, Noack I, Möller HJ, Rupprecht R, Baghai TC (2006) The influence of concomitant neuroleptic medication on safety, tolerability and clinical effectiveness of electroconvulsive therapy. World J Biol Psychiatry 7:162-170

Pogarell O, Hegerl U, Mulert C (2006) Electroconvulsive therapy and nonconvulsive status epilepticus - response to anticonvulsants might solve the dilemma. Pharmacopsychiatry 39:120-121

Pogarell O, Juckel G, Mavrogiorgou P, Mulert C, Folkerts M, Hauke W, Zaudig M, Möller HJ, Hegerl U (2006) Symptom-specific EEG power correlations in patients with obsessive-compulsive disorder. Int J Psychophysiol 62:87-92

Pogarell O, Koch W, Popperl G, Tatsch K, Jakob F, Zwanzger P, Mulert C, Rupprecht R, Möller HJ, Hegerl U, Padberg F (2006) Striatal dopamine release after prefrontal repetitive transcranial magnetic stimulation in major depression: preliminary results of a dynamic [123I] IBZM SPECT study. J Psychiatr Res 40:307-314

Pogarell O, Koch W, Gildehaus FJ, Kupsch A, Lindvall O, Oertel WH, Tatsch K Long-term assessment of striatal dopamine transporters in Parkinsonian patients with intrastriatal embryonic mesencephalic grafts. Eur J Nucl Med Mol Imaging 33:407-411

Preuss UW, Zill P, Koller G, Bondy B, Hesselbrock V, Soyka M (2006) Ionotropic glutamate receptor gene GRIK3 SER310ALA functional polymorphism is related to delirium tremens in alcoholics. Pharmacogenomics J 6:34-41

Rujescu D, Bender A, Keck M, Hartmann AM, Ohl F, Raeder H, Giegling I, Genius J, McCarley RW, Möller HJ, Grunze H (2006) A pharmacological model for psychosis based on N-methyl-D-aspartate receptor hypofunction: molecular, cellular, functional and behavioral abnormalities. Biological Psychiatry 59:721-729

Rupprecht R, Eser D, Zwanzger P, Möller HJ (2006) GABAA receptors as targets for novel anxiolytic drugs. World J Biol Psychiatry 2006; 7:231-237

Sato T, Bottlender R, Sievers M, Möller HJ (2006) Distinct seasonality of depressive episodes differentiates unipolar depressive patients with and without depressive mixed states. J Affec Disord 90:1-5

Schmitt GJE, Frodl T, Dresel S, la Fougere C, Bottlender R, Koutsouleris N, Hahn K, Möller HJ, Meisenzahl EM (2006) Striatal dopamine transporter availability is associated with the productive psychotic state in first episode, drug-naive schizophrenic patients. Eur Arch Psychiatry Clin Neurosci 256:121

Schüle C, Baghai TC, Eser D, Zwanzger P, Jordan M, Buechs R, Rupprecht R (2006) Time course of hypothalamic-pituitary-adrenocortical axis activity during treatment with reboxetine and mirtazapine in depressed patients. Psychopharmacology 186:601-611

Schüle C, Romeo E, Uzunov DP, Eser D, di Michele F, Baghai TC, Pasini A, Schwarz M, Kempter H, Rupprecht R (2006) Influence of mirtazapine on plasma concentrations of neuroactive steroids in major depression and on 3alpha-hydroxysteroid dehydrogenase activity. Mol Psychiatry 11:261-272

Schüle C, Zill P, Baghai TC, Eser D, Zwanzger P, Wenig N, Rupprecht R, Bondy B (2006) Brain-derived neurotrophic factor Val66Met polymorphism and dexamethasone/CRH test results in depressed patients. Psychoneuroendocrinology 31:1019-1025

Schüle C, Sighart C, Hennig J, Laakmann G (2006) Mirtazapine inhibits salivary cortisol concentrations in anorexia nervosa. Prog Neuropsychopharmacol Biol Psychiatry 30:1015-1019

Schwarz MJ, Krönig H, Riedel M, Dehning S, Douhet A, Spellmann I, Ackenheil M, Möller HJ, Müller N (2006) IL-2 and IL-4 polymorphisms as candidate genes in schizophrenia. Eur Arch Psychiatry Clin Neurosci 256:72-76

Seemüller F, Dehning S, Grunze H, Müller N (2006) Tourette's symptoms provoked by lamotrigine in a bipolar patient. Am J Psychiatry 163:159

Serretti A, Cusin C, Rausch JL, Bondy B, Smeraldi E (2006) Pooling pharmacogenetic studies on the serotonin transporter: a mega-analysis. Psychiatry Res 145:61-65

Shroff H, Reba L, Thornton L, Tozzi F, Klump KL, Berrettini WH, Brandt H, Crawford S, Crow S, Fichter MM, Goldman D, Halmi KA., Johnson C, Kaplan AS, Keel P, LaVia M, Mitchell J, Rotondo A, Strober M, Treasure J, Woodside DB, Kaye WH, Bulik CM (2006) Features associated with excessive exercise in women with eating disorders. Int J Eat Disord 39:6 454-461

Soyka M, Schmidt F, Schmidt P (2006) Efficacy and safety of outpatient alcohol detoxification with a combination of tiapride/carbamazepine: additional evidence. Pharmacopsychiatry 39:30-34

Soyka M, Schmidt P, Franz M, Barth T, de Groot M, Kienast T, Reinert T, Richter C, Sander G (2006) Treatment of alcohol withdrawal syndrome with a combination of tiapride/carbamazepine : Results of a pooled analysis in 540 patients. Eur Arch Psychiatry Clin Neurosci 256:395-401

Soyka M, Schmidt P, Franz M, Barth T, de Groot M, Kienast T, Reinert T, Richter C, Sander G (2006) Treatment of alcohol withdrawal syndrome with a combination of tiapride/carbamazepine : Results of a pooled analysis in 540 patients. Eur Arch Psychiatry Clin Neurosci 256:395-401

Soyka M, Penning R, Wittchen U (2006) Fatal Poisoning in Methadone and Buprenorphine Treated Patients - Are there Differences? Pharmacopsychiatry 39:85-87

Sterr A, Padberg F, Amann B, Mergl R, Mulert C, Juckel G, Hegerl U, Pogarell O (2006) Electroencephalographic abnormalities associated with antidepressant treatment: a comparison of mirtazapine, venlafaxine, citalopram, reboxetine, and amitriptyline. J Clin Psychiatry 67:325-326

Sunderland T, Hampel H, Takeda M, Putnam KT, Cohen RM (2006) Biomarkers in the diagnosis of Alzheimer's disease: are we ready? J Geriatr Psychiatry Neurol 19:172-179

Teipel SJ, Drzezga A, Bartenstein P, Möller HJ, Schwaiger M, Hampel H (2006) Effects of donepezil on cortical metabolic response to activation during (18)FDG-PET in Alzheimer's disease: a double-blind cross-over trial. Psychopharmacology 187:86-94

Teipel SJ, Pruessner JC, Faltraco F, Born C, Rocha-Unold M, Evans A, Möller HJ, Hampel H (2006) Comprehensive dissection of the medial temporal lobe in AD: measurement of hippocampus, amygdala, entorhinal, perirhinal and parahippocampal cortices using MRI. J Neurol 253:794-800

Teipel SJ, Hampel H (2006) Neuroanatomy of Down syndrome in vivo: a model of preclinical Alzheimer's disease. Behav Genet 36:405-415

Teipel SJ, Willoch F, Ishii K, Burger K, Drzezga A, Engel R, Bartenstein P, Möller HJ, Schwaiger M, Hampel H (2006) Resting state glucose utilization and the CERAD cognitive battery in patients with Alzheimer's disease. Neurobiol Aging 27:681-690

TozziF, Thornton LM, Mitchell F, Fichter MM, Lilienfeld LR, Reba L, Strober M, Kaye WH, Bulik CM, Price Foundation Collaborative Group (2006) Features associated with laxative abuse in individuals with eating disorders. Psychosom Med 68:470-477

Träber F, Block W, Freymann N, Gür O, Kucinski T, Hamman T, Ende G, Pilatus U, Hampel H, Schild HH, Heun R, Jessen F (2006) A multicenter reproducibility study of single-voxel 1H-MRS of the medial temoral lobe. Eur Radiology 17:1-8

Treutlein J, Kissling C, Frank J, Wiemann S, Dong L, Depner M, Saam C, Lascorz J, Soyka M, Preuss UW, Rujescu D, Skowronek MH, Rietschel M, Spanagel R, Heinz A, Laucht M, Mann K, Schumann G (2006) Genetic association of the human corticotropin releasing hormone receptor 1 (CRHR1) with binge drinking and alcohol intake patterns in two independent samples. Mol Psychiatry 11:594-602

van den Oord EJCG, Rujescu D, Robles JR, Giegling I, Birrell C, Busdzár J, Murelle L, Möller HJ, Middleton L, Muglia P (2006) Factor structure and external validity of the PANSS revisited. Schizophr Res 82:213-223

Wermke M, Teipel S, Fuchsberger T, Kretzschmar H, Westner I, Schroder M, Hampel H, Drzezga A (2006) Frontal diaschisis in a German case of fatal familial insomnia. J Neurol 253:1510-1512

Zetzsche T, Frodl T, Preuss UW, Schmitt G, Seifert D, Leinsinger G, Born C, Reiser M, Möller HJ, Meisenzahl EM (2006) Amygdala volume and depressive symptoms in patients with borderline personality disorder. Biol Psychiatry 60:302-310

Zill P, Buttner A, Eisenmenger W, Bondy B (2006) A possible impact of the neuroD2 transcription factor on the development of drug abusing behavior. Mol Psychiatry 11: 525-527

Index of Names

Z

Printing: Krips bv, Meppel, The Netherlands
Binding: Stürtz, Würzburg, Germany